DR. RICHARD MARRS'
FERTILITY
BOOK

DR. RICHARD MARRS'
FERTILITY BOOK

AMERICA'S LEADING FERTILITY EXPERT TELLS YOU EVERYTHING YOU NEED TO KNOW ABOUT GETTING PREGNANT

Richard Marrs, M.D.
and Lisa Friedman Bloch and Kathy Kirtland Silverman

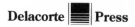
Delacorte Press

Published by

Delacorte Press

Bantam Doubleday Dell Publishing Group, Inc.

1540 Broadway

New York, New York 10036

Excerpt from *The Mommy Club* by Sarah Bird is reprinted with permission of Doubleday, a division of Bantam Doubleday Dell, copyright © 1991 by Sarah Bird.

Excerpt from *Newsweek* article, August 7, 1978, reprinted with permission of *Newsweek, Inc.* All rights reserved.

Excerpt from *Motherhood Deferred* by Anne Taylor Fleming, reprinted with permission of the Putnam Publishing Group, copyright © 1994 by Anne Taylor Fleming.

Excerpt from *Vital Signs* by Robin Cook, reprinted with permission of the Putnam Publishing Group, copyright © 1991.

Book design by Nancy B. Field

Library of Congress Cataloging in Publication Data
Marrs, Richard P.
    Dr. Richard Marrs' fertility book : America's leading fertility
expert tells you everything you need to know about getting pregnant
/ by Richard Marrs ; and Lisa Friedman Bloch and Kathy Kirtland Silverman.
        p. cm.
    ISBN 0-385-31436-1
    1. Infertility—Popular works. I. Bloch, Lisa Friedman.
II. Silverman, Kathy Kirtland. III. Title.
RC889.M367 1997
616.6'92—dc20   96-11350
                                                        CIP

Manufactured in the United States of America
Published simultaneously in Canada

January 1997

10 9 8 7 6 5 4 3 2 1

BVG

This book could not have been written without the many couples who experienced the pain and frustrations of being infertile. The strength and courage they demonstrated, enduring months and years of investigations and evaluations, makes them the true pioneers of this area of medical technology. Because of them, choices and chances have increased for all those who follow. To these pioneers, we dedicate this work.

We thank our children
—Ashley Marrs, Austen Marrs, Alexis Bloch,
Jordan Bloch, and Matthew Silverman—
for their patience,
and
Jonathan Bloch and Ron Silverman
for their love and support
during the writing of this book.

Acknowledgments

I would like to thank my former teachers, Dr. Phillip Thomson, Dr. Robert Franklin, Dr. William McGanity, Dr. Robert Girtanner, Dr. Val Davajan, Dr. Charles March, and Dr. Oscar Kletzky, for their efforts throughout my educational process.

And to all of my former fellows in reproductive medicine, who questioned and performed the various experimental protocols we developed in the early years of the Assisted Reproductive Technologies.

—RICHARD MARRS, M.D.

We would also like to thank the many patients who agreed to be interviewed, and who opened their hearts and re-lived their experiences for us.

We owe a debt of gratitude to the many experts who contributed both their time and their knowledge to our efforts. Among them are: Anita Aloia, L.V.N.; Jill Model Barth, Ph.D., B.C.D.; Carol J. Bennet, M.D.; Linda Callahan, M.A.; Elaine Gordon, Ph.D.; Michelle Leclaire O'Neill, Ph.D., R.N.; Dr. Daoshing Ni, D.O.M., L.Ac.; Kathy Parenicka, R.N.; Eva Ritvo, M.D.; and Carole Lieber Wilkins, M.A., M.F.C.C.

We would like to offer a very sincere and special thank-you to our editor, Marjorie Braman, who spent untold hours guiding us and helping us to turn our manuscript into the book it has now become. Your sensitivity toward this material, and your unwavering commitment to perfection, made an enormous difference.

Finally, our deepest gratitude goes to our agent Jillian Manus whose professionalism, knowledge, wisdom, friendship, and support helped us realize our dream, and see it to fruition. Thank you for always being there. Your dedication is immeasurable.

Contents

Introduction

Most of my adult life has been devoted to researching and treating infertility. It has given me moments of great joy and wonder. In 1982 I experienced the incredible excitement of initiating one of the world's first "test-tube babies." This IVF procedure gave doctors a true physiologic window through which we could observe the basics of human reproduction. Only four years later I helped to create the United States' first pregnancy produced from a frozen embryo. These early miracles still leave me in awe, even after thousands of successful births. Yet as I look back over the past fifteen years, I also remember the many, many other infertile patients I've treated. I think of how I held their hands through their suffering and listened to their hopes and their frustrations. My wish is to re-create these miracles of life for everyone who longs to have a child. If you are infertile, I understand what you're going through, and I want to help.

While it's hard to see anything positive when you're in pain, the comforting news is that you're not alone. You're fortunate to be living in an era when infertility has come out of the closet. Every day patients walk into my office with their own versions of the same thought: "Suddenly it's everywhere—on television, in newspapers and magazines. . . . Everyone knows someone who's having trouble conceiving." These patients are sharing in the new frankness about a problem that was hidden away during our parents' and grandparents' generations. Perhaps that's because there's exciting new technology to help us conquer it.

However open we may now be, infertility is still a heartrending problem: those of you who desperately long for a baby are still hurting. As you live each day, there's no way to ignore your problem and your sense of deprivation. This book will be a source not only of information but of comfort. Here you will learn about the incredible advances being made every day in the field of infertility and come to understand the new hope they hold out for you. You'll be able to inform and reassure people who are close to you and care about you that there *is* hope. And most of all you will learn how to query experts in the field—by doing that, you will learn too. Having worked with infertility patients for nearly twenty years, I know how knowledge can empower you when you feel hopeless and alone. You need to understand enough to become a partner in your own treatment instead of an "object of care." Every patient should be almost as knowledgeable as the physician who cares for them—the more knowledge, the less fear, and the more realistic hope they will have.

This is particularly important today because the cutting-edge technology that helps so many can also create confusion. It's becoming more and more difficult for patients to find accurate information and guidance. Over the years I've had the happiness of producing births for those who had all but given up hope. I've also had the pain and frustration of telling couples who came to me too late that their biological clocks had run out. They wasted precious months and years with ineffective treatment. Nothing is sadder for me. Patients are understandably angry when given such bad news. I would be too. That's why I have written this book. I want to make sure that you have all the information that's required to secure your best chance at success *right now.*

Ineffective treatment is not the only problem. The field of infertility is rife with old wives' tales and myths. Not long ago a patient named Mike grabbed me in the hall after I had finished scanning his wife. He showed me airline tickets and said, "I'm taking my wife to the Caribbean. Do you think it will solve our problem?" I told him to have a great time, but not to expect better results than if he stayed home. While it's true a vacation may relieve the stress that sometimes interferes with ovulation, it doesn't affect other aspects of fertility. Still, I encouraged Mike to skip a cycle of treatment and go on vacation. It could only help to bring enjoyment to his relationship. More often than not, infertile couples become so obsessed with getting pregnant that they lose any sense of the happiness they once had. This obsession can also affect their sex lives. Another patient confided to me that "since we're trying to get pregnant we're not having much sex. I save up my sperm for the big moment." I hear different variations of this thought in many of my initial consults. It's a widely held belief, but it's wrong. Your best chance of getting pregnant is with sperm that is ejaculated every 48 to 72 hours. After that, the quality may decline. As I said earlier, knowledge is key to your success.

Infertile people deserve a book they can trust in their time of need; as do the people who care about them, who have nowhere to turn for information. Even though I spend hours every day educating my patients, they invariably ask for something authoritative to read and consult later. They may have questions they don't think of when we are together, and sometimes there are things they aren't comfortable discussing out loud . . . at least not at first. I was always at a loss when asked to recommend a definitive reference book that would have all the answers. That's another reason my coauthors and I have written this book.

This work is complete in scope. It has always been my philosophy to treat the whole person, not just their clinical symptoms, to recognize the psychological and emotional problems created by infertility, not just the physical ones. In order to fully explore these issues, I have collaborated with a former patient and one of her close friends, each of them an informed and sensitive writer. They bring firsthand knowledge of the sometimes devastating emotional problems commonly faced in infertility. Together we examine known causes of infertility in humans. We explore diagnosis, as well as conventional and unconventional approaches to treatment, which we supplement with factual data. We look at the effects of treatment on patients, and on their friends and family. We give you true stories as a basis of comparison for your own problems. And we call on a number of well-known psychologists, who contribute insights based on their professional experiences. The result? A book of unparalleled scope, including specific advice you'll be able to adapt to your own fertility situation.

Our book will help you to:

- Understand the true nature of your infertility problems.

- Consult appropriate sources to find the best doctor for your treatment.

- Prepare for the physical and psychological side effects of being infertile by hearing about the problems of real patients.

- Understand the impact treatment can have on you and your relationships.

- Separate the myths from the facts about evaluation and treatment.

- Anticipate the financial aspects of treatment.

- Learn how to survive your pain if you don't conceive.

Not all problems are alike. This book will satisfy different needs for different people. The index will help you quickly find answers to your specific questions; the table of contents summarizes topics that will be discussed in each chapter. User-friendly charts and illustrations appear throughout the book to aid you in analyzing your changing feelings and goals at various stages of treatment. And there's a glossary of terms to help you through the technical medical information, and a list of resources—groups that work in various aspects of infertility and adoption—for you to call on if you need even more detailed information in a specific area.

Our goal in writing this book is to enable you to understand the advances made in the area of human reproductive disorders in order to help you aggressively seek solutions to your problems. We also want you to gain a realistic understanding of the emotional baggage that often accompanies the disorder, and how to deal with it. And we want you to realize that the fertility field is constantly changing, giving new hope to those who are trying to conceive.

—Richard P. Marrs, M.D.

DR. RICHARD MARRS'
FERTILITY
BOOK

1

Why You're Longing for a Baby

It's a Small World After All

It's around 8 o'clock. Your hostess, Sidney, a woman who seems to radiate confidence and a sense of accomplishment, carries the salad plates to her festive dining room table. Her husband, Gary, carefully refills the wineglasses and takes the drink orders of the dozen or so guests. The conversations shift between ballplayer trades and sneaky politicians, between irresponsible baby-sitters and finding the right preschool. Sitting there, quietly, you try to focus on one of them, but you can't. Why? Is it because they're not interesting to you? Is it because you can't relate to them? Or is it because you feel premenstrual symptoms, and you dread the thought of getting your period—proof that, once again, you're not pregnant.

Sara rattles on about the violence in the cartoons her four-year-old watches on television. She should only know how lucky she is to have a child. Mike, Evelyn's husband, argues about last Sunday's football game. Pamela and Steve arrive late; Sidney rushes over to greet them, and Pamela quietly nods to her with a hopeful glow. Isabelle, who's to your right, whispers something to Pamela. You overhear that Pamela arrived late because of an hCG shot, whatever that is. Suddenly you feel a wetness between your legs. It's like a knife through your heart. You sit there, numb. Then, in a daze, you excuse yourself and go to the bathroom.

It's a fait accompli once again. You stare in the mirror, not believing it, not understanding it. "Why me?" you ask, as tears well up. You reach for a tissue, but you're all out. You look around and finally discover some under the sink, next to a pregnancy tester and an Ovukit. Sidney and Gary? You thought they were totally absorbed in their successful careers and not at all interested in raising a family. The knowledge that you and your husband aren't alone brings a small moment of solace.

───────────── **YOU'RE NOT ALONE** ─────────────

It's not just you, your relatives, and your friends. *Everyone* can be affected by infertility . . . all races, religions, and socio-economic levels. In the United States today it is estimated that approximately five million individuals are considered infertile. What exactly does *infertile* mean? Clinically, the term is applied if a couple has difficulty getting pregnant after trying for six months. Approximately 40% of such infertility problems are attributable to the female. Another 40% are caused by the male. And the remaining 20% involve either a failure in the coupling, or remains unexplained.

You finish with your tissue. You pull yourself together by repeating what you've said so many times before: "There's always next month." You take a deep breath and walk back to the table with feigned confidence. Your eyes meet your husband's. He knows. And his poorly camouflaged look of disappointment makes your pain even worse. Then, to your dismay, the conversation at the table shifts to pregnancy. Should you remain detached? Or should you confide that you and your husband are trying, and risk completely coming apart at the seams, given that you just got your period, you're not pregnant, and you fear you may never be?

It's about now that you decide this is the worst party you've ever attended. The roast chicken tastes like cardboard. You gulp down wine, which suddenly has no taste. Then you notice Gary refilling your glass.

Alcohol and Infertility

Maybe that's the problem! You've read somewhere that alcohol isn't recommended if you're trying to get pregnant. Still, what's the difference at this point? You've already begun your period. It will be another 12 to 14 days before liquor can affect next month's ovulated egg.

But wait a second. . . . It takes two to tango. Could the alcohol your husband is consuming be the reason you haven't gotten pregnant? Could it be affecting his sperm count? Before Gary pours for your husband again, you reach out and cover his glass. He looks at you strangely. Nervously you whisper to him that maybe, under the circumstances, neither of you should overdo.

━━━━━━━━━━ **GOING . . . GOING . . . GONE!** ━━━━━━━━━━

While it's true that a man's reproductive system usually doesn't begin to decline until his sixth or seventh decade of life, certain things can temporarily impact his sperm's quality, their quantity, and their ability to penetrate an egg. Alcohol, recreational drugs such as cocaine and marijuana, smoking one to two packs of cigarettes a day, and high body temperature—produced, for example, by use of hot tubs—can all be linked to reduced fertility in the male. The good news is, sperm suppression is usually reversible. New sperm is created every 72 days. The speed with which a man's sperm get back to normal all depends on the magnitude of the abuse.

After Gary moves on, you redirect your attention to the conversation at the table. You realize it's no longer about who else *is* pregnant, but rather about how you can, with the correct guidance, *get* pregnant. Pamela seems well-informed. She says that she and her husband have been seeing an infertility doctor for some time. Now you really focus on the conversation, especially when she tells the group that the whole process of getting pregnant is much more complicated—and much less predictable—than we all have been led to believe.

Living Up to Expectations

If you're like most women, the concept of having babies was introduced to you at a very young age. As a toddler you were encouraged to carry dolls, push toy baby carriages, and care for a make-believe infant. It probably wasn't long before you and the little boy down the street started playing house. And before you went to sleep, your parents read you stories about families, passing on the implied assumption that having one is a right, not a privilege. It's no wonder that by the time you were in school, you were singing "First comes love, then comes marriage, then comes a baby in a baby carriage." By mirroring your parents' behavior, you learned the most commonly accepted version of the way life should be.

━━━━━━━━━━ **EVEN DISNEY TOLD YOU** ━━━━━━━━━━

Walt Disney reinforced our childhood views of family. In his world, even dogs played along. Take *101 Dalmatians*. Pongo, the dalmation hero, helps his master win over a lady friend, Anita. In the process, Pongo meets Anita's dog, Perdita. The two couples fall in love, and it

isn't long before puppies arrive. Babies, naturally, soon follow. The message to young children: Reproduction, for all species, is the natural course of events.

By the time you matured into a teenager, you were convinced that getting pregnant is an automatic and expected—even dreaded—event. For you, the focus was no longer on getting pregnant—that was a given. Instead it shifted to how *not* to get pregnant. Ideas from books and fairy tales were replaced by the kind of advice only movies and television can give. Scenes like the following infiltrated your life and convinced you that the danger of pregnancy was hard to avoid.

———— YOU'VE GOT TO BE CAREFULLY TAUGHT ————

In the 1970 movie *Summer of '42*, Hermie and Oscy, both 15, find a book detailing the twelve steps to sexual satisfaction. Hermie responds in a predictably worried tone: "I know the book means well, but what if she has a baby? I mean, if I follow these twelve points, she might just have a baby. And I can't afford a kid at this stage of my life." Oscy tells him not to worry, and sends him to the drugstore, where he experiences every teenager's worst nightmare as he tries to buy his first prophylactic.

Of course, you—all of us—feared the worst. Yearning for a sexual encounter, you'd suddenly be faced with the need to protect yourself against the otherwise inevitable disaster. So much energy was spent teaching you how *not* to get pregnant (as a teenager), it's no wonder you now feel confused, cheated, and depressed when it seems you're unable to anyway . . . as if you, and you alone, failed at what the rest of the world does automatically.

It's about now that you notice almost the entire dinner conversation is focused on the pregnancy issue. Why? Why is it the hot subject? Why is it that so many more people are infertile today?

The simple answer is that, because the baby boom generation is so much larger than the generations that came before it, there simply *are* more people these days. But these larger numbers of infertile people, resulting from a larger population, are misleading. As Pamela's husband, Steve, explains, while the causes of infertility may have changed, the *percentage* of people in each generation who are infertile has remained the same. That's because each generation has faced its own distinctive problems, which have been added to the varied causes of infertility. In the sixties, the IUD contributed. In the seventies, sexually transmitted diseases were a prominent cause of infertility. And in the eighties, women who might otherwise have had families with no problem had difficulty getting pregnant because they were trying at a later age, after pursuing careers. In other words, the woman who was potentially fertile in her twenties, may have lost that fertility by her late thirties, simply due to the passage of time. The fertility challenges we face in the nineties, which include the added impact of delayed childbearing and the possibility of factors in the environment that may affect the reproductive system, are merely the latest twists in the infertility story.

Changing Times, Changing Attitudes

In the fifties, things were perceived to be different. Women's attentions were focused on the family, the source of all domestic bliss. If women worked, it was because they had to. Given this mind-set, when most of our parents came of age they married young and got pregnant early. As a result, this period—roughly between 1945 and 1965—saw the highest birthrates and largest number of babies per family ever recorded in the history of this country. Early marriage contributed to this baby boom in two ways. First, since a woman can only get pregnant during a finite period of time—from roughly the ages of 12 to 45—women who married younger gave themselves more years in which to *be* pregnant. Today's generation, which starts pregnancy attempts later in life, has shortened that finite time period. In addition, marrying young helped women to avoid another problem—the decrease in fertility that follows as a woman ages. Today's woman, who puts off getting pregnant only to be faced with reproductive dysfunction, might have conceived easily had she followed her mother's example and tried at a younger age.

Pamela points out that in the sixties and seventies attitudes changed, and so did birthrates. Thanks in part to the invention of the birth control pill in the early sixties and the intrauterine device (IUD) in the late sixties, women began extending their education and becoming professionals . . . lawyers, doctors, and CPAs. They wanted careers, not just jobs. Striving to be the CEO of a corporation was suddenly acceptable. Family became secondary—standing in line behind "self." The seeds of a generation made up of highly competitive, goal-oriented, well-educated, success-driven people were sown. A group that, by its very definition, postpones having children to a later age.

Along with this goal-oriented mind-set, better birth control helped women to grow more free-spirited. They put off marriage and became sexually liberated. They began to experiment with multiple partners, increasing the incidence of sexually transmitted diseases. It wasn't until later on, when they wanted to have children, that the negative side effects of this sexual revolution—the hidden infections, tubal disease, uterine dysfunction, and ovarian abnormalities that had proliferated as a result of it—surfaced as fertility problems. The group that passed through the era of sexual freedom began to realize that they bore emotional and physical scars as a result.

It was about this time—in the beginning of the eighties—that the same women who had gotten the message to pursue careers as ambitiously as men, slammed into an emotionally charged conflict between career and family. A new message from society roared out at women: "You want to work . . . succeed . . . beat men at their own game? Go ahead. But don't expect to have a family too." Women were informed that they could opt for satisfaction in either the work realm or the family realm, but they couldn't have both.

Sidney understands this all too well. She pipes in that she feels she is a victim of today's society, where women are pushed to do it all, but never quite succeed. After years of determined commitment, she has a flourishing career. Now that she desperately desires children, and is looking toward family and motherhood, she feels she's being punished. Sidney's feelings of being overwhelmed are understandable. Today's society places a great burden on women, sending mixed signals about their place at home and in the workforce.

That's because things changed again as we approached the nineties. The economy was no longer booming, and the high-powered lifestyle it had funded was threatened. The need to have the biggest and the best was becoming, of necessity, less of a priority. Looking toward life's simpler pleasures became the in-vogue path to inner satisfaction. The media, as it so often does, brought this problem into sharp focus.

SHIFTING GEARS: THE '80'S

In the 1988 move *Baby Boom*, Diane Keaton plays a professional woman caught up in the world of power and success, who opts out of the rat race for the sake of a child. Her decision reflects the way society once again swung the pendulum of women's career paths back toward the family.

Infertility, the Social Disease of the Nineties

So now, in the nineties, "family" is it. The new boom is the family boom. Almost everything in life revolves around it . . . to such a degree that if you don't have one, you feel as if something is wrong with you. Of course you understand what Sidney is feeling. Women today who face infertility in their thirties and early forties become angry when they realize they bought into the idea of having a career first, instead of children. Some of their anger and frustration is directed toward the society that pressured them into a situation they would not necessarily have chosen on their own.

They're constantly reminded that having babies is now the "in" thing to do. The world of babies is suddenly an acceptable conversation piece for either sex in any situation, and that includes the workplace. Accessories and conveniences have been perfected to the point that babies are taken virtually everywhere, into public places as well as private ones. If women weren't faced with so much baby overkill, they might not feel so needy about having a child. The old adage "Out of sight, out of mind" may, for some, be truer than we realize.

The Media Won't Let You Forget

On the one hand, publications cite external factors that may explain why you are infertile in the nineties: certain foods, from caffeine to hormonally treated vegetables and meats; environmental toxins, from second-hand smoke to insecticides; electrical currents, from high-tension wires to electric blankets—to name only a few. And while these explanations may not directly help you solve your problem, the knowledge that they give can help you to feel a bit more in control of your situation.

On the other hand, the media dangles hope in front of you, even when it's not appropriate. Isabelle, a woman older than most at the table, offers that she has read incredible success stories in the magazines. Women over sixty are having babies using donated eggs. Other women have successfully achieved pregnancy from cryopreserved embryos. Someone adds that they heard doctors can now reconstruct fallopian tubes through laser surgery and achieve pregnancies. Fertility doctors can also help men with only a few sperm to fertilize eggs through high-tech micromanipulation. Because there's such a push to have children today, the media emphasizes every technological step forward in the world of infertility research. What it fails to point out is that none of these medical advances is equally effective for everyone. Announcing them serves to educate the general public. But for some, news of these new achievements offers false hope and unreasonable expectations. It all depends on your infertility disorder. Every person is different, and therefore it follows that every case will be too.

Obviously, the news isn't totally depressing. Keep in mind that while the same sort of infertility problems have been with us since the very dawn of man, and the ways we've tried to deal with them have shown some interesting similarities throughout the centuries, solutions *have* gotten better during the past few decades. As far back as the Old Testament, Abraham and Sarah were unable to have a child. It was with great trepidation, then, that Sarah brought her handmaiden to Abraham and told them to conceive. Nine months later Ishmael was born. Today, things might be easier for Sarah. We would very likely be able to help Abraham and Sarah create their child together, while keeping the handmaiden at a more comfortable distance.

But let's go back to Sidney's party. It's after 11 o'clock. By now you've learned a good deal more about the challenges you face. It doesn't matter what has influenced your desire to have children; all that matters is that you *do* want to get pregnant. And whatever your situation, the good news is that new fertility procedures give you greater hope of conceiving than ever before. Armed with this new knowledge, you feel like you can ask new questions, investigate avenues you hadn't known were there. But perhaps most important, you've learned you're not alone. You needn't feel stigmatized by infertility—it's not something to feel shameful or inadequate about. It's a condition that, for a variety of reasons, many couples face. It's also a condition you may well be able to have easily treated.

So continue to listen, to study, to ask questions, and to follow advice tailored to your needs—the kind of advice you'll find in this book. Our goal is to help those of you who for physical reasons would have needed help at any age, as well as those who put off planning a family and are now faced with some biological obstacles.

PART ONE

HOW BABIES
ARE MADE

2

A Woman's Role in Reproduction

Imagine this: You've come to your doctor's office for your first consultation. You're sitting in the two chairs across from his desk. You've never met a fertility specialist before, and you're nervous. You know the discussion you're about to have will hit on some of the most private and emotional aspects of your lives. Perhaps just making the appointment has already interfered with your emotional well-being, or with your connection as a couple. To keep it as safe as possible, you've rehearsed what you're going to tell him: "We've been trying to get pregnant for almost two years, and nothing has happened. It can't be the timing; we've been using a home ovulation predictor test, and following the instructions to the letter. Still, it's just not working. Something must be wrong with us."

Anyone Can Get Pregnant . . . Right?

"When she missed her first period, I begged her to get a pregnancy test, but she wouldn't. 'Why bother with a test? I know I'm pregnant.' She smiled an ironic I-told-you-so smile. . . . She had been knocked up by a West Point cadet friends had thrust on her late in the summer. So eager was he to make out that he had hardly pulled off her pants and lay on top of her before he'd come all over her legs. It had been their third, and, she had determined, their last date. It was a freaky impregnation, but, as they say in the hygiene books, all it takes is one sperm and one egg."
—*Alix Kates Shulman*
Memoirs of an Ex-Prom Queen
Copyright © Alfred A. Knopf, 1972

Remember the days when you believed that if you so much as looked at each other in the backseat of a Chevy you'd end up getting pregnant? And now you're sitting in a doctor's office trying to find out why nothing works. You wouldn't have worried so much as a teenager if you'd realized then the complexity of the process. So while your instinct on entering your doctor's office might be to ask for testing, probing, and use of the most recent high technology, an even more important first step is to learn exactly what normal human reproductive function is. It's the only way you'll understand how your doctor determines what abnormalities may be present, and what current medical technology might be used to correct them.

What Are the "Normal" Chances of Getting Pregnant?

To begin with, it might be of some comfort for you to realize that reproduction in even the most fertile human is inefficient compared with other animal species. If you really want to get pregnant, in your next life come back as a mouse, a cat, or even a fish. Lower species have all the luck. As a rule they ovulate multiple eggs, and their reproductive efficiency is extremely high. In fact, almost every time the females of lower mammalian species ovulate and have sexual activity, pregnancy results. One of the most common treatments for human infertility—using supraovulation therapy to produce multiple eggs during a single cycle—is an attempt to turn our evolutionary clocks back to what lower species do on a regular basis.

Normal Fecundity Rates

Age	Rate
15 years old	40%–50% per cycle
25 years old	30%–35% per cycle
35 years old	15%–20% per cycle
45 years old	3%–5% per cycle

Unfortunately for us, human beings and rhesus monkeys (our closest evolutionary counterparts) are the two primate species designed to be reproductively inefficient. Why we were singled out to evolve to this level of reproductive inefficiency, no one really knows. But in our case ovulation occurs just once each month, with a single egg, and then an incredible series of variables must all fall into place for a pregnancy to ensue. Because of this, the real expectation for pregnancy to occur in any given cycle, even under the best of circumstances with a fertile couple whose timing is perfect, is, on the average, just 25% per month. This percentage rate is called fecundity—the ability to conceive during any given cycle of ovulation—and it varies greatly according to a woman's age.

These fecundity rates assume that you are ovulating normally, and that you are having appropriately timed sex. As you can see, all women, even women who are fertile throughout their lives, have reduced fecundity rates as they age. This declining ability to conceive can't be changed by exercise, vitamins, or attitude, because it's totally related to the age of your eggs.

Not too many couples understand that a woman's body produces *all* the eggs she will ever have by the time she's a six-month-old fetus, still in her mother's womb. Your eggs are present at your birth, and they're exposed to every toxin and environmental condition that you encounter as you go through your life. Because they contain such sensitive genetic packages, this exposure may greatly affect them; as time goes on, your eggs become progressively less efficient at producing a fertilized embryo that can become a healthy baby. This breakdown of eggs as they age is one of the biggest problems women face in infertility treatment today, because there's simply no way to reverse it.

And fecundity is just one of the hundreds of variables that affect your ability to get pregnant. Of course, what makes things even more difficult is that a woman's reproductive tract, unlike a man's, isn't visible. The vagina, cervix, uterus, fallopian tubes, and ovaries are all internal, which makes it hard to observe and comprehend the many cyclical changes that occur during your reproductive cycle. (See Figure 2-1.)

Some Things Are Decided Even Before You're Born

Ovarian formation occurs between the fourth and fifth months of fetal life. Not only do the ovaries structurally form at this time, all the eggs you will ever have are made as well—on average, five to seven million.

Though this seems like a huge supply, you begin losing these eggs even as a newborn infant, more than a decade before your first ovulatory cycle. Throughout these early years, a girl's follicles degenerate in a

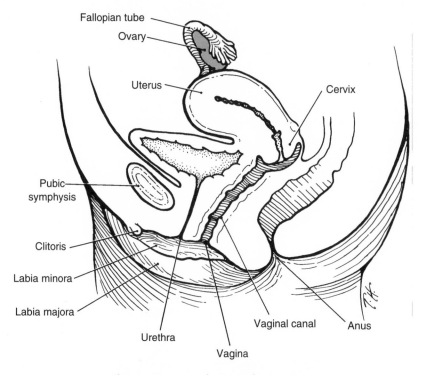

Figure 2-1: Female Reproductive Tract

rapid fashion. While they are not actually ovulated, this constant, day-to-day attrition uses up three million to five million eggs by the time you approach puberty and your first menstrual period (menarche). We don't completely understand why this happens, but we theorize that it may be due to a lack of certain protecting hormones, or to an inadequate level of the hormones that control follicle and egg maturity, such as follicle-stimulating hormone (FSH) and luteinizing hormone (LH). These hormones are produced by the pituitary gland, which is part of your brain. FSH and LH control the growth and development of the follicle and egg during the ovulatory cycle.

Whatever the reason, the net result is that most young women start menstruating between the ages of twelve and fourteen with just a half million to two million eggs remaining in their ovaries. The exact number depends upon the individual, and unfortunately we have no way of determining exactly what it is in your case (or in the case of *any* woman), either at the beginning of your reproductive years or as you grow older. Because we don't know the number of eggs that are actually available, it is hard to predict how many will mature if you are medically stimulated in preparation for in vitro procedures. This is a definite handicap when advising older women as to their possible success rate when they are considering infertility treatment.

How Your Reproductive System Matures

What we *do* know is that at or about the time of puberty, a specific part of your brain called the hypothalamus matures hormonally. This event is the catalyst that prepares the way for the beginning of ovulatory cycles and menstruation.

Within the human body, hormonal interaction and glandular function are cascading events that begin in the center of the brain, flow from gland to gland through a series of hormonal messages, and ultimately end up at a "target organ." During your ovulatory cycle the target organ is the ovary. For you, the process begins when your hypothalamus releases a hormone called gonadotropin-releasing hormone (GnRH), which signals the pituitary to release FSH and LH.

─────── **THE HORMONES THAT MAKE IT HAPPEN** ───────

You will be learning about FSH and LH throughout this book. These two hormones are manufactured in the pituitary gland beginning at birth. They are called "gonadotropins," because they target the primary sexual organs—the ovaries and testes—which are known as gonads. While these gonadotropins are continuously produced and released every 60 to 90 minutes, for our entire lives, their *sole function* is to stimulate normal ovulation in the female and produce functional sperm in the male.

In women, FSH and LH target the ovaries. As your ovaries receive these hormones they, or more precisely the follicles within them, respond. As the follicles respond, they make estrogens, which stimulate the maturation of your body. Regular ovulatory cycles usually begin within two to six months after your first menstrual period. At that point the brain and ovary will have achieved a balance, and you will start to ovulate and menstruate on a regular basis. (See Figure 2-2.)

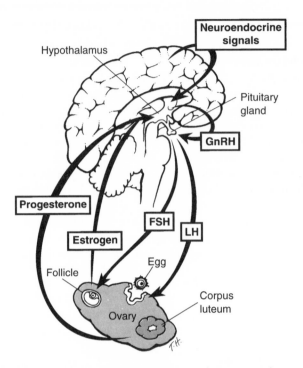

Figure 2-2:   Hormonal Balance Between the Brain and Ovaries

How Your Ovulatory Cycle Works

It's during your ovulatory cycle that an egg develops within the ovary until it's mature enough to be released and enter the fallopian tube. There it may come in contact with sperm, and fertilization can take place. Because of its many complex stages, ovulation causes some of the most common infertility problems, and therefore is an area where couples will most often receive initial evaluation.

CONVERSATIONS BETWEEN THE BRAIN AND OVARIES

Ovulation requires an extremely delicate balance between the ovary and the central nervous system. This connection isn't physical; rather, your brain and your ovaries talk to each other through a series of hormonal releases that act as signals which when correctly balanced, produce normal ovulation. But even balanced hormonal releases will fail unless your ovaries are correctly formed and structured. This ovarian makeup is developed while you are still a fetus in your mother's womb.

━━━━━━━━━ CAN YOUR EMOTIONS AFFECT ━━━━━━━━━
YOUR OVULATION?

The pituitary gland has often been called the master gland. It was once thought to control all hormonal function within the human body. We now know that the pituitary is merely a responder; it secretes hormones in response to signals from higher levels in the brain, such as the hypothalamus and the cortex. Because the cortex is the portion of the brain that contains our sensory functions, it can be influenced by emotional or other life experiences. These disturbances will then be passed down to the hypothalamus, which will in turn send them to the pituitary. The result may be changes in the levels of hormones the pituitary releases, and ultimately a change in ovarian function. Heaven only knows how many sleepless nights might be avoided if young women really understood this. The very act of worrying about the night her boyfriend's condom broke can often cause a woman to miss or delay her period. (See Figure 2-2.)

Since 40% of all infertility problems involve the female there's a good chance that your treatment will include correcting an ovulatory disorder, attempting to improve ovulation, or using various medications to supraovulate (produce multiple eggs in an already ovulating woman). To understand why your doctor uses certain methods and medications to accomplish these goals, you must develop a basic knowledge of how your ovulatory cycle works, as well as some understanding of the roles of the various hormones that control it. For a moment, visualize yourself as a microscopic organism in the bloodstream, and follow the path of the hormones that control ovulation and menstruation.

Ovulation, Day by Day

CYCLE DAY 1: MENSTRUATION MEANS STARTING ANEW

When you're part of an infertile couple, you have a natural tendency to consider the start of menstruation—the process during which the lining of the uterus sloughs off and passes out through the vagina along with menstrual blood—as the end of a cycle. To you, it is. The tissue that is being lost was intended to be the sheltering home for the fertilized egg. Losing it is the end of another month's dream, for an infertile couple. But medical professionals commonly refer to the onset of menstruation as the *first* day of a *new* cycle. To them, the end of the cycle was the point at which fertilization failed to happen.

When pregnancy doesn't occur, the levels of two hormones that built up in preparation for it—estradiol, which influences the lining of the uterus (the endometrium) to grow and develop, and progesterone, which triggers the receptivity of the endometrium for embryo implantation and attachment—fall rapidly, until their absence causes the uterine lining to break down and fall away. This is menstruation.

CYCLE DAYS 2–8: A WINNER EMERGES

When a pregnancy does not occur, your body quickly responds. By the second and third days of the menstrual cycle, pulses of FSH (follicle-stimulating hormone) are being released from your pituitary gland approximately every 60 minutes. Their role is to stimulate the follicles within the ovaries to begin their growth. As the pulses of FSH get larger and larger with each release, a group of follicles within the ovaries reacts. While we don't really know why a particular group of follicles is selected, and we can't really predict the number of follicles that will react in any particular woman, the same pattern always holds true. Over the next five to seven days of the cycle, the presence of FSH in the ovary will cause the follicles to grow and trigger the production of estrogen within them. Ninety-eight percent of the time, one follicle will emerge from the group during this period. This follicle overshadows the others because it manufacturers the highest amount of estrogen. It is this "dominant follicle" that will release an egg on approximately Day 14 of your cycle.

THE RIGHT RECIPE

What is happening within the follicles during this five-day period? Each follicle produces a group of important substances that cause multiple hormonal interactions to take place. Inhibin and folliclostatin are some of the substances that regulate the growth of one follicle over another. Oocyte maturation inhibitor (OMI) controls the final maturity of the egg before it leaves the follicle. And relaxin plays a major role in the actual mechanical release of the egg. All these substances can be found within the tiny sac that contains the egg. Whether they are there in appropriate or inappropriate amounts, and whether they are properly balanced, can affect not only the quality of the follicle but the quality of the egg. In fact, a mistake in this delicate recipe can even prevent ovulation during a given cycle.

As estrogen builds within the follicles, it also begins to enter your bloodstream, circulate to your brain, and reprogram your hypothalamus and pituitary gland. Initially, the rising estrogen causes an increase in

FSH release (positive feedback), but very quickly begins to suppress the amount of GnRH release and the ability of the pituitary to release FSH and LH (negative feedback). However, this rising estrogen does increase the production and storage of FSH and LH in the pituitary preparing for ovulation (positive feedback). Thus, as estrogen rises and negative feedback begins, there will be smaller amounts of FSH and LH in the pulses that occur every 60 to 90 minutes. This gradually, over one or two days, leads to less estrogen production within the follicle prior to ovulation.

This communication between the brain and ovary is called a positive/negative feedback loop. The balance it produces is an important and delicate one; if anything is out of kilter, a number of infertility conditions can result. In fact, if a woman doesn't ovulate, it's most often due to an imbalance between GnRH, FSH, LH, and estradiol, a form of estrogen that is produced by the ovarian follicles, the four basic hormones of the ovulatory cycle. (See Figure 2-3a and 2-3b.)

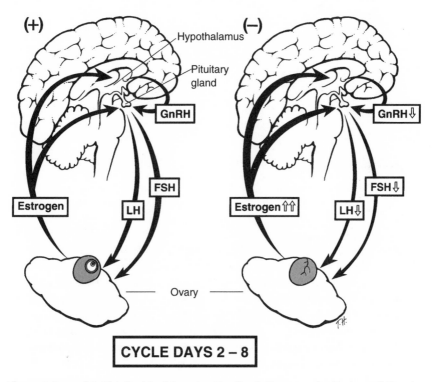

Figure 2-3a and 2-3b: Positive/Negative Feedback Between the Brain and Ovaries

CYCLE DAYS 9–13: OUT IT GOES

In the normal ovulation process, not only does rising estrogen decrease the amounts of GnRH, FSH, and LH that are released by your hypothalamus and your pituitary, it also stimulates another major event—the increased production and storage within the pituitary of LH and, to a lesser extent, FSH. As this happens the follicle begins to enlarge. The egg it contains also begins to change, becoming surrounded by cells called granulosa cells. Usually by Days 8 to 10 the fluid in the follicle has built up to the point at which the follicle is visible through the use of ultrasound. However, the egg still cannot be seen. Because it's a submicroscopic structure with an outer diameter of approximately 160 microns (the approximate size of a pinpoint), an egg that is developing in the follicle is not visible to the naked eye or via any currently available imaging equipment.

As the follicle enlarges, the egg is also becoming mature, or capable of being fertilized. Although your eggs are all formed while you are still a fetus, they reach only a certain point in their genetic maturity and then stop developing. When they stop, each of them still contains 46 chromosomes, the same number of chromosomes as all the other cells in your body. Your eggs remain that way unless they are exposed to a high level of LH during follicle dominance and before actual ovulation. This "LH surge" causes a resumption of their maturation process. Because of it, the egg that is in the dominant follicle prepares itself to release half of its chromosomes when it comes in contact with a sperm. When fertilization successfully takes place, the remaining 23 chromosomes will then combine with the sperm's 23 to regain a total of 46 chromosomes. (See Figure 2-3c.)

HORMONAL CURVE BALLS

Anything that throws off the balance between the LH release and the response of the egg in its final maturity—be it stress, competitive physical training, or chronic illness—can affect fertilization and normal genetic competency. This process can be interrupted in other ways too. An egg that is mechanically removed, or inadvertently released from a follicle that has not had an LH surge, will not be mature, and won't be capable of being fertilized. That is why the removal of eggs for procedures such as in vitro must be perfectly timed, and must follow the eggs' final maturation.

By the time the follicle reaches its maximum growth, normally about an inch in diameter, your estrogen levels have also reached their highest

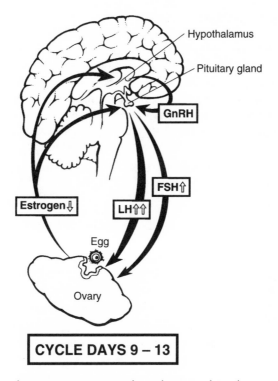

Figure 2-3c: Hormonal Mechanism of Ovulation

point of the entire menstrual cycle. This usually occurs around Cycle Day 12 or 13. (See Figure 2-3c.) These high estrogen levels create such sensitivity within your pituitary gland to the pulses of GnRH that your hypothalamus is sending out, that one of them causes a huge release of stored-up luteinizing hormone. This is the LH surge. The LH surge signals the follicle to begin thinning out in one area. Within 24 to 36 hours after the beginning of the LH surge, the follicle opens like an eggshell and its stored up fluids are released.

Contrary to what most people believe, the ovary doesn't fire the egg toward the end of the fallopian tube in the same way that Nolan Ryan pitches to his catcher. Instead, fluid dribbles slowly from the follicle over a short period of time, and the egg oozes out onto the surface of the ovary.

─────────────── **LOSING IN OVERTIME** ───────────────

The LH surge, which takes place just before the egg is released from the follicle, is what you measure when you use a home ovulation predictor test. Couples who've educated themselves about reproduc-

tion react to a positive test result by having intercourse 24 to 36 hours later—by "doing everything right." However, this is another case where a little knowledge can be dangerous. Ovulation is variable. It can occur with different timing in different women. Some women ovulate the same day the predictor becomes positive. Waiting 24 to 36 hours to have intercourse may actually prevent these women from conceiving. While the predictor technology is good, it may require some time spent with your obstetrician/gynecologist or reproductive endocrinologist to understand how it should be interpreted in order to be effective with your individual system. Even with the help of these experts, finding the correct timing can be complicated. Hundreds of hormonal interactions take place from the time the LH surge occurs until the moment the follicle opens and releases the egg. Scientists have spent their entire careers analyzing the hormonal action within that short period of time. And although they can measure it hormonally, and can see it through ultrasound, they still don't completely understand the complex series of events that triggers ovulation.

Although the dominant egg emerges, the sac that contained it remains behind in the follicle, where it continues to receive pulses of luteinizing hormone. This LH causes it to undergo a transformation. It turns into a small cyst, called a corpus luteum, whose job is to produce the hormone progesterone.

CYCLE DAY 14: THE EGG'S JOURNEY

The egg, which is now sitting on the surface of the ovary, is flattened and surrounded by granulosa cells, the sticky cells that were forming as the follicle and egg were getting closer to ovulation. This mass of gummy material surrounding the egg is called cumulus oophorus. The cumulus oophorus plays a crucial role in what happens to the egg after this point. It makes it possible for the fallopian tube to pick up the egg.

Your fallopian tube is connected at one end to the inside of your uterus. The other end, which is closest to the ovarian surface, widens and opens up like a funnel. The end of the funnel has hundreds of little fingerlike projections which are called fimbria. The fallopian tube isn't a passive structure. Muscle fibers within it cause it to contract and move toward the egg and the ovary. Anything that interferes with this tubal movement can disrupt its ability to pick up the egg, and in the process, prevent fertilization. When the fimbria on the end of the funnel come in contact with the cumulus oophorus surrounding the egg, it sticks to them

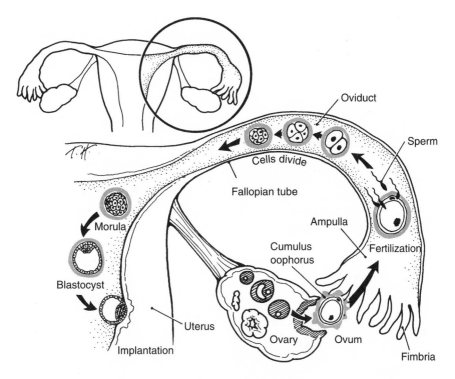

Figure 2-4: Interaction of the Fallopian Tube and Ovary During Ovulation

and the egg is picked up and moved into the fallopian tube. (See Figure 2-4.)

Once the egg is inside the tube, the sticky mass of cumulus cells and the egg stay in what's called the ampullary portion of the fallopian tube (its widened funnel-like area) for one to two days. Here the egg is nurtured and supported, and if fertilization occurs within 24 to 36 hours, normal embryo growth should begin. The egg has a limited period of time to live—whether on the surface of the ovary or within the fallopian tube—before fertilization occurs. While we're not totally sure how long eggs can survive, our experiences with in vitro culturing suggest that fertilization should occur within 24 hours of ovulation for a viable embryo to result.

How Your Body Prepares to Receive the Egg

While all of this is going on, several other things must be happening outside the area of your ovary and follicle if fertilization is to occur. As you recall, a woman's estrogen builds to its highest level just before ovulation occurs. Your estrogen level on Day 1 of the cycle, during menstruation, will be, on the average, somewhere between 40 and 50 units. Each unit represents one picogram per milliliter of serum. By the time of ovulation it will have increased tenfold, reaching 400 to 500 pg/ml. Not only does this massive increase modulate the hormonal interactions controlling ovulation, it has direct effects on other target organs as well. The cervix is one example.

As you can see in Figure 2-1, the cervix is the opening to your womb at the top of the vaginal canal. It is here that sperm gain entrance to your reproductive tract. Although there is a clear opening between your cervix and your uterine cavity, sperm cannot pass through it unless cervical mucus is present. And if the sperm have no way to enter the cervical canal, and ultimately the inside of the uterine cavity, they will die in the acid environment of your vagina within 20 to 30 minutes after ejaculation. Luckily, as ovulation approaches, the rising estrogen level triggers the production of mucus from glands in the first part of your cervical canal. This mucus is the source of the watery vaginal discharge that most women experience one to three days prior to ovulation.

If your estrogen is inadequate, or if the mucus-producing glands in your cervix are damaged or nonresponsive, there will not be enough mucus produced for sperm to be picked up out of the vaginal canal after ejaculation. Moreover, this mucus production continues for just a short period of time. Once the follicle, which has been producing larger and larger amounts of estrogen up to this point, ruptures and releases its egg, it becomes a corpus luteum and begins producing small amounts of progesterone. Progesterone is extremely important in preparing your uterine lining for the acceptance of the embryo during the initial stages of implantation; it's the primary hormone that supports the early pregnancy through its twelfth week. But it also causes the cervical mucus to become very thick and viscous, which will actually block sperm movement.

This thickening of the cervical mucus is another reason an ovulation predictor test should not always be relied upon. If you are one of those women who ovulates on the day the test turns positive—rather than 24 to 36 hours later, as the test instructions would lead you to believe—but you wait that additional 24 to 36 hours to have intercourse, your thickened mucus won't allow sperm to enter your cervix. Even though your and your partner's systems may otherwise be normal, the timing the test advised you to use will have dramatically interfered with your ability to conceive. *One way to ensure this doesn't happen is to have intercourse the day your test is positive, as well as on the day following a positive test.*

Assuming intercourse is properly timed, millions of sperm are deposited in the vagina, where a few thousand are then picked up by the cervical mucus. After a few minutes—or at most a few hours—in the cervical mucus, the sperm move upward into the uterine cavity and toward the opening of the fallopian tube. They quickly enter the tube, and if the egg has been picked up from the surface of the ovary, they meet it approximately an inch and a half from the end of the fallopian tube that is closest to the ovary. The sperm then gather on the sticky mass formed by the millions of granulosa cells that surround the egg, and begin working their way through.

Once egg and sperm meet, fertilization will occur, if it is going to, within about six hours. After the egg is penetrated by a sperm, mechanisms that are built into the egg allow no further penetration, no matter how many sperm continue to be available in the fallopian tube. Approximately 16 to 24 hours after penetration, the egg develops different cellular characteristics. A tremendous amount of cellular and genetic activity goes on in a very short period of time during this process. It's at this point that some genetic disorders can occur. This is particularly true in the case of older women, because the mechanism of gene replication in a consistantly normal pattern doesn't take place in older eggs.

If the Egg Is Fertilized

During the first one or two days of its development process, the embryo remains where it was when fertilization occurred in the fallopian tube. At that point the tube begins its second important function, moving the embryo down toward the uterus in time for it to attach and implant. The normal fallopian tube has an intricate network of tiny hairlike projections (cilia) that wave in an undulating fashion. These cilia carry the embryo through the fallopian tube and into the uterine cavity. If your tubal environment is damaged and these cilia are not present, or if they are markedly reduced in number, a tubal pregnancy can result. Also, if the cells within your fallopian tube have been damaged—through infection or surgery, through the use of an IUD, or any other type of trauma—the embryo may not receive adequate nutritional support during its growth and journey through the fallopian tube, and it may die before it has a chance to implant. Doctors have no way of knowing if damage has occurred. There's no outward sign; you would, like so many others, simply appear to be unable to conceive.

"We have lived through the era when happiness was a warm puppy, and the era when happiness was a dry martini, and now we have come to the era when happiness is 'knowing what your uterus looks like.' "

—*Nora Ephron*
Crazy Salad
Published by Alfred A. Knopf
Copyright © 1975, Nora Ephron

How the Egg Implants

While it seems as if everything has been taking place in the fallopian tube, your uterus has also been at work, readying itself to receive the embryo. This preparation of the uterine lining starts as early as the fifth or sixth day of the menstrual cycle, when the dominant follicle is selected and your estrogen level starts rising. This estrogen also influences the lining of your uterus—the endometrium—to grow and develop. The endometrium is almost nonexistent at the beginning of the cycle, having been sloughed off like a snake's skin during the prior menstrual period. But after your estrogen starts to rise, a new growth of endometrial lining begins. This endometrium thickens and proliferates until ovulation occurs. Since both ovulation and endometrial growth are estrogen dependent, they happen in tandem; the trigger for ovulation also helps the uterus to prepare to receive the embryo.

During the four to five days following ovulation the endometrium not only continues to thicken into a spongy, receptive lining, it also grows new blood vessels. This final maturing of the uterine lining is generated by the secretion of progesterone. It is progesterone that triggers the receptivity of your uterine endometrium for implantation and attachment. Under its influence the endometrium softens and develops a web of new blood vessels to nourish the implanted embryo. As you can see, the hormones controlling fertilization, embryonic growth, and the final preparation of your uterine lining must be precisely synchronized for implantation to occur. (See Figure 2-5.)

When the embryo enters the uterus, it floats in the fluid of the cavity until it finds a place to attach in its spongy and protected environment. This attachment is complicated by the fact that the embryo is surrounded by a protein membrane called the zona pellucida. The zona pellucida shields the egg from penetration by multiple sperm or sperm of another species, and after fertilization its membrane holds the growing

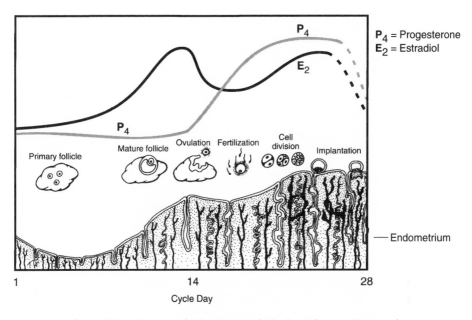

P_4 = Progesterone
E_2 = Estradiol

Endometrium

Cycle Day

Figure 2-5: Hormonal, Ovarian, and Uterine Changes During the Ovulatory Cycle

cells together in a cluster and prevents them from floating away in different directions. Once the embryo forms into a blastocyst—the final stage of embryo development in which the cells separate themselves into fetal cells and placental cells—it has to break out of the zona pellucida membrane in order to implant in the uterus. This process is called "hatching." During hatching, the membrane surrounding the developing embryo cracks open like an eggshell, and the embryonic structure squeezes out, burrows into the endometrium, and attaches to the wall of the uterus.

Once the embryo has attached, its placental blood vessels very quickly link up with the tiny blood vessels that have grown in the endometrium, and form a link between the mother's uterus and the embryo.

CAN MY TUBAL PREGNANCY BE SAVED?

One of the most common questions I hear in situations in which a woman has a tubal pregnancy is: "Why can't we take the implanted embryo and move it into the uterine cavity?" Unfortunately, the embryo will die. While the embryo is still far too small to see at the time it implants—even with a microscope—and its connection to its mother is even smaller, this connection is pivotal. Once it takes place, whether in the uterus or in the fallopian tube, the embryo will die

within milliseconds if its blood supply is interrupted in an attempt to place it somewhere else.

CYCLE DAYS 23–24: FAILURE

If you haven't become pregnant by this point in your cycle, the corpus luteum, which is programmed to release estrogen and progesterone for just 14 days after ovulation, will stop producing these two hormones, and will disintegrate. Your levels of estrogen and progesterone then fall rapidly, reaching their lowest point at the end of the monthly cycle. In response, the positive/negative feedback loop will play itself out yet again. Because it's no longer receiving estrogen from the ovaries, your hypothalamus will once again increase the amount of gonadotropin-releasing hormone (GnRH) being released every sixty minutes. This GnRH will cause your pituitary gland to release follicle-stimulating hormone (FSH), as well as a small amount of luteinizing hormone (LH), both of which will be picked up by blood vessels that run through your pituitary gland. From the pituitary, this hormonal message will be carried out into your bloodstream.

CYCLE DAYS 24–28: TRY, TRY AGAIN

As this hormone-rich blood circulates through your body, molecules of FSH come in contact with your ovaries, and with the follicles that are contained within them. The FSH begins to stimulate, or preselect, a group of follicles, calling them up for the next ovulation, which will take place about two weeks later. As this is happening the lining of your uterus, which is no longer receiving estrogen and progesterone, will begin to break up, leading once again to menstruation.

Success—The Planted Seed

If pregnancy *has* occurred, and the embryo is solidly implanted in the endometrium, the changes of early pregnancy proceed at a fantastic pace. Estrogen and progesterone levels begin to rise, causing you to experience breast sensitivity, tenderness, and fluid retention even before your menstrual period is missed. Human chorionic gonadotropin (hCG) also begins to be produced once the placenta attaches to the maternal system. This is the hormone that we measure to confirm a pregnancy. The reason it's so difficult to accurately predict a very early pregnancy is that the embryo has to build to a certain point in cellular mass before enough hCG is produced to be detected in your bloodstream. Even with the most sensitive blood analysis currently available, this usually doesn't happen until around the tenth day after ovulation. And while hCG in a woman's blood is an indication that an embryo has implanted, it still can't tell us whether it's located in the uterus or in a tube. We'll be discussing the ways in which your doctor can tell whether your pregnancy has implanted in the tube in Chapter Eight.

───────────── **WILL IT WORK?** ─────────────

The viability of a pregnancy can be predicted early on by watching the pattern of hCG production. We know today that if a healthy embryo has implanted in the uterine cavity, the hCG level will double approximately every 48 hours during the first six weeks, and about every 72 hours throughout the next two to four weeks. At that point the pattern flattens out significantly. When measuring hCG every two to four days in an early pregnancy, we're comforted if we see that the level is doubling during that interval. It isn't until hCG levels reach approximately 2,000 IU/ML that we can perceive the pregnancy sac in the uterus using vaginal ultrasound. Shortly thereafter we can usually see the early fetus within the pregnancy sac, and observe the pulsation of fetal cardiac activity. While would-be parents might think this is a long wait, it's actually relatively early. Only a few years ago, prior to the advent of vaginal ultrasound, this confirmation would have taken another one to two weeks, and a pregnancy would not have been confirmed until it reached its sixth to eighth week.

Implantation and the Immune System

We've described a number of the things that happen after implantation, but we have yet to touch on one significant component of pregnancy: the response of your immune system to the early stages of embryo formation. This is a territory that is only recently being explored by fertility specialists, and knowledge about it is growing at a tremendous rate. The more we learn about immunologic responses to implantation, the more we realize that they might cause some women who conceive fairly easily to continually lose their pregnancies. While the area is complicated, it is worthwhile to spend a few moments reviewing it, since we will be referring to it later in this book.

When the sperm enters the egg, a completely new and unique cell is formed. Half of this cell consists of the characteristics of the female egg cell, the other half has the genetic components of the male sperm cell. When they unite, the resulting cell is not exactly like either.

In most cases, if we were to inject cells of a different genetic makeup into our bodies, our immune systems would reject them. For instance, if you received a skin graft from your partner, you would reject it. Histologically and genetically those cells would be different from yours, and your immune system would respond to them as foreign bodies. Only if the donor had identical histologic types (identical cellular makeup of their tissues) and identical genetic characteristics, would the graft be accepted.

This is similar to what takes place in the vast majority of pregnant women when the sperm cell and the egg cell unite. The embryo that is formed is a totally new cell. As it moves into the uterus, its mother's immune system initially perceives it as a mass of foreign cells. The embryo's attempt to attach to her uterine lining is met by rejection from her immune system.

Normally, during this initial rejection by its mother's immune system, the embryo responds by sending back signals to tell her immune system that it's meant to be there. When the mother's immune system receives this message, it stops trying to reject the embryo, and begins producing "blocking antibodies." These antibodies protect and support the implantation and growth of the embryo throughout pregnancy.

In order for a woman to conceive, her body first has to view her own embryo as foreign and try to get rid of it. If she doesn't do this, the blocking antibodies that protect the embryo throughout the pregnancy won't be produced, and the normal process of implantation won't take place. If a couple is too closely related, or if they have common histological characteristics, they may produce embryos that are so similar to the mother's makeup, they won't be recognized as foreign and pregnancy will fail.

So, It's Not as Simple as It Seems

By now you understand that a simple comment like, "We've been doing everything right, why aren't we pregnant?" is simplistic. There are hundreds of variables in your reproductive system that have to fall into place within seconds and minutes for conception to take place. When you truly understand the process, it's mind-boggling to consider that pregnancy occurs so often.

While you don't have to master every detail, having this general understanding of how babies are made will be a tremendous help to you when you're going through your infertility treatment.

Terms We Used in This Chapter

Ampullary: the outer or distal end of the fallopian tube. It is also the widest part of the fallopian tube.

Blastocyst: the time in embryonic development where the embryo consists of the cells that will make the placenta and those which will form the fetus.

Blocking antibodies: protective antibodies that are formed by the mother's immune system in response to her embryo during implantation.

Cervix: a narrow opening that connects the uterus to the vagina and produces mucus that allows the sperm to enter into the uterus.

Chromosome: the structure in each cell's nucleus that holds the parent's genetic information in the form of DNA (deoxyribonucleic acid).

Cilia: the hairlike projections inside the fallopian tubes that move the egg and or embryo toward the uterus.

Corpus luteum: the cyst that forms after a follicle releases its egg. It produces estrogen and progesterone during the second half of the ovulatory cycle.

Cumulus oophorus: a sticky mass of cells in a cloudlike pattern that surrounds the egg at the time of ovulation.

Dominant follicle: the largest follicle of a follicle group; the dominant follicle contains the egg which will ovulate.

Embryo: a term used to describe the time from the fertilization of the egg until the eighth week of pregnancy.

Endometrium: the lining of cells inside the uterus which is sensitive to estrogen and progesterone stimulation.

Estrogen: a category of female hormone that is necessary for female characteristics.

Fallopian tube: a narrow tubular structure connected to the uterus that carries the egg from the ovary into the uterus after fertilization.

Fecundity rate: the ability of a woman to become pregnant during any given month that ovulation occurs. It is described as a percentage figure, i.e., 25% per month.

Fertilization: entrance or penetration of the egg by the sperm cell.

Fimbria: fingerlike projections on the end of the fallopian tube that pick up the egg after ovulation.

Follicle: a small fluid-filled sac contained within the ovary that prepares the egg for ovulation. The follicle is also the estrogen-production factory in the female.

Follicle-stimulating hormone (FSH): a protein hormone produced and released by the anterior pituitary gland. FSH stimulates follicle growth in the female and sperm production in the male.

Gonadotropin-releasing hormone (GnRH): a small protein hormone produced in the hypothalamus responsible for controlling the production and release of FSH and LH.

Gonadotropins: the protein hormones FSH and LH, which stimulate ovarian function in the female and testicular function in the male.

Granulosa cells: the cells within the ovarian follicle that make estrogen and progesterone during the ovulation cycle.

Hatching: the final event that the embryo must complete before implantation can occur. Hatching of the embryo is a breaking out of the zona pellucida in order to implant in the endometrial cavity.

Human chorionic gonadotropin (hCG): a hormone produced by the placenta during pregnancy. It is used as an LH replacement during ovulation-induction therapy to cause egg release.

Hypothalamus: the midportion of the brain which produces GnRH and other hormones that control the pituitary gland.

Inhibin: a protein hormone that interferes with the activity of FSH.

In vitro fertilization and embryo transfer (IVF-ET): the procedure in which the egg is removed from the ovary, fertilized in the laboratory environment, and the resulting embryo placed into the uterine cavity.

Luteinizing hormone (LH): protein produced and secreted from the anterior pituitary gland which is involved in ovulation.

Menarche: the onset of menstrual function.

Menstruation: the cyclic shedding of the endometrial lining of the uterine cavity, indicating lack of pregnancy.

Morula: a fertilized egg after 4 or 5 days of growth. This fertilized egg (embryo) contains 16 to 32 cells.

Oocyte: another term for egg.

Oocyte maturation inhibitor (OMI): a protein found in the follicular fluid that keeps the egg from maturing.

Ovaries: the female organs responsible for the production of sex hormones and eggs.

Ovulation: the release of the egg from the follicle.

Pituitary: a small gland at the base of the brain that secretes hormones that control our endocrine organs.

Placenta: a spongy structure surrounding the fetus that serves as a conduit between the mother and fetus during pregnancy.

Progesterone: the hormone produced from the corpus luteum after ovulation. It is also the hormone responsible for maintenance of early pregnancy.

Prolactin: the hormone produced from the pituitary that prepares the breasts for lactation.

Pronuclear oocyte sperm transfer (PROST):   another term for ZIFT.

Relaxin: a hormone that may be involved in uterine muscle activity.

Supra ovulate: the stimulation of multiple eggs to ovulate.

Tubal embryo transfer (TET):   the placement of the embryo into the fallopian tube after in vitro fertilization.

Ultrasound: an instrument that emits pulsed sound waves which are reflected off solid tissues, to give an image of internal body structures without the use of X ray.

Uterus: a muscular organ with a hollow cavity lined with a layer of cells called the endometrium. The function of the uterus is to protect and nourish the developing embryo/fetus.

Vagina: a canal in the female that connects the external sex organs with the cervix and uterus.

Zona pellucida: the outer protein covering of the egg that the sperm first comes in contact with during fertilization.

Zygote: a fertilized egg.

Zygote intrafallopian transfer (ZIFT):   placement of a fertilized egg into the fallopian tube; see PROST or TET.

3

A Man's Role in Reproduction

You may be thinking: What could be simpler than a man's reproductive system? A man gets sexually excited, has an erection, has intercourse, ejaculates—what else is there to know? Woody Allen may have summed it all up for you.

———

"WHAT HAPPENS DURING EJACULATION!"

A group of sperm is lined up along the tubular sides of a B-29–looking tunnel.
SPERM ONE: I'll see you guys in the ovary.
SPERM THREE: Save me an egg!
SPERM TWO: I'll wind up with twins yet!
LOUDSPEAKER: Fire sperm!
SPERM ONE: Geronimo!
He goes, and they all rush out after him.

  —*Woody Allen*
    Everything You Always Wanted to Know About Sex but Were Afraid to Ask

———

If you're entering the world of infertility, you'll quickly learn that the male reproductive system is far more complicated and delicate than Woody makes it seem. That's why many couples find themselves facing a "male factor problem." Knowing how the normal male reproductive system works is a great help in understanding the steps your doctor will take to correct the many things that can go wrong with it.

As we explained in Chapter Two, hundreds of precisely timed elements have to fall into place during a woman's ovulatory cycle for pregnancy to occur. One of the most important variables in this intricate mix is the condition and functional ability of the male's sperm. Every step in the sperm's maturation, in its development, and in its journey through the reproductive tract can affect its quality and its ability to move efficiently through the female reproductive tract toward the ultimate goal of meeting and fertilizing the egg.

Hormones, for Him

The interaction between the central nervous system and the testicles governs the male reproductive process in much the same way the relation between the central nervous system and the ovaries directs that of the woman. And, as in the woman, hormones are the catalysts.

There are certain similarities between the hormonal processes of men and women. In both sexes, the hypothalamus releases gonadotropin-releasing hormone (GnRH) into the system every 60 to 90 minutes. In both cases this GnRH triggers the pituitary gland to release two additional hormones—FSH (follicle-stimulating hormone) and LH (luteinizing hormone). However, the FSH and LH that are released produce very different effects in the two sexes. In a woman, they stimulate the production of estrogen and progesterone in the ovary. In a man, the FSH that is released from the anterior pituitary stimulates cells in the testicles to grow, mature, and release male germ cells (sperm). Concurrently, the LH secretion from the pituitary stimulates unique cells in the testicles—Leydig cells—to produce the primary male hormone, testosterone. It's testosterone that causes normal male sexual characteristics such as facial hair, muscular development, and deepening of the voice. While women's ovaries also produce small amounts of testosterone, the amount is so minimal that it doesn't cause these physical changes, except in certain abnormal situations, which we will discuss later.

Because FSH and LH serve two entirely different purposes in the male, it's possible for one to cause problems, while the other does not. For example, if only the release of FSH—which directs the growth of sperm—is deficient, a man can have an infertility problem, yet not have any change in sexual characteristics such as normal ejaculatory function, beard growth, body shape, or sex drive. He will still be fully "male." The truth is, a man's ability to reproduce rarely has any relation to the traits we commonly think of as "masculine." It is only when LH, which directs the production of testosterone, is also affected (a condition similar to having the testicles removed completely) that these secondary sexual characteristics will be affected.

Another important difference between the sexes is that while the release of FSH and LH from the pituitary gland into the male system is chronic—in other words, both hormones are produced at an even rate throughout the month—the release of these hormones in a woman's system is cyclical. By this we mean that GnRH received by a woman's pituitary during the first half of the month stimulates predominantly the production of the hormone FSH, which in turn stimulates the maturation and then—after an LH release—the release of an egg. But during the second half of the month, GnRH will cause a woman's pituitary to produce predominantly the hormone LH, which triggers the corpus luteum to produce progesterone and estradiol to prepare the uterus for implantation. The chronic release of both FSH and LH means that a man is fertile, or producing sperm cells, on a constant basis. But if woman's pituitary released both FSH and LH chronically, her reproductive system would be at a stalemate. Follicles and eggs would not grow and mature, and the uterus would not develop a receptive lining (endometrium).

While the chronic release of hormones in the male system sounds simpler, on the surface, than a woman's cyclic pattern, it relies on a

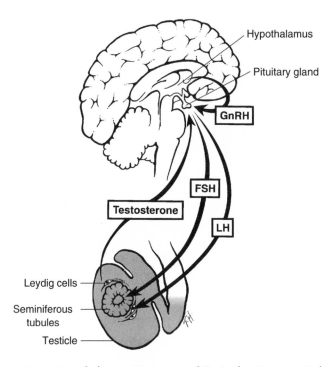

Figure 3-1: Hypothalamic, Pituitary, and Testicular Hormone Balance

perfect balance between FSH and LH being maintained at all times. To fully appreciate the importance of this balance in the male, you first need to understand how the testicles and the male reproductive tract are designed, and how they produce and release sperm into the female reproductive system. (See Figure 3-1.)

The Testicles

The testes are external organs approximately the same size as the ovaries.

─────────── **THEY THINK WITH THEIR *WHAT* . . . *???*** ───────────

Some—in particular the female members of society—would say that a man's brain is controlled by his testicles. In fact, the opposite is true. A man's testicles are controlled by his brain. Without the brain, and the release of FSH and LH it stimulates, the Leydig cells wouldn't produce testosterone, and the male wouldn't have any male secondary characteristics or sex drive.

Anyone who's ever worn a jockstrap has had cause to wonder from time to time why the testicles are on the outside of the body. Like so many of nature's decisions, this one was made for a good reason. Temperature and sperm production (spermatogenesis) go hand in hand. Sperm cells don't develop or function well when their temperature is higher than 93°F to 94°F. Your normal core body temperature is 98.6°F. By placing the testicles in a scrotal sac outside the body, nature keeps them at the cooler temperature that's required for normal sperm production.

─────────────────── **RULES TO LIVE BY** ───────────────────

Will a man who exercises regularly—goes to the gym, plays basketball, rides a bicycle for twenty miles—have sperm problems because he's become overheated? No! His body's natural air-conditioning, the sweat glands, will dissipate heat and cool down his testicles. But the man who sits in a hot tub or Jacuzzi for extended periods of time is tempting fate. The water is heated as high as 101°F and recirculates constantly, leaving the testicles with no way to dissipate the heat. Having "cooked" his sperm cells, he should expect to see a decrease in his sperm count, as well as deficiencies in his sperms' motility, shape, and size. Will he recover? I'm happy to report that the answer

is yes. In 1982 a group of six postdoctoral fellows—all recently proven fertile males—worked with me in my laboratory at the University of Southern California. As there was much discussion at the time concerning the effects of hot tub exposure on sperm production and function, I set up a controlled study using the seven of us, each of whom had fathered a child within the prior two years. We were all tested with routine semen analysis and sperm penetration tests three days prior to hot tub exposure; the sperm parameters for the group were above normal, including sperm penetration rates of 80% to 100%. On the day of exposure four of us sat in a hot tub with a water temperature of 101°F for an hour, while the other three (the control group) sat at poolside. The parameters for all four of us became abnormal within three days after this single hot tub exposure. Our sperm motility was zero, and our sperm counts were severely depressed. This remained constant for two weeks, but gradually returned to pre–hot tub exposure levels within four to six weeks—with one exception. The parameters for one of my fellows (who now is a well-known reproductive endocrinologist) remained abnormal after six weeks. He was sure that we had "overcooked" him, and that he would never be the same. I'm happy to report that slowly, over time, he regained his normal parameters. He's had two more children since the time of that experiment.

INSIDE THE TESTICLE

The internal structure of the testicle is made up of two primary systems: the seminiferous tubules and the epididymis.

The seminiferous tubules are a series of tiny, convoluted tubes . . . so tiny, in fact, that there are hundreds coiled up inside each testicle. These tubules are lined with millions of Sertoli cells, each of which is intended to support and nurture a single spermatocyte as it develops and grows. The spermatocyte starts out as an immature cell without a head or tail—an amoebalike mass, each contained within its own Sertoli cell. Under the influence of pulses of FSH, the Sertoli cell makes the nutrients and raw materials that are necessary for the spermatocyte to mature. Over a 72-day period it will slowly begin to develop separate components: a head, which contains genetic material; a middle piece, containing energy materials for movement; and a tail, which will propel it forward. If you could look inside the seminiferous tubule with a microscope during this period, you would see each spermatocyte attached to its own Sertoli cell, like a tadpole with its head attached to the cell lining and its tail floating toward the middle of the tubule. (See Figure 3-2.)

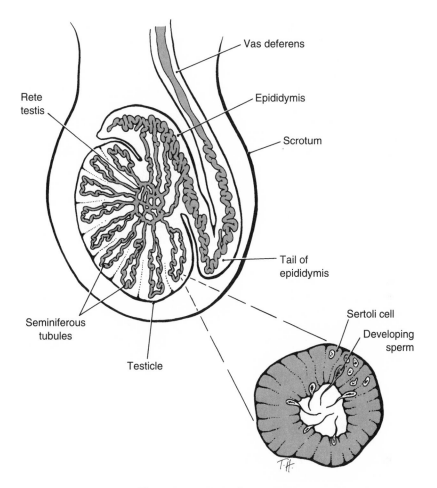

Figure 3-2: Testicular Anatomy

SAFETY SHIELD

In the material of the testes between the seminiferous tubules there are cells called Leydig cells. These Leydig cells manufacture the hormone testosterone. Infections within the seminiferous tubules can damage the Sertoli cells and create a problem with sperm production. But because the Leydig cells are outside the sperm-producing area, the production of normal amounts of testosterone won't be affected. Once again, infertility and "maleness" are separate considerations. Only if the infection is actually within the testicular tissue will the production of testosterone, which controls secondary male sexual characteristics, be affected.

At the completion of its growth, the spermatocyte detaches from the Sertoli cell and floats out into the seminiferous tubule, which leads it toward the center of the testes and into a collecting station called the rete testis. (See Figure 3-2.) Prior to this, pituitary hormones influence it to reduce from a 46-chromosome cell to a 23-chromosome cell, the correct number of chromosomes for fertilization. After remaining in the rete testis for a short period of time, it moves into the head of the epididymis. Because it is not yet motile, it will be carried along on this journey by various mechanisms within the rete testis.

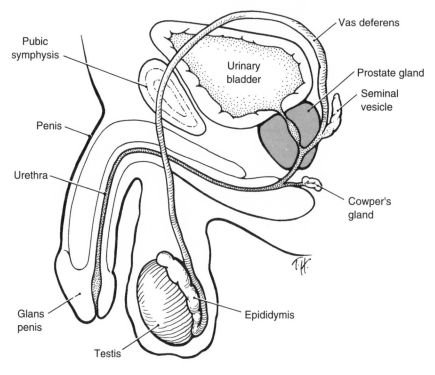

Figure 3-3:   Male Reproductive Tract

QUALITY IS JOB ONE!

Most people assume that sperm cells form and develop properly; they look normal, and have normal genetic components. But in fact, sperm development is not unlike the assembly line in most manufacturing plants. On any given day, one of the workers may perform below par. If he's working at General Motors he may miss a bolt in the chassis. At General Electric he may forget to connect a wire in the blender. And so the product goes down the assembly line with deficient parts that may not be recognized until it reaches the consumer. Quality control is a problem with sperm too. Some may be missing microscopic particles that are necessary for their genetic material to be normal. Some may have abnormal heads, or maybe even multiple heads. In fact, "normal" ejaculate, when visually examined under a microscope, will contain as much as 40% abnormal sperm—a failure rate that would quickly put General Motors out of business. Fortunately for us, millions of sperm are produced in each 72-day cycle. Even if only 60% are normal, there are still more than enough to complete the task.

The epididymis lies outside the testicle, alongside the testicular process. (See Figures 3-2 and 3-3.) If you run your fingers across the top of the testicle, you can actually feel this very small, coiled structure. In reality, the tubules within your epididymis are approximately twenty feet in length, but they're so tiny ($^{1}/_{300}$th of an inch in diameter) they can still fit into this very small space.

NORMAL IS AS NORMAL DOES

Can a man who manufactures normal sperm still have a problem? Yes. Infections of the seminal vesicle, the prostate gland, the urethra, or the penis can all harm previously normal sperm. If the infection is located where the fluid component of the ejaculate is manufactured, white blood cells may be found in the ejaculate, which will affect sperm motility as well as the sperms' ability to fertilize an egg. Infections within the urethra and the penis can also affect sperm quality, even though the sperm cells were normal prior to entering these areas. Males whose prostates have been removed can also have problems. Their ejaculate may not contain the nutritional components that are necessary to keep the sperm alive during their journey into the mucus of the cervical canal.

After completion of its growth in the seminiferous tubule, the sperm enters the head of the epididymis, and over a period of one to three days it moves through its entire length down to the epididymal tail. It is within the epididymis that the sperm becomes mature. It grows motile: the beat-to-beat action of its tail begins, enabling it to move on its own, rather than relying on contractions of the tubules to propel it. It also becomes more directional in its movement. Sperm that are removed from the head of the epididymis have some ability to swim, but they tend to move in circles rather than in a straight line. Sperm that come from the middle portion or the tail of the epididymis have matured to the point that they can swim in a straight line—they have what we call "directional motility."

Having reached the tail of the epididymis the mature sperm move into the vas deferens—the ejaculatory duct. There they wait for ejaculation to send them out through the penis. The initial contractions during orgasm come from the epididymis and the vas deferens. They move the sperm up into the area of the prostatic urethra. There the accessory glands of the male reproductive tract, the seminal vesicles, contract violently and expel a large amount of seminal fluid, which then pushes the sperm through the prostatic urethra. Along the way the prostate gland contributes additional fluid, which combines with the seminal vesicle fluid to form "ejaculate," a thick, gooey substance that moves the sperm into the urethra of the penis. It is there that the muscular contractions of the penis itself move the fluid ejaculate out through the end of the penis in a very forceful fashion and into the vaginal canal. (See Figure 3-3.)

Mr. Sperm's Wild Ride

When the sperm cell—which is accustomed to balanced acidic/alkaline conditions with a pH of 7.2—enters the vagina, it faces a hostile environment. The vaginal canal is extremely acidic. Its pH ranges between three and four. One of the jobs of the ejaculate is to maintain a balanced pH. Unfortunately, this protection is short-lived. The coagulum is attacked by the acidity of the vagina, and by the higher temperature of the vaginal canal, and the thick fluid becomes liquefied within three to five minutes. Once that occurs, the sperm, which have the ability to swim, quickly begin searching for a protected environment. That protected area is the cervix—the opening to the uterus—which connects the vaginal canal to the uterine cavity.

If intercourse and ejaculation occur close to the ovulation period, cervical mucus provides a way for the sperm to swim out of the ejaculate and into the cervical canal. If normal cervical mucus is not present, due to a problem in the female reproductive tract or to the fact that intercourse did not take place around the time of ovulation, the sperm won't be able to enter the cervix and they will die in the vaginal canal. Assuming the mucus has been prepared properly, due to rising estrogen prior to ovulation, the sperm cell will fight its way toward the uterine cavity accompanied by several million other sperm. They have just 15 to 20 minutes from ejaculation to reach their target.

───────────────────── **BOTTOMS UP!** ─────────────────────

Most women who are trying to get pregnant become concerned when
they stand up after intercourse and feel a drainage of fluid from the
vaginal canal. Some prop themselves up on a pile of pillows. Others
go so far as to have their husbands pick them up by their ankles and
shake them. Are they right? Are sperm really falling out? Not if the
woman has stayed in a reclining position for fifteen to twenty minutes. All the sperm that are going to enter her cervical mucus will
have entered it during that time. The drainage she feels is just liquefied seminal fluid, which was never intended to move up into her
upper reproductive tract. If, however, the woman has intercourse and
gets up . . . moves around . . . takes a shower . . . goes to the
bathroom . . . within a few minutes of ejaculation, ejaculate and
sperm may very well drain from the vaginal canal, making it difficult
for sperm migration to take place. Certainly any type of bathing,
douching, or washing of the vaginal canal within fifteen to twenty
minutes of ejaculation could severely affect the ability to conceive.

The mucus in the cervical canal works as a filter to eliminate abnormal sperm. It contains a series of channels whose width is precisely the
width of a normal sperm head. Sperm whose shape and size is standard
will fit the canals as comfortably as a train fits its track, and will quickly
migrate through the mucus. Abnormal sperm will be left behind, and
won't move on to the upper levels of the female reproductive tract. Some
of the normal sperm that move into the cervical mucus will migrate up
into the uterus and fallopian tubes within five to ten minutes. Others will
be held in the cervical mucus, as if in a reservoir, for as long as 24 hours
before moving on. We don't know why some are selected earlier than
others. It may be as simple as the fastest swimmers being the first to
move on.

Sperm reach the uterine cavity in groups of thousands. Once there,
they face a daunting task. The uterine cavity is huge in comparison to
the size of the sperm. A sperm making its way from the opening of the
uterine cavity all the way to its upper lateral edges, where the openings
of the fallopian tubes are located, covers as much territory as we would if
we swam across Lake Michigan. The sperm, which can swim just 25 to
50 microns per second, must now cover inches. They manage to do so
quickly because they're propelled by muscle contractions in the uterus,
as well as by their own power. Channels, or furrows, lead them up the
lateral sides of the cavity in much the same way that freeways lead us to
our destinations. Once the sperm reach the opening of the fallopian
tube, they begin the final phase of their journey.

Fertilizing the Egg

Assuming it is not obstructed, the fallopian tube will allow the sperm to enter. Hundreds of them now begin racing for the honor of reaching the egg first. They're helped along their way by tubal contractions. Chemical and hormonal signals from the egg may also aid in bringing sperm closer. This combination of factors guarantees that any egg that is residing in the fallopian tube after ovulation will be found, as surely as iron filings are found by a magnet. At this point the sperm will begin interacting with the egg's protective coating—the cumulus.

The stripping away of the cumulus is the first phase of the fertilization process. The cumulus is such a massive group of cells that hundreds of sperm will have to interact with it before it is broken down and the

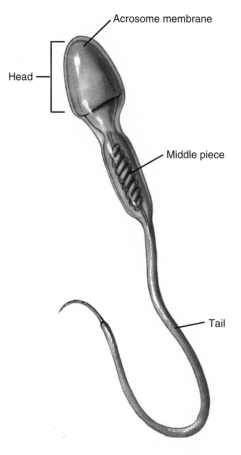

Figure 3-4: Diagram of a Human Sperm Cell

protective membrane surrounding the egg is exposed. The cumulus cells are held together by hyaluronic acid bonds. Each wave of sperm that reaches the egg attacks it from all angles, like sharks in a feeding frenzy. As they do, they release an enzyme called hyaluronidase, which breaks down these bonds. Individual cumulus cells then fall away from their partners, until, in a matter of a few hours, the egg is stripped clean. Thousands of sperm die in the process. Their places are taken by new groups that migrate up through the fallopian tubes, like wave after wave of troops landing on the beaches on D-Day.

After the first assault removes all the cumulus cells, the sperm begin to interact with the membrane around the egg, the zona pellucida. Hundreds of sperm attach themselves to the protein membrane of the zona, until one finally penetrates and fertilizes the egg.

What makes this sperm different from the several hundred others that are trying to punch a hole through the membrane of the egg? In order for a sperm to penetrate the membrane and fertilize the egg it must be "capacitated," or "activated."

As we said earlier, the sperm consists of a head, a middle piece, and a tail. The head is basically a protein carrier for the genetic package that fuses with the genetic material of the egg when fertilization takes place. It's surrounded by a double-layer protein membrane, the acrosome membrane. In order for the sperm to attach to, and then break through, the membrane of the egg, enzymes between the two protein layers must become "activated." This is known as an acrosome reaction. (See Figure 3-4.)

WHEN DO SPERM BECOME ACTIVATED?

There's a wide variation of timing for this. Certain percentages of sperm become activated as early as when they enter the cervical mucus. Others become activated as they move through the uterus and fallopian tube. Most frequently the acrosome reaction occurs when the sperm encounters the cumulus mass surrounding the egg, or when it meets with the zona pellucida. But acrosome reactions can take place even outside the female reproductive tract. Sperm that come into contact with an egg in the laboratory, or have been "washed" or prepared in other technical ways, have no problem becoming acrosome reacted, or capacitated.

In order for penetration and fertilization to take place, a high percentage of sperm must be acrosome reacted by the time they reach the outer membrane of the egg. As the acrosome membrane breaks down,

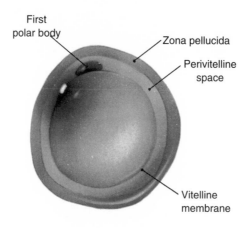

First
polar body

Zona pellucida

Perivitelline
space

Vitelline
membrane

Figure 3-5: The Egg Cell

the enzymes it contains will allow the sperm head first to fuse with the membrane of the egg, and then ultimately break through it to get inside the zona pellucida. Once inside the zona pellucida, the sperm enters the perivitelline space.

The perivitelline space is the area between the zona membrane and the vitelline membrane—the final layer separating the sperm from the nucleus of the egg. Once a single sperm breaks through the zona pellucida, it quickly attaches to the vitelline membrane, and within a matter of minutes fusion of the sperm's acrosome membrane and the egg's vitelline membrane takes place. During this process the sperm head is actually incorporated into the nucleus of the egg. This process has been followed through time-lapse cinematography, both in animal and in human egg interactions. Photography reveals the sperm being engulfed and surrounded by the egg's cytoplasm; the sperm is pulled in as if it fell into quicksand. Once the head of the sperm enters the cytoplasm or the nucleus of the egg, fertilization begins to take place. (See Figure 3-5.)

While the sperm is fusing with the egg and undergoing fusion with the outer membrane of the zona pellucida, the egg is undergoing a reduction of its chromosomes to become a 23-chromosome cell, rather than a 46-chromosome cell. This set of 23 chromosomes is released in a small blister called the first polar body. The sperm head that enters the nucleus of the egg already contains 23 chromosomes. Therefore the fertilized egg cell will contain a total of 46 chromosomes, half from the female and half from the male. Within 8 to 12 hours after the sperm has penetrated and incorporated into the nucleus of the egg, its head disintegrates. It is during this breaking apart that the genetic material from the

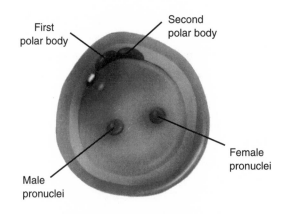

First
polar body

Second
polar body

Female
pronuclei

Male
pronuclei

Figure 3-6:   Fertilized Human Egg

male partner interacts with the female's chromosomes. During in vitro fertilization we can visually confirm the fertilization event when two small craterlike structures appear on the surface of the egg. These are called the male and female pronuclei. (See Figure 3-6.)

Over a period of 12 to 16 hours, the male and female pronuclei come together in the cytoplasm of the egg, the chromosomes form a single packet, and the fertilized egg cell divides into a two-cell embryo. Each cell of the two-cell embryo contains 46 chromosomes, which are identical to the 46 that the fertilized egg contained prior to its division. As the embryo continues to develop, it divides every 16 hours or so—from two cells to four, from four to eight, and so on throughout embryonic development. The chromosomes will also continue to double themselves, so that each cell will always contain 46 chromosomes that are identical to the original 46. This is why all cells in the body, be they liver, brain, skin, contain chromosomes identical to those in the undivided fertilized egg cell. The 23-chromosome component of the single sperm that reaches and fertilizes the egg lives on in every cell of the new life that is produced.

The fact that a single chromosomal package duplicates itself millions of times is just one aspect of the miracle of reproduction. Think of it. Each of us began as a single cell from our mother's body, and a single cell from our father's body. As a fertilized egg we were a mere $1/100$th of a millimeter in diameter. Yet within nine months we emerged screaming and kicking, weighing as much as ten pounds, measuring 19 to 22 inches in length, fully equipped to develop into a mature human being.

The very intricacy of this process should make it clear how easy it is for problems to arise—be they sperm problems, egg problems, cervical mucus problems, or others. Because there are so many possibilities, it is extremely important to try to understand precisely why problems are happening, and what we can and can't do to correct them. Most important of all, you should realize that given the many ways reproductive function may be interfered with, blame shouldn't be placed on one partner or the other. Once you understand the variables involved in achieving pregnancy, you can move on to correcting disorders or enhancing the resources that do exist. While this approach is rational, unfortunately it isn't always easy.

A NEW WAY TO LOOK AT THINGS

When a man has a borderline or subnormal sperm function, physicians often try to achieve a pregnancy by making the woman suprafertile, instead of aggressively approaching the male's problem and dealing with it. Doctors should do everything they can to enhance a man's sperm, before focusing on promoting a higher level of fertility in the woman's already fertile system, as a way of overcoming a male factor disorder.

If this is your situation, keep in mind that your doctor can suggest ways to improve the quality of the sperm your partner's producing in order to better the odds of fertilizing your eggs, before—and quite possibly without—having to put you through painful and invasive treatments.

Emotions and Erections

Stress and Sperm

Can a man become so emotionally distraught from the fact of infertility itself that the stress will diminish his sperm production and sperm function? While it is possible to find out through tests whether depression or other emotional factors are making a woman stop ovulating, and to correct her ovarian balance through medication such as clomiphene citrate, this approach is not possible for men. The fact that there is so much fluctuation in sperm production from day to day and week to week makes it difficult to demonstrate a cause-and-effect relationship between stress and poor sperm production. And even if one could be shown, there is no simple medication approach that would stabilize or normalize sperm production in the way that the drug clomiphene citrate corrects ovulation in women.

While it's not possible to demonstrate a cause-and-effect relationship between stress and poor sperm production, emotions can still play a big part in a man's ability to get his partner pregnant. A woman doesn't need to actively perform in order to receive sperm. But a man does; he has to achieve an erection and reach orgasm to move sperm from his body to hers. Any type of emotional struggle—troubles at work or with close relationships, for example—can temporarily interfere with a man's performance in this regard. Imagine how much more easily an infertility diagnosis, with all of the questions about ego and performance that accompany it, can inhibit his ability to reach orgasm. When this is the case, it makes it physically impossible for him to impregnate his partner. This physical barrier, brought on by a man's emotional state, can turn a possibly insignificant problem into a real crisis. Frustration, anger, and feelings of failure can then begin to escalate as the man feels he's losing ground in his struggle toward his goal. A man in this situation should take a moment to reexamine the situation, to refocus on himself and his partner, and to work to regain the feelings of confidence and security he previously felt within his relationship. Once he accomplishes this, he can put them back on track toward their goal of having a baby.

Terms We Used in This Chapter

Acrosome membrane: a covering over the head of the sperm which contains enzymes that, when released from the membrane, will allow the sperm to penetrate the egg.

Acrosome reaction: the breakdown of the acrosome membrane that changes the sperm into a cell that can penetrate the egg.

Capacitation: a change in the sperm cell that occurs after ejaculation and during the passage through the female reproductive tract, which enables the sperm to penetrate the egg.

Cervical mucus: a mucus secretion produced by glands in the cervical canal under the influence of estrogen.

Cervix: a narrow opening that connects the uterus to the vagina and produces mucus that allows the sperm to enter into the uterus.

Chromosome: the structure in each cell's nucleus that holds the parents' genetic information in the form of DNA (deoxyribonucleic acid).

Coagulum: nonliquefied ejaculate that is present upon emission.

Cumulus oophorus: a sticky mass of cells in a cloudlike pattern that surrounds the egg at the time of ovulation.

Cytoplasm: the material within the cell that is fluidlike and contains the microscopic structures that relate to cell function.

Directional motility: a term used to denote sperm that can move in a straight line.

Ejaculate: the fluid (semen) that carries the sperm cells out of the male's reproductive tract.

Ejaculatory duct: the tubes that connect the testicular system to the urethra in the penis for the release of sperm during orgasm.

Epididymis: the coiled tubules attached alongside the testicles that act as a storage system for the sperm prior to ejaculation.

Estradiol: an estrogen formed and released by the ovarian follicle during ovulation.

Estrogen: a category of female hormone that is necessary for female characteristics.

Fallopian tube: a narrow tubular structure connected to the uterus, which carries the egg from the ovary into the uterus after fertilization.

Follicle-stimulating hormone (FSH): a protein hormone produced and released by the anterior pituitary gland. FSH stimulates follicle growth in the female and sperm production in the male.

Germ cell: the precursor of other cells, i.e., the spermatid is the precursor cell of the sperm cell.

Gonadotropin-releasing hormone (GnRH): a small protein hormone produced in the hypothalamus, responsible for controlling the production and release of FSH and LH.

Hyaluronic acid: the bond, or glue, that holds granulosa cells in a tight mass around the mature egg cell.

Hyaluronidase: an enzyme that is found in the sperm membrane, which is released during fertilization so that the sperm can separate the granulosa cells from the egg.

Hypothalamus: the midportion of the brain that produces GnRH and other hormones that control the pituitary gland.

Leydig cells: the cells in the testicles that manufacture testosterone.

Luteinizing hormone (LH): protein produced and secreted from the anterior pituitary gland which is involved in ovulation.

Nucleus: the part of the cell that contains the genetic profile.

Penis: the male sexual organ.

Perivitelline space: the space between the zona pellucida and the surface of the egg cytoplasm.

Pituitary: a small gland at the base of the brain that secretes hormones that control our endocrine organs.

Polar body: an extrusion of material from the cytoplasm of an egg. It usually contains unused sets of chromosomal material.

Progesterone: the hormone produced from the corpus luteum after ovulation. It is also the hormone responsible for maintenance of early pregnancy.

Pronuclei: structures that look like moon craters on the surface of the egg; the presence of pronuclei indicates fertilization.

Prostate gland: a walnut-shaped gland that provides fluid for semen during ejaculation.

Prostatic urethra: the portion of the male urethra that goes through the prostate gland.

Rete testis: a network of canals that drains the sperm from the seminiferous tubules.

Scrotal sac: a saclike structure that cradles the testes.

Seminal fluid: the liquid that carries the sperm out of the male reproductive tract.

Seminal vesicles: the glands that produce the majority of the seminal fluid.

Seminiferous tubules: the tiny tubules within the testes that are necessary for sperm production.

Sertoli cell: the cells within the testes that are involved in sperm cell production.

Sperm: the male reproductive cell.

Spermatocyte: an immature sperm cell.

Testicle: the male reproductive organ.

Testis: singular for testicles.

Testosterone: the male hormone.

Urethra: a small tubular canal that carries urine in the female, and urine and seminal fluid in the male.

Vas deferens: the tube that connects the epididymis (sperm storage area) to the prostate gland; the pathway for sperm to leave the testicular area.

Vitelline membrane: the membrane that surrounds the egg cytoplasm, which the sperm fuses with prior to penetration of the egg cytoplasm; located under the zona pellucida.

Zona pellucida: the outer protein covering of the egg that the sperm first come in contact with during fertilization.

PART TWO

FACING INFERTILITY

4

Infertility and Its Treatment—
Are You Ready?

How do you begin infertility treatment? The first thing you have to do is admit that you need it. That sounds so simple on the surface, and yet so often it's not.

Me? Couldn't Be

Infertility is an interesting word; it represents different things to different people. To those who don't want children, it's a positive concept, offering a sense of personal and sexual freedom that would otherwise be lacking. But that isn't the case with most of you who are reading this book. To you *infertility* means that you're "sterile"—that you may never have a baby. You shudder at the thought. Some of you try to deal with it by simply changing the concept. It's just too hard to call yourselves that frightening word *infertile*. You find you have an easier time accepting the concept if you refer to yourselves as subfertile, or temporarily infertile, which implies that with some medical assistance you will still be able to reproduce. This is a reassuring idea, which you can embrace more easily. Others of you may deal with infertility by becoming caught up in denial. Denying it's a possibility, let alone a probability.

Denial is one of most common side effects of infertility. It's also one of the most harmful. It eats up precious months and years during which a problem might have been successfully dealt with. If you're an older patient, they may have been the only months and years when treatment would have been effective. Two patients, Mary and Joe Evans, were just such a case. As Mary describes it:

We'd been happily married for six years before we even thought of having a baby. I developed my legal practice, and Joe kept moving up as an executive in a major computer company. Neither of us felt the time was right; we wanted to be secure in our careers first. We never worried about having a family. It was a given. Our focus was just on when to start the process.

After my 36th birthday I felt the clock ticking. I'd built the thriving practice I'd always said I wanted. But when I looked at the different life experiences of my friends, many of whom had children and enjoyed parenting, my need to have a family took hold. It probably helped that a lot of my professional friends were feeling the same way. When I told Joe I was ready, he was quick to agree. I threw away my diaphragm and immediately began preparing for our new family. It didn't occur to me that I might not have one—a family was my birthright. I'd found success in almost everything I'd done in life. Why should this be different?

Ten months later I still wasn't pregnant. When I told Joe I was concerned—even a little afraid—he reminded me that the past months had been pressure packed. We'd been apart a lot because of his business trips. He wasn't surprised we weren't pregnant. He told me he knew in his heart that we would be soon. He reminded me that I hadn't had any gynecological problems. And he certainly didn't have any trouble ejaculating. I accepted his explanation. I wanted to. I just wasn't ready to concede that we had a problem. I guess that's when the denial took hold.

After six more unsuccessful months, I had to admit that we needed help. I approached my gynecologist. He'd known me since I was a teenager. It was comfortable, and I trusted him. He assured me it was too soon to worry. He told me I probably just needed to pinpoint my ovulation every month using a basal thermometer, and to have intercourse at two-day intervals right before and after I ovulated. I was eager to accept this; it didn't sound too serious. And so we followed his advice for another six months, while our obsession with having a baby became part of our everyday life.

It wasn't until after my 38th birthday that we discussed more advanced methods with our doctor. He prescribed a very basic fertility drug to be taken with each cycle, and for the next twelve months I used it. Still no success! Instead of facing the fact that it just wasn't working, Joe and I kept telling each other that we were satisfied with our medical care, and that a pregnancy would eventually happen. Three years after we'd made the decision to create a family, we were still childless.

Worse yet I was hitting 40, and something we hadn't considered to be that important had become the very thing that drove all of our thoughts. I began to read articles, to talk to friends and family . . . even to strangers, if the subject came up. I was finally willing to acknowledge to people who were close to me that we were having a problem and we needed help. By the time one of my friends sent me to a specialist, we were afraid that our window of opportunity had passed, and that at this point, maybe nothing would give us the children we so desperately desired. To our horror, our new doctor told us that having wasted four precious years, there was now a chance that we were right.

Looking in from the outside, it's easy to see that Mary and Joe were in denial. But how do you know if *you* are? As we said earlier, pregnancy should occur within six months of actively trying to conceive. If it doesn't, then it probably won't without some kind of help. Giving it more time is rarely the answer, especially if you're over 35. So why do we sometimes fall back on denial when this happens, instead of immediately going for help? Denial is the protective coping mechanism we use when a truth is simply too painful to face.

SIGNS THAT YOU MAY BE IN DENIAL

- **You find yourself feeling anxious for no obvious reason.**
- **You find yourself keeping busy just so you won't have to think.**
- **You're not willing to discuss your infertility problem with anyone else.**
- **You find yourself having "pro and con" discussions about your problem in your own head.**
- **You react defensively when the subject of infertility is brought up.**
- **You find yourself taking a normal behavior—such as eating or drinking—to extremes.**

While talking to friends and family is fine, you might want to consider seeing a professional if you suspect you're in denial. A trained psychologist or psychiatrist will not only understand your situation, they'll be careful not to strip your denial "defenses" away before you're ready to face your infertility.

JOIN THE GROUP

If you are in denial, don't feel alone. It's the rare couple that quickly accepts the situation, and immediately moves toward appropriate treatment. For most of you, the idea of not being able to have a baby the old-fashioned way is unthinkable. Mary and Joe's pattern of denial is typical. As you saw, it went through several stages during the course of their four-year journey. At first they were reluctant to admit they had a problem at all, preferring to blame their childlessness on circumstances and lifestyle. Once they began to acknowledge the possibility, their denial insinuated itself into their choice of a caregiver. Staying with their familiar ob/gyn made the problem seem less serious. It also caused them to lose 18 irreplaceable months.

ACCEPTING IT

Let's assume that you've now gotten past your denial, and you've accepted the reality of your situation. That's good, right? Well . . . almost. Accepting your situation and starting treatment, without understanding ahead of time what you're committing yourself to, can be another prescription for disappointment.

Most couples facing infertility have no realistic idea of what infertility treatment is like. As they are thrust into diagnosis and treatment, they become aware of the physical, emotional, and financial traumas that are associated with it, by experiencing them firsthand. No one ever told them what we're telling you now; you can spare yourself some of the pain by preparing yourself, both mentally and physically, for what lies ahead.

Think of infertility treatment as a journey toward having a baby. You probably got ready for your last big trip by becoming acquainted ahead of time with the territory you were about to visit. You gathered information through your travel agent, and from guidebooks and maps. You estimated expenses and prepared yourself with plenty of travelers' checks. And you found out about hidden pitfalls by talking to friends and acquaintances who'd actually been there. All this for a vacation? Imagine how much more important it is that you be well-informed and fully prepared for a treatment you hope will change your entire life.

It's not unlike that trip you took. As you plan your infertility journey, you need to learn how to choose *the best possible doctor to guide you through your particular problem.* You need to have some minimal *understanding of the various tests and treatments* that may be used in helping you.

And you need to truly be aware of the *commitments of time, money, and emotion* you'll be expected to make. For in almost all cases, infertility treatment will alter your daily life. It will intrude on your career, your personal relationships, and your emotional stability in ways you can't possibly anticipate.

Maybe you think none of this matters. Your desire to be pregnant pervades every aspect of your life. You're so desperate to have a child, you're willing to do whatever it takes, no matter the consequences. Think again. Even if you feel you're at your emotional limit and you can't bear to wait another day, take some time to learn at least a little about your condition and the infertility process as a whole. By being prepared, you can ease the pain and limit the negative impact infertility may have on your future. You'll learn to avoid the sort of mistakes that can prevent you from ever conceiving. And if nothing else, you'll satisfy your need to be doing something . . . hopefully the *right* thing.

You should embark on the initial leg of your journey with three major goals. First, to arm yourself with some general knowledge of infertility. Next, to select the correct doctor to guide you. And finally, to work with him or her in coming up with a "game plan" for your treatment.

Getting General Knowledge

You can't overestimate the importance of general knowledge. It's one of the few things that can help to give you some feeling of control in an otherwise out-of-control situation. Where can you go to obtain a basic education in infertility? One source is books like this one—a complete guide that helps you to understand the cause of your specific problem, the various alternatives that are available to treat it, and the impact infertility can have on your everyday life.

Your local community hospital's medical library, or the medical library at a nearby university that offers medical training, will offer a number of sources that can assist you in your hunt for knowledge. Articles on infertility are published on a monthly basis in professional journals such as *Fertility and Sterility*, the *Journal of Reproductive Medicine and Genetics*. Most of them are written in such a way that with some basic knowledge you will be able to understand them and learn from them.

In this age of the information superhighway, it's also worth your while to search for information through such on-line services as CompuServe, America On-Line, and the Internet. Not only can you find references to published data and gain access to information about what is happening in federal agencies, you may also come across computer bulletin boards being used by your fellow infertility patients. This will give you a chance to find out about their latest firsthand experiences, as well as to ask questions of them. This is a good way for you to make contact with people either within or beyond your immediate geographic area, whose experiences may offer you both information and support. If you don't have access to the Internet in your own home, you can often gain entree through a local university or in some states, through your public library.

Looking toward other sources, there are a number of organizations that speak directly to the various issues involved in infertility. Resolve is a support group for couples suffering from infertility. It has offices nationwide, in most major cities. It is an excellent source of both factual information and emotional support. It offers written materials, support groups, and networking.

The American Society for Reproductive Medicine (ASRM), is located in Birmingham, Alabama. Founded in 1944, it currently has approximately 11,000 physician members nationally. ASRM produces numerous educational brochures and booklets concerning all aspects of fertility and infertility treatment, which it will furnish to you upon request.

The Society for Assisted Reproductive Technology (SART), a division of the ASRM, was organized in 1985, and I served as its president for its first two years. SART is made up of approximately 260 centers throughout the U.S., which do specialized work in assisted reproductive technology to aid infertility patients. SART will gladly provide you with informational sources and statistical outcomes of various types of infertility treatments. All of these avenues will continue to be helpful to you throughout the various stages of your treatment—whether you're in the beginning, in the middle, or toward the end of your journey.

Finding the Right Doctor

Had Mary and Joe recognized early on that they had a real problem, they might have handled their choice of physician differently. They would have learned the important differences between an ob/gyn who incorporates infertility as just one minor area of his general practice, and a true subspecialist in the field. That distinction might have saved them two precious years on Mary's time clock. For you, as well, it is important that you make the distinction between doctors who are truly trained and who specialize in the treatment of infertility, and those who are merely treating infertility as an adjunct to their general obstetrics and gynecology practice.

─────────── **MOST COMMON COMPLAINT** ───────────

"Why did I waste so much time with my ob/gyn before coming to this center? . . . I can't believe how stupid I've been. . . ."

WHAT MAKES AN INFERTILITY SPECIALIST?

Try this . . . walk into any medical office building in any major city in the U.S. and look under the listing "Obstetrics and Gynecology." These days you'll find that nearly every doctor who's practicing obstetrics and gynecology will list his specialties as "Obstetrics, Gynecology, *and Infertility.*" This is a misleading phenomenon, given that among the approximately 28,000 obstetrician/gynecologists practicing in the U.S., only about 500 are board-certified subspecialists in infertility (known as "reproductive endocrinologists"). While all of these physicians are gynecologists, reproductive endocrinologists' practices are set up *solely* to assist in reproduction. Because of this, they have specialized ultrasound equipment, expanded office hours for the cycling patients, and the necessary surgical and laboratory facilities to accommodate their infertile patients' daily needs.

These specialists can be hard to find. Although the American Society for Reproductive Medicine will give you a listing of "infertility specialists" in your geographic area, their list doesn't discriminate between the true specialists and ob/gyn general practices. Resolve is a better source for narrowing down the field of ob/gyn physicians that claim to be infertility specialists. Before a physician is listed as an infertility subspecialist by Resolve, his education and credentials are reviewed by an independent board. If you call your local chapter or the national office, they will give you a listing of physicians that includes their credentials, their educational backgrounds, and their areas of specialization within the infertility treatment process.

Maybe this process sounds like a lot of trouble to you. Maybe you're even wondering if it's really all that important to see a subspecialist for your treatment. The answer depends on a number of issues.

First, how much experience and training does your regular ob/gyn have in reproductive medicine? Many gynecologists have gained good expertise in infertility through hands-on experience, even though they haven't had subspecialty training or been board certified.

Next, is a subspecialist readily available? In some small metropolitan areas and rural communities, subspecialists are nonexistent. If that's your situation, you might want to go to a competent ob/gyn for your basic evaluation, rather than driving three or four hours for routine infertility testing by a subspecialist in a city. If this is the course you take, you probably will still want to make some preliminary contact with a subspecialist, and be prepared to move on to that subspecialist for advanced care if your local ob/gyn feels your situation warrants it.

If, on the other hand, you do live in an area where subspecialists are readily available, your choice not to move on may be complicated by something else—separation anxiety. The fact that Mary's ob/gyn had cared for her during her entire adult life clouded her decision to move ahead to more appropriate treatment, or to second-guess the treatment she was receiving from him. Even when his treatment wasn't producing results, she stayed bonded to him with a false sense of loyalty.

The "loyalty excuse" often crops up because patients know that when they separate from their settled doctor-patient relationship, they'll have to reveal themselves to a stranger. Or it may be that your physician doesn't want to lose you. Even if you're ready to move ahead to a subspecialist, your gynecologist, the person you've trusted for so many years, may lead you to believe you are already getting the best care available. So you continue under his care until he finally admits that your problem has advanced beyond his abilities, and that you need a subspecialist. For certain patients this can be particularly dangerous.

- If you're over the age of 35 and you don't conceive within the first six to twelve months of trying, don't waste time! Go to a subspecialist!

- If you're known to have preexisting tubal damage, go to a subspecialist!

- If you're aware of sperm abnormalities, go to a subspecialist!

- If you don't know the reason for your inability to conceive, and your ob/gyn can't schedule testing at appropriate times in your cycle due to the fact that his office isn't open seven days a week, or his obstetrical practice interferes with your infertility testing, go to a subspecialist!

- If your ob/gyn continues to prescribe fertility drugs without regular scans of your ovaries—checking for cysts that could block your ability to conceive, or cause unnecessary harm—go to a subspecialist!

Time is important. Treatment is expensive. Don't waste either one.

Once you've decided you want a subspecialist, remember that Resolve can recommend physicians in your area and help you narrow the choices by explaining the particular area within infertility that each physician specializes in. You will find that some reproductive endocrinologists work primarily with endometriosis. Others work only with in vitro fertilization. And some specialize in male factor problems. If you have some basic idea of what your problem is, you may be able to use Resolve to link up with the appropriate expert.

Using the friends you have in the medical community is another possibility. Talk to the practitioners you trust about who has the best reputation, and who would be most suitable for you. Cross-reference their opinions with the physicians recommended by Resolve and, if you want, with the suggestions offered by the American Society for Reproductive Medicine.

And finally, learn from friends who've had infertility problems and who've undergone care. Find out what doctors they used. Ask if they were satisfied with their care. If they changed subspecialists, find out why. If they're seeing a new doctor, ask why he's a better match for them.

If this seems like a lot of work, keep in mind that while the relationship you have with your subspecialist will hopefully be short-term, in many instances it's not. The quest to have a baby may become a day-to-day, month-to-month, even a year-to-year ordeal, so you'd better believe your "guide" is the right one for you. You have to feel comfortable discussing your most personal secrets with the physician you choose; after all, infertility may involve some of them. You have to have a sense that he's listening to you carefully, and that he's answering your questions fully. And, of course, you have to feel confident that he's offering you the most appropriate care for your individual situation. Maybe you'll decide he isn't. The knowledge you've already gathered from the sources around you will help you to make that decision.

Interviewing Your "Guide"

After you've done your research and have chosen the physician you believe is the best one for you, you should schedule an initial consultation. This visit will cost you between $150 and $400. It's money well spent: it's your chance to interview him face-to-face. Because he'll be giving you a number of complicated facts that might be hard for you to remember accurately later, you'd be well-advised to bring a tape recorder. Start by asking your potential doctor about his qualifications, his educational background, and how long he's been practicing infertility. Don't be embarrassed to do this; your future depends on the doctor you choose.

"Everyone is ignorant, only on different subjects."

—*Will Rogers*

While your interview may lead you in a number of directions, there are two basic questions you should always be sure to explore.

First, find out how his specific practice is run. In some subspecialists' offices, the initial visit might be the only time you will see the doctor unless you require surgery. In these offices, nurse practitioners and paramedical personnel provide the bulk of your care. This system can be efficient, and allows the patient base of the office to be large, but it doesn't permit you to talk to your doctor on a regular basis—and as an infertility patient, you'll have questions almost daily. Your guide should be there for you regularly to provide the answers, thereby reducing the frustration that inevitably comes with infertility treatment.

Next, ask about the rate of success your prospective doctor and his center have experienced using various treatments. If you're familiar enough with your own problem to anticipate that you'll be facing one of the more advanced infertility treatments, which falls into the category of assisted reproductive technologies (which we'll describe later in Chapter Twelve), ask for his statistical results. And be sure the figures he gives you represent live birthrates, not just pregnancies that were initiated by him or by his clinic. Not only should you find out about his statistical outcomes for assisted technologies, but also for tubal surgery and ovulation induction with inseminations. You could take these statistics and compare them to the national statistics—for example, those provided annually by SART. The following table is a sample showing how SART's statistics are presented for two different procedures—GIFT and IVF. While you may not be familiar with these two procedures yet, you should familiarize yourself with the way in which their success rates are explained. The SART table tells you how often a particular procedure was performed during the year, the number of pregnancies that resulted, the number that were lost through miscarriage or because they were ectopic (implanted in the fallopian tube instead of the uterus), and the number that were successfully delivered.

SART Results of Gamete Intrafallopian Transfer (GIFT) and In Vitro Fertilization–Embryo Transfer (IVF-ET) in Patients Under 40 Years of Age and with No Male Factor Problems*

	IVF-ET	GIFT
#Procedures	16,158	3,199
#Pregnancies	3,947 (24%)	1,210 (38%)
#Deliveries per Procedure	3,198 (20%)	992 (31%)
#Miscarriages and/or Ectopics	749 (19%)	218 (18%)

*Modified from *Fertility and Sterility,* December 1994

Procedures such as insemination, ovulation induction, tubal surgery, and uterine surgery are normally not reported in any published or national format. If you're anticipating having any of these procedures, you'll have to question your physician carefully in respect to his success rates. Don't assume that because these percentages aren't reported on an annual basis, his figures aren't important. If any of these is the procedure you'll be undergoing, you really do need to know his level of expertise.

The five most important questions to ask your doctor prior to entering into any type of treatment are:

1. What is your background and training?
2. How many of these procedures do you perform annually?
3. What is your pregnancy rate per procedure?
4. What is your "baby rate" per procedure?
5. Who does more of these procedures annually than you do, and how do their success rates compare to yours?

Question number five is your "lie detector test." A physician who misrepresents his success rates can be exposed simply by calling your local Resolve chapter and requesting current data on the physicians in your community who perform the various procedures that are of interest to you. Use these figures as a reference, and keep in mind that a physician who fudges on question five is probably stretching the truth on one through four as well.

If Mary and Joe had asked their ob/gyn these tough questions, they would have realized they were wasting their time. If the doctor you're interviewing has any problems with the questions you've asked, move ahead to the next physician on your list. You must always keep in mind that infertility treatment can drain you of your time, your money, and your mental health. Given all these potential problems, it's vital that you feel comfortable with your choice of caretaker.

A SHORT INTERVIEW

The first doctor I saw hated my asking so many questions. His answers were vague, and he knew it. Finally, he blurted out, "Look, I'm the doctor here. I ask the questions. You'll just have to learn to trust me. If you don't like it, there's the door." I used it, and I haven't seen him since.

—Susie, age 32

Not only was Susie's doctor intimidated by her questions, his defensive reaction told her that she would never feel comfortable with him, or respect him and his medical practices. His bedside manner would definitely have clashed with her personality during treatment. Susie had read enough to understand that infertility treatment is not an exact science; your doctor may have to experiment with a number of different recipes before he finds the one that gets you pregnant. The process can take longer than you anticipate. If your physician keeps you in the dark, it will not only be painful, but extremely frustrating as well.

Hopefully, the physician you're interviewing won't behave the way Susie's did. Hopefully, he will answer your questions fully and clearly, and treat you as a partner in your own care. If he does, and if you're still satisfied that you've chosen the appropriate guide at the end of your interview, you're ready to move ahead. If that's the case, your new guide will plan the first steps in your treatment with you. If you're like most patients, you'll be facing a series of tests.

Tests Before Treatment

"Anxiety is the space between the 'now' and the 'then.'"

—Richard Abell
Own Your Own Life, 1976

It's hard to wait when you want something to happen *now*. But tests are a necessary prelude to your infertility treatment. Your physician will be performing a series of them in hopes of closing in on your possible problem areas and determining the exact cause of your infertility. Each individual test asks a specific question and looks for an answer. Each one is a possible step toward your diagnosis. Without them, your treatment can't follow.

The good news is that in most infertility practices, the testing process is somewhat standardized; if you've already had some preliminary infertility treatment, your work is partially done. That's why at our offices, we require all new patients to send us their prior medical history and records *before* coming in for their initial consultation. The doctor you're meeting with will probably do the same. We review these records carefully in advance of our first meeting with the couple. Because we're familiar with the tests that have already been done, we can move quickly to the next step should our patients decide to go forward . . . without wasting time and money duplicating answers that are already available. If no prior tests have been performed on you, a complete evaluation—a basic workup—will have to be completed. Your doctor should discuss with you what these tests are, the order in which they will be done, and what the results will tell him. He should also answer any questions you may have about them. If you don't have access to a doctor who will explain them to you, don't worry. We'll be giving you a complete description of the basic workup in Chapter Five.

Unfortunately, not all causes of infertility can be determined by a standardized series of tests. In these cases, the line between tests and treatment becomes blurred, because treatment is often prescribed in order to serve as a test. If a pregnancy doesn't result, it helps your doctor to determine your problem, and teaches him how to alter the recipe so there's a better chance of success in the future.

Formulating a Game Plan

Before you take a big vacation, you work with your travel agent on an itinerary. You know where you are going and when. You know approximately what it will cost. And you know what physical conditions to expect once you get there. That doesn't leave you much to worry about, does it?

Wouldn't it relieve many of your fears about infertility treatment if you and your new guide came up with a similar overview of what to expect? We agree. We think it's imperative that every couple has a game plan. Because treatment can be an intrusion into your lives, your game plan needs to be thorough. It should make you think about the cost of the treatment that's being recommended, and whether you can afford it. It should help you to understand the amount of risk and possible pain that is involved. It should help you to anticipate how the recommended treatment will intrude on your work life and your sex life. It should make you consider the treatment's religious ramifications, if this is important to you. And it should help you to take an honest look at the effect it might have on your relationship as a couple.

The goal of a game plan is not to scare you, but rather to prepare you with a realistic picture of the future as you set out to try to have a baby. Much like an itinerary, a game plan will reduce the possibility of wasting time and money, something all infertile couples desperately try to avoid.

The game plan you make with your doctor during your initial visit won't be set in stone. If the results of the tests he performs are different from what he anticipated, your course of action may change—and with it, your game plan. Ask your doctor ahead of time what modifications may have to be made to your initial plan. The alternatives can and should be discussed, so there's little or no surprise in the future. Being informed will help you adjust and be flexible if these new alternatives do have to be faced.

You should be prepared to make a new game plan as you reach each plateau in your treatment. You'll need to meet with your doctor as you finish the phase you've previously agreed on, and come up with a realistic analysis of the problems, costs, and timeline associated with the next treatment he is recommending.

The Time Factor

Time takes on two meanings when dealing with infertility. Probably one of the reasons you've opted to go into treatment is because you've been watching your biological clock race forward. Like Mary and Joe, most couples who are infertile eventually learn about the decrease in fecundity rate that occurs with the passing months and years. So as you continue to be unsuccessful each month, you may become increasingly obsessed with time.

Once you're actually in treatment, you may find yourself constantly examining the calendar. Each cycle has a built-in clock of its own. In order to succeed, you have to become attuned to what happens with each tick. Some of them dictate tests or treatments that you'll have to respond to immediately. The timing of ovulation tests, injections, and procedures isn't necessarily predictable. Planning for these things is just not possible, so if you're entering infertility treatment, prepare to be flexible with the clock, no matter how clumsy or out of character it may seem.

Fitting the Family Death Around Infertility

When my husband's favorite uncle, Ted, died suddenly, we realized how important our infertility treatment had become, both to us and to our extended family. The funeral was in another city, and it was critical that my husband be there. When we informed Dr. Marrs of the death, he reminded us that we were almost halfway through a cycle of Pergonal, and we wouldn't be able to adjust the cycle around the funeral. The extended family quickly decided to move the funeral back a couple of days to allow for our IUI cycle, offering that Uncle Ted would have wanted it that way.

—Karen, age 40

Treatment can also demand daily and weekly commitments of several hours during parts of your cycle. Not only will this have to be allowed for, it must take precedence over everything else in your life, including family and work-related responsibilities. One missed step during a month's cycle could be the cause of a failed attempt. It's too expensive to dabble. You have to commit to your treatment one hundred percent. Given this, a factor to consider when choosing your doctor is whether his office is conveniently located, relative to your home and office. If it's not, you'll have to set aside additional time to get there.

Periodically, larger blocks of time may also be called for. If you're facing one of the assisted reproductive procedures, you'll have to be able to spend several hours the day before your outpatient surgery preparing, and possibly spend several days afterward recuperating.

Living with these pressures month after month, maybe even year after year, will sometimes become too constrictive. That's one of the reasons it's recommended you stop treatment occasionally, and return to some of the other priorities in your life. Taking a break will not only help to bring normalcy back to your body, it will help you to center your thinking and bring your obsession with infertility back into perspective.

Physical Costs: Getting Ready
—What to Expect

If you're entering infertility treatment, you should anticipate experiencing varying degrees of pain and inconvenience throughout the process. The standardized tests that are performed prior to treatment may give you some temporary physical discomfort. During treatment, the male partner may have to collect sperm several times every month and deliver it to the doctor's office. If you're the female partner, you may be placed on medications that substantially alter your normal attitudes and emotions. The side effects may leave you feeling out of control and your partner may, at times, feel it would be easier to live in a locked ward at the state mental hospital. Daily intramuscular injections may also become a part of your life; you and your partner will have to agree on how to administer them. And regular blood tests may have to be performed to evaluate hormone levels. Picture yourself as a pin cushion; that's how most female infertility patients start to feel. If you have a needle phobia, and you want to push ahead in treatment, you'll have to learn to fight your fears.

You may eventually find that your best hope for a pregnancy lies in assisted reproductive technology. If that's the case, prepare yourself for medically invasive treatment, including surgical intervention, laser intervention, and anesthesia. If you have difficulty in any of these areas, you may need to take time away from your treatment to think it through or to work with a professional—a counselor or therapist—who can help you with your fears.

Monetary Costs: The Price Tag Can Be High

EXPLORING YOUR INSURANCE COVERAGE

The costs for a diagnostic workup, and for the treatment that follows, have the potential to rise surprisingly high. That's why it's important that you develop a general understanding of costs as one part of the preparation for your journey. Initially, you'll want to know what charges to anticipate for your diagnostic workup. And once you've been given a diagnosis, you'll want to have a clear understanding of what the costs could be for your specific treatment regimen. To develop a rough budget, refer to Chapter Thirteen, where you'll find a complete breakdown (as well as a nationwide comparison) of costs for the diagnostic workup and for various types of treatments.

Determining the price tag for your journey is a very important part of your game plan because coverage for infertility disorders by private insurance carriers is spotty, at best. The Health Insurance Association of America conducted a study in 1987 that found half of the top 20 commercial carriers pay for IVF in their typical policy, and seven of the remaining ten carriers reimburse for IVF under some of the policies they offer. And a report issued by the Congressional Office of Technology Assessment stated that private insurance is covering 70% of non-IVF infertility expenditure. But when you enter treatment, and explore with your present carrier whether you are covered for infertility procedures, you may find those figures hard to believe. Don't give up hope. There are certain carriers that provide coverage specifically for infertility treatment, as well as for assisted reproductive technologies. Among these, at present, are Prudential, New York Life, Travelers, Aetna, and a number of the new managed care groups such as Pacific Care, Health Net, and Cigna.

You have additional ammunition if you live in one of the ten states that currently mandates coverage for infertile couples as of this writing: Maryland, Texas, Illinois, Massachusetts, Hawaii, Colorado, California, Arkansas, Connecticut, and New York. Each of these states has directed that coverage be provided for infertility diagnosis. Treatment, including assisted reproductive technologies, may also be partially or completely covered. You're particularly lucky if you live in Massachusetts, Rhode Island, or Illinois, the three states that require coverage of all diagnosis and treatment approved by the American Society for Reproductive Medicine.

Unfortunately, the mandate to cover doesn't guarantee that coverage will actually be provided. In California, for instance, there has been a law on the books since 1990 requiring all insurance companies to offer coverage for infertility treatment, including some assisted reproductive technologies. But there has never been any instance of enforcement of the mandated law against a group or employer who refused to offer this coverage. So while the mandate exists, it has never been tested or utilized. If you're not familiar with your state's requirements for mandated coverage or its enforcement procedures, you should call or write your state insurance commissioner and ask for information specifically related to infertility coverage.

Health maintenance organizations (HMOs) are a form of coverage that's definitely worth exploring. As competition in the managed care field becomes increasingly aggressive, HMOs and other managed care organizations are more and more frequently providing infertility coverage, including coverage for assisted technologies, as a way to entice patients to sign up. That's why it's important that you shop around. One consideration in choosing a doctor may be whether he or she eases your financial burden by being part of a managed care group or an HMO.

Spending beyond your limits magnifies the stress you're already under as you try to get pregnant. In the world of infertility treatment, there are no guarantees, other than the high cost. If your treatment fails, the severe emotional fallout is compounded by your financial loss. So be sure you clearly understand what your financial commitment is, given your diagnosis, and discuss up front with your doctor exactly how much treatment you can realistically afford.

Life Isn't Perfect

Even with the best of treatment, not all infertility disorders can be corrected. You should face the possibility right from the start that the end result of your efforts may not be a child that is genetically linked to both—or even one—of you. Some of you may have to look at other alternatives in order to establish a family. Understandably, this can be difficult to accept. But once you do, the end result can be very rewarding.

For instance, if you are diagnosed with premature ovarian failure and can't produce your own eggs, you may choose to use an egg donor to conceive. You will remain the biological mother, and carry the baby to term. While the baby won't have your genetic makeup, it will have your husband's. Such egg donations have helped thousands of couples. In conjunction with IVF, they demonstrate a high success rate. They have certainly become a viable alternative for women Mary's age or older, who may otherwise have waited too long to carry a child. Similarly, donor sperm may be necessary if your sperm production is either nonexistent or abnormally low. If using a third party as an egg or sperm donor isn't an acceptable alternative for you, you can look toward the option that adoption offers. At the very least, you should become informed as to your choices, and find out what each one entails. You may also want to look for professional counseling to help you work through your feelings with respect to your alternatives.

Hopefully, by now, you've gained great insight into the world of infertility treatment. You've learned where to go for information, and how to choose the right guide. You've gotten a sense of the commitments you'll be making in order to undergo treatment—its financial costs, its practical aspects, and its formidable demands on your time. With this newfound understanding, and a willingness to forge ahead, you are now ready to begin your journey toward trying to have a baby.

Terms We Used in This Chapter

Assisted reproductive technologies (ART):   a term used to identify procedures such as IVF, GIFT, and ZIFT.

Clomiphene citrate: a synthetic hormone that stimulates a woman to ovulate. Clomiphene citrate can also be used in men to improve sperm production. The brand names of this substance are Clomid and Serophene.

Endocrinologist: a physician who specializes in diagnosis and treatment of problems relating to hormones or endocrine gland abnormalities.

Gamete intrafallopian transfer (GIFT):   a surgical procedure whereby the egg and the sperm are laparoscopically placed into the fallopian tube.

Human menopausal gonadotropin (hMG):   one of the "fertility drugs," consisting of FSH and LH. HMG is made from the urine of postmenopausal women.

Hysterosalpingogram (HSG):   an X-ray study in which a dye visible by fluoroscopy is injected into the uterine cavity to determine the shape of the uterus and patency of the fallopian tubes.

Infertility: the lack of conception after six months of unprotected intercourse.

In vitro fertilization and embryo transfer (IVF-ET):   the procedure in which the egg is removed from the ovary, fertilized in the laboratory environment, and the resulting embryo placed into the uterine cavity.

Laparoscopy: a surgical procedure in which a telescope is inserted through the abdominal wall to view the inner organs.

Laparotomy: a surgical procedure in which an incision is made through the abdominal wall in order to view the inner organs.

Pergonal: a mixture of FSH and LH that is used to stimulate ovarian follicle activity. The most common source for production of this drug is postmenopausal women's urine.

Postcoital test (PCT):   a test used to determine whether sperm/mucus interaction is normal, i.e., whether the sperm can move properly through the cervical mucus.

Ultrasound: an instrument that emits pulsed sound waves which are reflected off solid tissues to give an image of internal body structures without the use of X ray.

5

The Basic Workup

The elevator door opens, and Linda and Tom nervously step into the corridor. Linda checks the suite numbers and quickly turns left. Tom lags a few steps behind. They feel strangely distant from one another, but at the same time, closely bonded by the painful sense that they're the only people in the world who've been reduced to this fast-approaching appointment. Tom catches up to Linda as she reaches the door to the doctor's suite. Their eyes meet. She takes a deep breath, calming her pounding heart, while collecting her strength. Tom opens the door, and they walk into a world they dread calling their own.

Linda examines the carpet as she nervously moves toward the receptionist's window to announce their arrival. She's greeted with kindness, which goes unnoticed. Tom quickly grabs a magazine and finds a seat. Linda joins him, getting a faint smile from another person in the room. She barely reciprocates, too self-conscious to help break the ice. Once seated, she studiously takes in the office decor. Informational pamphlets stare back at her, as do the notices on the bulletin board for emotional-support group sessions. Her own shoes seem to be the only comfortable thing to look at. Nothing is said between her and Tom; they are too caught up in their own thoughts.

While we're describing Linda and Tom, this could be any couple on the day of their first appointment with an infertility expert. If he's just a doctor, why is it so hard to approach him? Once you put yourself in their position, the answers are obvious.

First There's Fear

If you're seeking professional help, then something must be wrong with you, and not knowing what it is can be petrifying. You wonder . . . you imagine the worst . . . soon you find yourself fearing the answer almost as much as the problem. Could it be that after your doctor runs all of his tests, you'll find out that either you or your husband is sterile? God forbid! You quickly put the thought out of your mind, hoping the problem isn't that serious or difficult to treat. Still, your mind races uncontrollably. What *could* the trouble be? Will this doctor actually be able to determine it? You've heard from friends that not understanding the cause of your infertility can be the most frustrating experience of all. What if you and your doctor *are* lucky enough to figure it out? Will it be too expensive to treat? Will you need surgery? Will your medical treatment be painful? And how much will it interfere with your life? It's about now you start feeling sorry for yourself. Why are so many people out there having children easily when you are having such difficulty?

You begin to conjure up all sorts of scenarios. Was it because you had sexual intercourse for the first time at the age of 16? Was it that abortion you had when you were 21? How about the sexual partners you were with before you got married? Were there too many? Or maybe it's that vaginal infection you got years ago . . . the one you thought was properly medicated and corrected? What if it really wasn't? What if it's spread to your fallopian tubes and affected their ability to function? What will your husband think when he learns the reason the two of you aren't conceiving is an infection you got from another man? And what about the women in your husband's past? He never impregnated any of them. Why? Is something wrong with his sperm? Maybe he'll never be able to get you pregnant.

You may feel all of this, and more, as you enter into the diagnostic phase of your infertility treatment. Don't worry, these are all normal fears; it would be odd if you didn't have them, or some like them. What's worse, look where you're starting this process—in a stranger's office. So what if he's a professional? You're about to have one of the most intimate discussions in your life with a person you've never met. No wonder your anxieties are growing by the second. Who is this person, really? You've been referred to him through good sources . . . his credentials seem to be up to par . . . but what is he really like? Will he be young or old, alert or tired? And even more important, can he be trusted with the personal information you and your husband are about to give him? Will he answer your questions? Will he instill confidence? Will you walk out of his office feeling as if a healthy baby is just around the corner for you? When all is said and done, will he be the one who will help you to bring a child into this world—a feat you and your husband have been unable to accomplish on your own? Please God, let the answer be yes!

There's so much riding on this, you're afraid to move. How could you possibly focus on a magazine when you're this busy trying to control your desperate fears and hopeful expectations?

Then the nurse announces, "The doctor will see you now." As you walk down the corridor, you pass by hundreds of baby pictures on the wall, infants obviously produced by the doctor you're about to meet. "Ouch!" Who wants to see newborns held by happy parents? Twins and triplets, no less. And yet it's proof that this stranger *is* successful. Shouldn't the pictures make you feel good? Someday you and your new family could be there for all to see too. And wouldn't that be wonderful?

Your Initial Appointment— Knowledge Is Power

Let's take a step ahead in time and assume that having escaped the terrors of the waiting room, and having met your doctor, your interview goes well. He seems to meet all the criteria for a guide, which you learned about in Chapter Four. You're feeling more comfortable as he clearly describes the process you're about to embark on. It begins with identifying the cause, or causes, of your infertility. The first two steps in accomplishing this are:

- Reviewing your previous medical evaluations, and
- Completing your medical history

In most cases, you'll be doing this during the course of your first appointment. Once these steps are completed you will, in all likelihood, move on to the basic workup, a complete evaluation of your and your partner's reproductive systems.

REVIEWING YOUR PREVIOUS MEDICAL EVALUATIONS

One thing that you will absolutely want to bring with you to your initial meeting with your infertility subspecialist is a complete set of any previous medical records that pertain to your gynecologic history, as well as the results of any tests that have been done during prior infertility evaluations. Allowing the infertility subspecialist to review these records instead of putting him in the position of creating your history from scratch will prevent delays and repetition of testing, and will save you both time and money. The physician who performed your prior tests may have told you they showed that everything was normal, but the subspecialist could possibly see different things as he reviews them, and may have a different opinion based on them.

When reviewing previous medical records I have often found misinterpretation of testing. In cases too numerous to count, an appropriate therapy instituted after correct interpretation resulted in a pregnancy without doing any further evaluation.

Your new subspecialist should *want* to be cognizant of your former testing. If he doesn't ask to review your former records during your initial appointment, think again as to whether he is going to be your best choice for your infertility treatment.

COMPLETING YOUR MEDICAL HISTORY

After reviewing your prior records, your subspecialist may feel that he needs to have additional questions answered. This may include fleshing out in more detail the areas your prior physicians already went into. Or it may involve discussing areas that weren't explored previously. Be patient if this seems repetitious. Your new subspecialist, who has a deep knowledge of infertility problems, may be looking into possibilities that weren't obvious to your prior doctor.

In order to complete your medical history, your physician may spend time with you talking about past events. Have you ever been pregnant? Has your husband ever been involved in establishing a pregnancy? Do either of you have a past history of any type of chronic medical condition such as thyroid disease, adrenal disease, high blood pressure, or other similar disorders that might in some way affect your ability to get pregnant? Do you take medication for long-standing medical conditions like hypertension or diabetes? Do either of you have a history of exposure to environmental toxicity? For example, are toxic chemicals or radioactivity present in your workplace?

———— CAN CHEMICAL EXPOSURE AFFECT YOUR CYCLE? ————

Current research points to a number of common chemicals as possible reasons for menstrual irregularities. These include organic solvents such as paint thinners and dry cleaning fluids, as well as ethy-

lene glycol ethers, such as those found in varnishes, fingernail polishes, and some dyes, inks, cleaners, and degreasers. Exposure to benzene also seems to be linked to an increased incidence of menstrual irregularities.

Your answers to these questions may help your physician to pinpoint some obvious areas of concern, which will then dictate where your testing should begin. For instance, if your husband works in a nuclear power plant, he should be tested first. Your doctor will look for abnormalities in sperm production, as well as for problems with sperm function that might compromise the sperm's ability to penetrate an egg. If, as a young girl, you had a ruptured appendix, you may have had a pelvic inflammation as a result. Your evaluation would begin with a check of your fallopian tubes to see if they're clear, as well as with a check of your pelvic environment to confirm its status. These are just two examples of how a thorough medical history can help you and your physician to short-cut your search for the cause of your infertility.

Once your medical history has been completed to the satisfaction of your subspecialist, he may or may not want to do an additional routine physical exam or ultrasound. This will probably depend on whether he found new information while expanding your medical history, or on the timing and extent of the last exam your primary care physician gave you. Also, if your partner's prior semen testing indicates that a male factor problem is possible, he may be referred to a urologist for evaluation at the time of your initial appointment.

As you can see, in some cases your doctor will be able to hone in on your problem and to move toward treating it based solely on your medical history or on abnormalities which have been found in a prior physical examination. If so, you will have saved both time and money—a rare and welcome phenomenon in the realm of infertility treatment. More frequently, you will need to continue with a third diagnostic step—the basic workup.

The Logic of the Basic Workup

There are various ways to approach this basic infertility evaluation. If your medical history or physical examination *did* indicate an obvious problem area, your doctor will naturally start his testing by concentrating on it. But when no specific abnormalities that are considered suspicious are found, your doctor won't have such a definite direction to move in.

When this happens, different doctors have different approaches. Some start by doing a laparoscopy to evaluate the pelvic environment. Others perform a hysterosalpingogram to determine whether the fallopian tubes are formed normally and are clear. Some use semen analysis as their first step in the evaluation of the couple.

While each of these approaches meets with some degree of success, the best option for you, as a patient, is to be given a workup that is designed to find your problems in the fastest and most cost-efficient manner possible. To do that your doctor should:

1) Test for the most common infertility problems first; we're about to tell you what they are. Only when those problems have been eliminated should he move on to testing for less common, and finally for the least common, problems.

2) Use the least physically invasive and least painful testing approaches first, and advance to more intrusive tests, or to surgical intervention, only as they seem necessary. We'll be describing the most common infertility tests for you in this chapter, so that you'll understand the degree of invasiveness of each of them.

3) Use the testing method that is least expensive but will still tell accurately whether or not you have a problem. We'll be giving you a complete list of costs in Chapter Thirteen, so that you can check on this prior to your testing.

This approach has been developed through many years of experience, training, and evaluation of infertile couples. If you are concerned with saving time, money, and pain, you should study it and insist on it.

As infertility specialists have gained experience in diagnosing infertile couples, they have discovered that some disorders have certain patterns of frequency. Looking at the universe of infertile couples, difficulties with ovulation and/or sperm account for approximately 40% of the problems that are found. Therefore, your doctor should first question you about ovulation problems, and problems with sperm production or sperm function. Then he should observe your ovulation cycle, and do a semen analysis. If he finds abnormalities in ovulation at that time, he should stop at that point and fix the abnormalities, without moving on to more invasive testing. And if he finds a problem with sperm function, he should use one of the several methods that have been developed to assist subnormal sperm to accomplish fertilization.

What Are the Most Common Infertility Problems?

A Quick Guide to the Frequency of Infertility Problems

Ovulation and/or Sperm Problems	40%
Sperm/Mucus Interaction	15%
Fallopian Tubes and/or Uterus	15%
Pelvic Environment	15%
Unexplained	15%
Total	100%

If your doctor can't detect a problem with your ovulatory cycle or with your husband's sperm production and function, he should then consider whether there is a deficiency in your cervical mucus, or with the interaction between your cervical mucus and your husband's sperm. Another 15% of infertile couples will fall into this category.

If problems still haven't been found, the next thing he should do is question whether there are any structural abnormalities of the fallopian tubes or of the uterus, or whether there are any obstructions within the uterine cavity or fallopian tubes. These areas account for another 15% of all infertility problems.

Assuming no abnormalities are found, the final step your doctor should undertake is to look at the interior of your pelvic cavity to determine whether any adhesions or pelvic endometriosis are present. About 15% of the women in infertile couples have some type of pelvic problem that restricts their ability to conceive.

While it appears that the last three steps are interchangeable—each one locating 15% of infertility problems—they're actually not. These tests have been arranged for you in order of invasiveness, moving from the least physically difficult to the most challenging.

Following this logical and patient-friendly plan, there are five steps in the basic workup.

- ovulation testing
- male testing
- cervical function testing
- testing the reproductive tract
- testing the pelvic environment

The Tests in the Basic Workup

STEP ONE: OVULATION TESTING

Testing Your Past Ovulation
   Menstrual Cycle Length
   Basal Body Temperature
Predicting Your Upcoming Ovulation
   LH Surge Testing
   Blood Hormonal Tests
   Cervical Mucus Tests
Confirming Your Ovulation
   Ultrasound
Testing Luteal Phase Function
   Blood Hormonal Tests
   Endometrial Biopsy

STEP TWO: MALE TESTING

Basic Semen Analysis
   Visual Testing
   Computer-assisted Semen Analysis
Advanced Semen Testing
   The Hamster Test
   In Vitro Mucus Penetration Test
   Electron Microscopy
   The Hemizona Assay Test

STEP THREE: CERVICAL
FUNCTION TESTING

The Postcoital Test (PCT)

STEP FOUR: TESTING THE
REPRODUCTIVE TRACT

   The Hysterosalpingogram
   The Carbon Dioxide Test
   Computerized Axial Tomography
   Magnetic Resonance Imaging
   Ultrasound HSG (sonohysterogram)
   Hysteroscopy

STEP FIVE: TESTING THE
PELVIC ENVIRONMENT

   Laparoscopy

These five steps consist of a number of different tests. We've summarized them in the above table, and will be discussing them in detail for you throughout this chapter.

Step One:
Ovulation Testing—Are You or Aren't You?

A basic workup normally begins with an evaluation of your ovulatory cycle. The tests that you take during this evaluation will focus on four important things.

1) They will tell you whether you have been ovulating on a regular basis in the past.

2) They will attempt to predict the exact timing of your upcoming ovulation.

3) They will confirm whether you actually did ovulate during the cycle currently being tested.

4) They will test whether your luteal phase—the part of the cycle when your uterus prepares to receive a fertilized egg—is functioning properly.

Unfortunately, in order to determine whether your cycle is working, you will have to take more than one test. That's because every ovulation test is only an *indirect marker* of whether correct biological function is taking place. For example, an ultrasound of your ovaries can show whether your dominant follicle for the month has shrunk or not. If it has, it's likely that an egg has been ovulated and released. But since your doctor can't actually see the egg, this remains an assumption, not a certainty. Every other ovulation test is like this—an indirect marker of appropriate function. In much the same way that the jury in a murder case adds up a number of items of circumstantial evidence to decide whether the defendant is guilty or innocent, your doctor will look for appropriate responses to a combination of these tests to conclude whether you are ovulating correctly.

Another thing for you to remember is that—as we described in Chapter Two—your ovulatory cycle has a series of different phases. Like a piece of machinery with multiple moving parts, where the failure of one can stop the whole apparatus, each phase of your cycle must also be working correctly in order for the whole to function.

HAVE YOU BEEN OVULATING?

Establishing after the fact whether you have been ovulating regularly can be accomplished inexpensively and noninvasively. You doctor should look at a combination of two things in order to make this determination.

Your Menstrual Cycle

Have you had regular menstrual periods in the past? From a clinical standpoint, women are thought to have regular ovulatory cycles if they have a history of menstruating at 28- to 32-day intervals. It would be rare for you to have abnormal ovarian function if you fall into this group.

Basal Body Temperature

BURN YOUR CHARTS

I still see two or three new couples a month who come into my office for their initial consultation carrying two or three years' worth of daily temperature charts for my review. Their previous physicians had led them to believe that these BBT charts are vitally important in their quest for conception. Relying on these charts to time their intercourse, and then still failing to conceive, can in itself be responsible for an undue amount of stress on these couples. When I tell them to throw away their basal thermometers, we take the first big step in reducing some of the pressure involved in their infertility treatment.

Basal body temperature is a much misunderstood test. Many couples think that they can use their BBT charts to determine the best days on which to have intercourse in order to conceive. They don't realize that a BBT chart is of historical value only. It can indicate, *after the fact*, that you *did* ovulate. Over a period of months it can show you whether your ovulation is more or less regular. But what it can't do is predict when ovulation is about to occur. If your goal is to have intercourse, or precisely timed fertility testing, that coincides with ovulation, a basal body temperature chart is not an accurate indication of when it will occur.

The reason for this is that, as the name implies, it's based on body temperature. After an egg is released from its ovarian follicle, a woman begins to secrete progesterone. This hormonal change triggers an increase in her basal (or core) temperature. In order to do a BBT chart, you take a resting basal temperature at the same time each morning for several days prior to the day you anticipate your ovulation will occur. At the time of ovulation, or shortly thereafter, your basal body temperature will elevate 0.6°F to 0.8°F over the baseline that you've established.

While it sounds good in theory, the basal body temperature method is fraught with inaccuracy. For starters, the change in temperature is usually so slight, it can be misidentified. And your sleep patterns can also make a difference. Maybe you'll have a restless night's sleep, or get out of bed during the night. Either of these things is enough to impact a basal body temperature reading the next morning.

PREDICTING UPCOMING OVULATION

Three tests are commonly used to tell you when you are going to ovulate. Each of them will help to predict this with varying degrees of accuracy and at varying expense.

LH Surge Monitoring Kits

The most precise predictor of ovulation is a hormonal change, which occurs immediately preceding follicle rupture. As we discussed in Chapter Two, just before the egg disengages from its home within the ovary, there is a release of stored-up luteinizing hormone, which is called the LH surge. Because of this, the concentration of luteinizing hormone found in a woman's urine is a good indicator of approaching ovulation.

Over the past ten years a noninvasive and inexpensive testing system has been developed specifically for this purpose. LH surge monitoring kits are simply urinary tests that measure the concentration of luteinizing hormone in a woman's urine. They can be performed in about five minutes in your home or office, saving you the time and expense of going to your doctor's office to be tested.

While a number of brands are on the market, and all of them have been tested by their respective manufacturers, Ovukit has also been checked in clinical studies by objective gynecological practitioners. It can easily be found over the counter, at a cost of approximately $60.

THE SURGE GUIDE—CURSE OR BLESSING?

With the development of the home LH monitoring systems, a new-found predictability and control over ovulation timing was accomplished. For the patient, this precise timing is reassuring; for the physician, it is scientifically sound; but for your husband, it can be a nightmare. There have been many a board meeting, business presentation, or golf game, that have been cancelled due to the appearance of a blue dot, pink stick, or blue line appearing on one of the test systems used today.

To determine when your LH is surging, you should use your kit to check your urine beginning two to three days prior to the midpoint of your cycle, the time at which most women are expected to ovulate. If you have kept a basal body temperature chart of your past cycles, you should have a good idea when this midpoint will be. When luteinizing hormone reaches a measurable concentration in your urine (greater than 25 mIU/milliliter), you know that you are going to ovulate within 24 to 36 hours.

These tests of LH elevation, or "surge guides" as they are sometimes called, indicate very reliably and accurately when ovulation will occur.

Blood Tests

Some doctors do blood tests on their patients, and have their hormonal levels analyzed, as a means of predicting ovulation. In our opinion this predictor is overly expensive, and too physically invasive for this particular use. In order to pinpoint in this way exactly when ovulation is going to occur, tests must be taken, and hormone levels have to be performed, on a daily basis. The cost of this serum analysis for estrogen, progesterone, and luteinizing hormone runs about $150 a day, and the information about upcoming ovulation that is gained is almost identical to that which you can get much less expensively with an LH surge monitoring kit.

Mucus Changes

In the past, before it was easy to measure hormone levels, physicians used the appearance of a woman's cervical mucus as an indicator of approaching ovulation, and as a marker of adequate amounts of estrogen in her bloodstream.

As you approach ovulation, from about the sixth or seventh day of your cycle, your estrogen begins to increase at a steady rate. This estrogen rise triggers the production of mucus from glands in the outer part of the cervical canal. This mucus is the source of the watery vaginal discharge that most women experience a day or two prior to ovulation. If you are about to ovulate, it should seem stretchy, and generous in amount.

Even though we now have more accurate tests of hormone levels, some physicians still use changes in cervical mucus as their sole predictor of ovulation. Beyond the fact that this is very subjective and not very accurate, there is another reason why it is not usually recommended. In certain cases a patient can be ovulating normally but still have poor cervical mucus production. Some examples of this are women with cervical infections or prior cervical surgeries, such as cryosurgery or cervical conization. Using mucus production as an indication of ovulation for these women could be very misleading. At best, cervical mucus should be used as an additional, indirect marker, which confirms more accurate tests.

CONFIRMING THAT YOU OVULATED

The tests we've just discussed have been ones that predict when you are about to ovulate. Yet another test helps to confirm that you actually *did* ovulate. A simple test that can confirm your ovulation is ovarian ultrasound.

Ultrasound

This type of testing is important because some conditions exist in which your ovaries prepare to ovulate, but then don't—luteinized unruptured follicle syndrome (LUF), for example.

An ultrasound machine bounces sound waves off solid and fluid-filled masses within the pelvis, and projects their images onto a screen. It can be used to find abnormalities within the pelvis, to look at uterine and ovarian size and position, and to spot uterine cavity defects or ovarian cysts. It also can discern a pregnancy. It is also commonly used to detect ovulation.

Originally, ultrasound pictures of a woman's developing follicles were taken externally. The abdomen was covered with a kinetic gel, which helped conduct sound waves, and a probe was passed over the abdomen. Today, almost all infertility specialists use vaginal ultrasound, in which a probe covered with kinetic gel is actually inserted into the vagina. The process is simple and painless, and because its pictures are taken internally, a vaginal ultrasound is considerably more accurate.

▬ THE INVENTION OF VAGINAL ULTRASOUND . . . ▬ OR, FULL BLADDERS WEREN'T FUN

As late as 1982, if you had come into my office for an ultrasound to determine your ovulation timing, you would have found it to be a very uncomfortable process. The biggest problem with ultrasound in those days was that doctors placed probes on the outside of the abdominal wall, then tried to see ovaries that were hidden well down in the pelvic cavity. The only way we could get a reasonable look at them was by asking patients to overfill their bladders. Once distended, the bladders pushed the ovaries closer, giving the physician a better look at the follicles and their development. In those days, waiting rooms were filled with women praying their doctors wouldn't run late. They'd still be there praying if it weren't for one of my patients—Mary Beth.

It all started when I received a call from a research engineer. He'd spent his company's time and money developing an ultrasound probe that could be inserted into the vagina, for use on women with bladder problems. To his dismay, it didn't work. He asked me to give the probe a try before they scrapped it. Most of my patients took one look at that vaginal ultrasound probe and said they'd rather not have it used on them. The few who agreed might as well not have. All that it revealed was the outline of a full bladder; seeing their ovaries was even more difficult than with abdominal ultrasound.

Luckily, before I returned the probe, Mary Beth came in—late, as usual. And of course, as usual, she had an empty bladder. Since I was about to go into surgery, I told her I couldn't wait for her to fill up, and she responded by starting to cry. As an act of desperation, I told her we could try the experimental probe. To my amazement, this attempt with vaginal ultrasound gave me a picture of Mary Beth's ovaries and uterus that was better than I had ever gotten with any other patient. It was then that I realized my patients' full bladders had been pushing their ovaries out of sight. Thanks to Mary Beth, the era of vaginal ultrasound (and empty bladders) had begun.

Using ultrasound, your doctor will be able to see the size and shape of your ovary, and detect whether your follicle has begun to rupture and collapse, indicating that ovulation has occurred. While the ovary can be clearly seen through this method, ultrasound is still an indirect marker of ovulation, because the egg is microscopic in size, and ultrasound can't actually see it within the follicle. The follicle's collapse leads us to believe that the egg has emerged, even though we haven't really seen it. That's why combining ultrasound with an LH surge monitor, and getting a positive result on both tests, gives the most accurate possible diagnosis of ovulation.

Generally, the best time to start ultrasound is right after your LH surge. At this point your doctor can look at your ovary, observe its size, and see whether a follicle has begun to swell in preparation for ovulation. (See Figure 5-1.) He can then continue to use ultrasound to confirm whether the follicle has collapsed, signaling ovulation. This change in the follicle's size and shape is the best visual indication of ovulation we can get. (See Figure 5-2.)

Once probable ovulation has been seen, ultrasound can be used to measure the thickness of your uterine lining (the endometrium), and see whether it seems to be growing at a rate that will make it adequate for implantation of a fertilized egg.

If you are worried about safety factors with ultrasound, don't be. Ultrasound does not involve radiation; it's merely soundwaves. It's been used since the early seventies, multiple studies have been done on it, and no soft tissue effects or other abnormalities of eggs, fetuses, or reproductive organs have been demonstrated as a result. For this reason you should feel comfortable having an ultrasound done at any time during a pregnancy, without concern for any possible effects on your reproductive tract or your developing fetus.

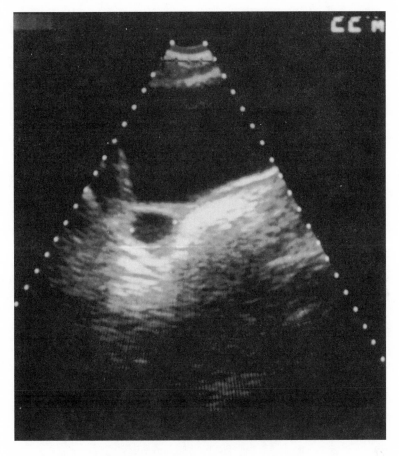

Figure 5-1:   Follicle Prior to Ovulation

TESTING THE LUTEAL PHASE

In order for your ovulatory cycle to be normal, each individual phase must function well. Even if you have tested positively for ovulation, you could have a luteal phase abnormality—a problem in the way your uterus prepares itself to receive and carry the fertilized egg. There are two different ways to test for this.

Blood Tests

While we don't recommend them as a marker for ovulation, blood tests *are* valuable for testing the luteal phase of your cycle. If your ovulation appears to be normal, but you are still not getting pregnant, it might

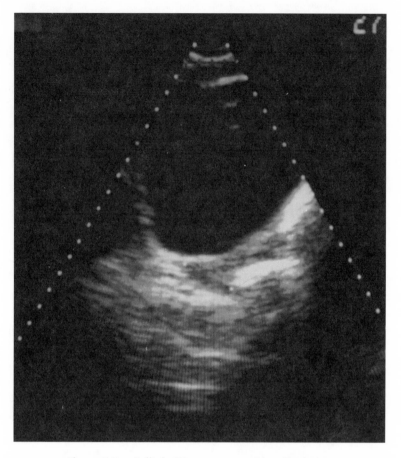

Figure 5-2:   Follicle Disappearance After Ovulation

be due to some irregularity in the production of estrogen, which influences the lining of the uterus to grow, or of progesterone, which triggers the receptivity of the lining for implantation. The levels of these hormones can be checked through blood tests. To do this, your doctor will take a blood test seven to ten days after your LH surge. He will look at the amounts of estrogen and progesterone in your blood, and confirm whether the levels of these two hormones have elevated. If they have, he can tell whether you have ovulated, whether the timing of your ovulation was as expected, and whether normal amounts of estrogen and progesterone are being generated.

Endometrial Biopsy

Your doctor will probably follow up your blood tests with an endometrial biopsy. Under the influence of estrogen and progesterone, the interior of your uterus should be thickening into a spongy, receptive lining, and growing new blood vessels in order to support a fertilized egg. By taking an endometrial biopsy, your doctor can confirm that this is actually happening.

Perhaps you are wondering why an invasive test like this is needed. After all, an ultrasound can let your doctor see whether your uterine lining is growing. That's true, but simply seeing the size of the lining can't tell him whether it, and the blood vessels that are a necessary part of it, are developing quickly enough and well enough to be ready for a fertilized egg at the precise time it arrives. By looking at the hormones in your blood sample, your doctor will know whether the corpus luteum is producing normal hormones. A sampling of the cells of your endometrium can tell him this. A reading of these cells by a pathologist can tell your doctor exactly what phase the uterine lining is in. If the timing of the lining's development, when compared to the timing of your ovulation, is off—perhaps by as little as two days—it could result in a failed pregnancy attempt. Therefore, if he's at all suspicious that your lining may not be properly prepared, your doctor will want to perform an endometrial biopsy.

The good news is that while the biopsy is an invasive procedure, and therefore not usually called upon until late in the testing process, it sounds worse than it actually is. When you're told you need a biopsy, your likely first worry is "Will it hurt?" After all, a biopsy usually involves a cut or incision. You'll be happy to hear there are none in this test, so you needn't be afraid. In order to do an endometrial biopsy, your doctor will insert a small catheter through the opening of your cervix. Using a syringe that's attached to the back of the catheter, he'll apply suction to collect a sample of the endometrium. Usually, women describe the experience as a sharp cramp at the moment the catheter is inserted, with another bit of cramping accompanied by a tugging sensation when the endometrial tissue's being taken. Afterward, you may have some slight cramping for a few more minutes, and a little spotting that can last up to a day or two.

While it's accompanied by some discomfort, an endometrial biopsy takes only about 60 seconds, and for a woman with unexplained infertility, it's diagnostically essential. If you have a low threshold of pain, or are extremely anxious about the biopsy, you might want to ask for medications to help you through the test. Narcotic analgesic medications like

Valium, Vicodin, codeine, and others can aid you in relaxing. And antiprostaglandin medications such as Motrin, Advil, Naprosyn, or Anaprox can be taken 45 minutes before the procedure to dull any pain.

Step Two:
Everything You Wanted to Know About
Sperm but Were Afraid to Ask

When Antonie van Leeuwenhoek invented the microscope in 1677, one of the first things he chose to examine through his crude instrument was human seminal fluid. While he may not have fully understood the function of the sperm he saw there, he felt that somehow he was looking at the seed of life. And since there were no female physicians in that day, who was going to argue with him?

Despite this early interest, there is still a great deal of confusion about sperm. Are they fragile or hardy? Do they like their environment hot or cold? What can you do to enhance their survival? These questions are common, but they probably stand second to what really worries you—can your husband's sperm actually impregnate you? After your doctor's completed the tests that make up the second step of the basic workup, you should have a pretty good idea of the answer.

PREPARING FOR YOUR SEMEN ANALYSIS

Collecting Sperm

Before the semen can be analyzed, a specimen will need to be collected. Sounds simple? Not always. While every couple that goes through the basic workup has to collect sperm, the problems with doing this are rarely discussed openly. First you're told not to be embarrassed . . . good luck! Then you're told it's a simple procedure. Perhaps it is physically, but the psychological side is a whole other question. Once that kicks in some men can't masturbate to provide a semen specimen for analysis to save their lives. Others can, but with extreme difficulty. That's because while it is disguised as a medical test, collecting sperm is actually a sexual act that's being forced to happen at a specific time and under enormous pressure. If you fail to accomplish it, your sperm can't be analyzed, and your prospects of having a baby are slim.

Religion can also be a deterrent, in that some faiths don't allow masturbation for any reason, even for collection of sperm. Orthodox Jews and Catholics, for example, have to get the approval of their rabbis or priests in order to proceed with this aspect of the basic evaluation of male fertility.

Even if no religious roadblocks exist for you, you shouldn't discount the way in which the test invades a very personal and private side of your life. Too many men anticipate the same sort of bleak picture of the proceedings that Sarah Bird painted in her book *The Mommy Club*.

HOW NOT TO GIVE A SEMEN SAMPLE

"Are you sure?" she asked plaintively. *"Even if I helped?"*

"Even if you pumped me full of Spanish fly and did the Dance of the Seven Veils." Victor's whisper was a strained hiss. *"It is just not going to happen. Not in here. Not in that goddamned test tube. I mean, a test tube, for chrissake. I'm supposed to be a sharpshooter on top of champion stud? Not with Wiegand and that gum-snapping nurse breathing down my neck. Jesus, I played the guy last fall in the club racketball tournament. Hopeless serve."*

"I hadn't noticed the gum."

"Did he beat you?"

"What has that got to do with anything?"

"Just trying to isolate the inhibiting factors here."

"Goddammit, Hillary, don't go psychotherapeutic on me. Here. You try coming in a Pixie Stick with the fluorescent lights buzzing overhead, someone snapping their Juicy Fruit on the other side of the door, and a couple dozen drooling babies flashing their gums at you. See how hard it is then to 'isolate the inhibiting factors.' Here. Take it." The tinkle of glass breaking could only mean that Hillary had not taken the test tube.

"Are you certain you're not trying to sabotage us?" she asked calmly.

Victor made a strangled sound. *"I'm leaving before I say something I might regret."*

Obviously you should do whatever you can to move through the test as easily as possible. First, make sure your surroundings are optimum. Traditionally, men have been handed a cup, then told to go into a room and produce a specimen. In some cases the "room" has been a public bathroom in an office building or hospital. To avoid this extremely difficult situation, you should make sure ahead of time that your doctor provides a comfortable place, appropriately set up for semen collection.

Some men have difficulty collecting specimens unless their wives are present and participating in the collection. The room provided in your doctor's office should be designed to accommodate both of you. Otherwise, you should be allowed to do your collection in the privacy of your own home. Some men can collect a semen specimen only through sexual intercourse. In these cases nonspermicidal, nonlatex condoms need to be provided.

After collection, many men worry whether the amount of fluid in the container is enough. In most cases, they shouldn't. The containers that are most often provided for semen collection are sterile cups that were actually developed for urine cultures. The average volume of a semen sample is anywhere from one to two cc's, and the urine culture containers normally hold anywhere from 50 to 100 cc's of liquid volume. They are obviously not meant to be filled up when used for a semen sample.

If the semen is collected at home, you have approximately 30 to 45 minutes to get your specimen to your doctor's office or laboratory for analysis. This is another instance when the location of your doctor's office is important: you shouldn't have to drive a hundred miles an hour to get there within the time limit.

Beating a Ticket the Hard Way

I had twenty minutes left. I was racing through the streets to get to the doctor's office, when I heard a siren. Sure enough, a policeman pulled me over for speeding. If I waited for him to write me up, my husband's precious sperm would no longer be viable. So I pulled the sperm out of my bra and begged the officer to let me go. I'll never know whether he was sensitive to my situation, or simply shocked. It doesn't really matter. He let me go immediately. And fortunately my husband's sperm was still fresh when I reached the laboratory.

—Dana, age 38

Don't transfer your sperm in a cool environment. It's a commonly held belief that cold sperm live longer. The opposite is true. Some patients have used coolers to transport treasured specimens, only to discover they're dead on arrival. Staying at body temperature is optimum for sperm survival. To keep them warm during the trip from your home to your doctor's office, you can carry your specimen next to your body inside your clothing. This will ensure maximum survival rate.

Those men who have difficulty collecting sperm will be sorry to hear that a single semen analysis is usually not adequate to determine potential fertility. In order to confirm an abnormal or normal semen profile, one to three semen analyses need to be performed over a period of a month to six weeks. And if the semen profile is abnormal, additional semen will then be needed for more advanced tests of sperm function.

Since it's important to provide the laboratory or the doctor with a sample that reflects the man's optimum sperm population, he will need to wait from two to four days between ejaculations. These intervals are absolutely necessary. So even though the patient may normally have intercourse on a daily basis, he will most likely be asked to abstain for two to four days prior to a semen analysis. This will give his doctor the best representation of the patient's sperm production and motility characteristics.

Checking the Laboratory

The accuracy of a semen analysis is directly related to the expertise of the laboratory that performs it. Every laboratory that's licensed to do clinical work is permitted to perform semen analyses, yet not all laboratories that have approval to do this work perform the test frequently enough to do it well. Don't be afraid to question your doctor about the lab he's using, or about his own lab if he's doing the analysis himself. If they do one a month, they probably won't be adequately experienced or equipped to give you an accurate assessment of your sperm's potential. In that case, you should move on to a lab that does at least 50 to 100 semen analyses a month. Don't be afraid to push on this point. An inaccurate semen profile won't help your treatment, and might even hold it back.

The routine semen analysis that the lab will do to confirm the sperm's quantity and quality may be accomplished in one of two ways.

The CASA Method   Today, most laboratories use computer-assisted semen analysis (CASA). In this method of testing, a computer-programmed instrument accurately counts the sperm cells and determines not only how many of them there are, but also how many are active, the velocity of the active sperms' movement through the ejaculate, and whether the shape of the sperm is normal. If at least 40% of the sperm are moving normally, the semen is considered adequate. Because CASA doesn't rely on a human being's visual abilities or judgment, this method of testing provides you and your doctor with an extremely accurate sperm analysis.

The Visual Method   In the visual method of semen analysis, a laboratory technician places a semen sample on a slide that has been divided into a grid. He manually counts the number of sperm per microscopic field, and multiplies his count by several factors to produce an estimate of millions of sperm per cc of fluid volume. He then visually determines the sperm's motility by estimating the percentage of the sperm that are moving, and noting the quality and speed of their movement. This is an older method of semen analysis, which is obviously subject to human error. It's most often used by laboratories that don't have computerized testing equipment—usually those whose volume of semen work isn't great enough to justify it. You should keep in mind that if this is the method being used by your doctor, the skill and experience of the individual technician who runs the test is of paramount importance.

More Advanced Testing

Certainly the first approach to determining male fertility is the routine semen analysis we have just described. In one out of three cases it is normal, and no further male testing is required within the basic workup. However, if the semen analysis demonstrates low sperm count (oligozospermia), low sperm motility (asthenospermia), or abnormal sperm shapes (teteratospermia), additional testing will need to be done to determine the overall functional ability of the sperm. These tests of sperm function are somewhat controversial, and are not used by all centers. However, if your doctor is familiar enough with them to know what answers each test can appropriately be expected to yield, and to ask only those questions, they can be very useful in pinpointing specific sperm problems.

Advanced sperm testing consists of four commonly used tests, each with varying degrees of accuracy and usefulness. Not all infertility doctors perform all of them, for good reason. You should understand the questions that each test asks, and make sure that the appropriate tests are performed to diagnose the source of your problem.

The Hamster Test   Some men who appear to have normal sperm when their semen analysis is done, still cannot fertilize an egg. One of the possible reasons for this is that their sperm don't become capacitated— they don't properly complete the acrosome reaction, the interaction that must occur between the two protein layers that surround the head of the sperm in order for the sperm to be able to break through the outer membrane of an egg and then fuse with the egg cytoplasm.

For many years doctors were unable to test for this sperm malfunction. The only way to definitely demonstrate the sperm's ability to penetrate an egg was to actually watch it do so, and it was both painful and impractical to harvest women's eggs for this purpose. But in 1975 a doctor in Hawaii, Dr. Yaginamachi, came up with a novel idea. He suggested that if researchers were able to strip the zona pellucida membrane away from animal eggs—the membrane that makes eggs species specific—they could then be used to test human sperm. Nearly all mammalian egg species were tried, and shown not to work . . . rabbit, mouse, dog, cat, and frog eggs, to name a few. Then Dr. Yaginamachi tried the golden hamster egg. When he washed and prepared three zona-free hamster eggs and put them into a solution with human sperm, normal fusion took place, and a new test was born.

The sperm penetration assay (SPA) or the hamster penetration assay (HPA), as it is commonly called, was considered to be a breakthrough in male fertility testing. Its use spread quickly, and it became the standard that was employed to test for the fertilizing ability of men's sperm. Unfortunately, its misuse spread quickly too. In their enthusiasm, doctors misled themselves into believing that the hamster test could be a predictor of pregnancy in a couple. Their efforts to use it that way, and the test's failure to accurately predict pregnancy, resulted in a controversy that surrounded the SPA until 1982. What doctors failed to take into account was that while the hamster test can accurately tell you whether sperm has the ability to penetrate an egg, there are countless other factors that may prevent the couple in question from producing a pregnancy.

Today the SPA has weathered the test of time. Infertility centers that are advanced in their diagnostic and treatment abilities now know how to properly use it. It can pinpoint those men with a high sperm count who still aren't effective because their sperm don't become capacitated. One in ten men with normal semen profiles falls into this category; once their problem is identified, their sperm can often be treated, and its ability to fertilize an egg can be enhanced. Conversely, it can also tell men with a low sperm count that they may still be able to produce a pregnancy, because the sperm they have *do* become capacitated.

If your partner's sperm is being tested through SPA, or through the hemizona assay test, which we will be discussing later in this chapter, it is important that you ask your doctor or lab for two separate results—your own results, and the results for the "donor control sample." Reputable labs will run such a control, using proven fertile sperm, to verify that tests results aren't affected by the quality of the eggs that are being used, or by the environment in which the sperm and eggs are placed. Because these factors can vary, the only way for you to really know that your results are valid is to compare them to a proven fertile control.

In Vitro Mucus Penetration Test   The in vitro mucus penetration test (IVMP) is another test that was developed in the seventies. Doctors began to use this test in an attempt to see whether a man's sperm had the ability to move through a column of mucus, theoretically establishing the sperm's ability to fertilize his partner's egg.

In order to do the test, a sample of cervical mucus either from a normal woman or from the man's partner is placed in a small capillary tube, and the sperm being tested are placed at one end. After a period of time the tube is examined under a microscope to see how many of the sperm managed to migrate through the tube.

There are several problems with this test. First, if mucus from a normal woman is used, all that will be established is the ability of the sperm to move through that particular mucus in a laboratory setting. This may have no bearing on the sperm's ability to move through the actual partner's mucus. Second, even sperm that can move through mucus may not have the ability to penetrate and fertilize an egg once they reach it.

Despite these shortcomings, the IVMP test is still used by doctors to demonstrate sperm's ability to migrate. If, for some reason, your doctor decides to run this test on your partner's sperm, you should bear in mind that the results have no significant bearing on the sperm's ability to fertilize your egg.

Electron Microscopy   While some doctors do electron microscopy as a standard part of the basic male workup, we don't suggest it. It has limited use in establishing whether sperm function is normal; it's best reserved as a follow-up test to locate specific structural abnormalities within the sperm and to explain an abnormal finding that's already been made through other tests. Most of the abnormalities that will be found with electron microscopy are congenital defects that would otherwise be impossible to see. And, unfortunately, most of them are not correctable.

A typical example is the absence of mitochondria, the energy packets within each sperm cell that allow it to move properly. If sperm appear to be immobile during the basic semen analysis, electron microscopy—which can magnify them up to 100,000 times their normal size—would let your doctor see whether an absence of mitochondria is the cause.

Another syndrome that can be definitely diagnosed only by electron microscopy is the lack of an acrosome membrane. It would be appropriate to use electron microscopy as a follow-up test for sperm that appear motile but still fail to penetrate the egg during the hamster penetration test. If the lack of an acrosome membrane is confirmed, these men will be able to fertilize an egg only with the help of mechanical insertion of the sperm cell directly into the egg cell. For them, only the most advanced technology available for in vitro fertilization should be considered. Quickly establishing this problem through electron microscopy lets them proceed directly to this high-tech level of treatment, without wasting time and money on less extreme possibilities that would never be effective for them.

The Hemizona Assay Test   The latest development in sperm function testing is the hemizona assay test, which was developed in the late eighties at the Jones Institute in Virginia. This test goes one step farther than the hamster test by using human eggs, which were extracted for use in in vitro cycles but were not implanted because they were too immature to be used or because they failed to fertilize. Rather than discard them, these eggs are frozen and stored for use in hemizona assay testing. Unlike the eggs that are used in the hamster test, those used in the hemizona assay test still have their zona pellucida membranes intact.

To do a hemizona assay test, these frozen eggs are thawed and then sliced in half. The halves are then put in an environment similar to that used for in vitro fertilization. The patient's sperm are placed with one half of the egg. Proven donor sperm are placed with the other half to serve as a control test.

While the hamster test shows whether a sperm can become fused with the egg once it is inside its outer membrane, the hemizona assay test shows whether the sperm has the ability to penetrate that outer membrane.

The Best Sperm Test—It's Two Tests in One!

The best way to test sperm function is by combining the hamster penetration assay with the hemizona assay. By doing this, your doctor can confirm both of the primary sperm mechanisms that are necessary for fertility. First, the ability of the sperm to pass through the zona membrane of the egg is shown by the hemizona assay test. But because the human eggs that are used in the hemizona assay test are dead, the hamster test is then needed to demonstrate whether the sperm have the ability to fuse with the egg's inner membrane, and to actually fertilize the egg once they've entered its cytoplasm. Using both of these tests together is the most thorough means of determining how well sperm will function when they come in contact with a human egg, whether in a glass petri dish or within the human body.

Step Three:
Testing Cervical Function—
It Takes Two to Tango

If no problems are detected during the first two steps of the basic workup, your doctor will then ask you and your partner to come together and perform an interactive dance that's meant to tell you whether your cervix is functioning correctly. Unfortunately it won't involve tap shoes or music, and it won't help you to practice your movements ahead of time. This is one maneuver where you've either got it or you don't.

THE POSTCOITAL TEST

The postcoital test (PCT) tells you, among other things, whether your bodies are in rhythm. First it tests whether your cervix is producing adequate and serviceable mucus. Then it shows whether there is any problem in the interaction between that mucus and your partner's sperm.

As we explained earlier, many doctors check mucus production during the ovulation phase of a basic workup. The postcoital test is a much more specific look at your mucus. Not only does it tell you whether your cervix is producing enough mucus in response to the estrogen that peaked prior to the release of your egg, it also tests the mucus biochemically to confirm that it has the right properties to assist in sperm transport. This test might show that your mucus is inadequate in amount, possibly due to damaged mucus-producing cells. Or it might show that it is inadequate in quality—possibly because it contains white cells from an infection that are lethal to your partner's sperm; or that it has an acidity problem; or that it contains antibodies that block sperm from moving through it.

To prepare for a PCT, you should begin using an at-home LH surge monitoring kit two to three days before you expect to ovulate. Once the stick in your kit turns blue, indicating your LH surge, you and your husband should have intercourse the next morning. Following intercourse, you should go to your doctor's office to be tested. He'll give you an ultrasound to determine whether you've ovulated. Assuming you haven't, he will remove a sample of your cervical mucus for testing. The process during which he does this will feel much like a routine pap smear examination.

Your doctor then looks at your mucus sample under a microscope. He gauges its stretchability, and he checks for cellular debris. He counts the number of your partner's sperm that maintain their motility while in it, and watches how they move. If his microscopic examination doesn't look favorable, he'll probably discuss other issues that may be affecting the postcoital test. If your postcoital test does look favorable, your doctor will move on to the fourth stage of your basic workup.

STEPPING OUT A NORMAL CYCLE

Since there's no single test that can clearly establish whether you have a normal ovulatory cycle, or whether your cervical mucus is receptive to your partner's sperm, let's summarize the multiple tests that you and your doctor should use. In doing so, let's assume that you are having fairly regular menstrual bleeding intervals, and that your partner's sperm profile is normal.

1. Two to three days before you expect to ovulate, you should begin to use your at-home LH surge monitoring kit. Once you get a positive indication of the LH surge, you should plan to have intercourse the following morning, and then see your doctor.

2. He will take a sample of your cervical mucus, and see whether the mucus-sperm interaction is appropriate and functional.

3. Your doctor will then do an ultrasound of your ovaries and uterus. The scan of the ovaries will indicate whether an egg is still present inside a matured follicle, or whether that follicle has released the egg. By visualizing your uterus through ultrasound, your doctor will be able to tell whether your uterus's endometrial lining is appropriately developed. As we said earlier, the estrogen rise prior to ovulation not only prepares your cervical mucus for sperm penetration, it also stimulates the growth and maturation of the endometrial lining.

4. If the appearance of the follicle indicates that the egg did not yet ovulate, the scan should be repeated the following day. It is important to verify that the follicle actually collapses and disappears, to ensure that you are actually, mechanically releasing the egg.

5. Final confirmation of a normal ovulatory cycle comes seven to nine days later, when you return to your doctor's office for a blood test that will measure your estrogen and progesterone levels to confirm that you have, in fact, ovulated. If you have, your follicle will have turned into a corpus luteum, which will

be producing adequate amounts of estrogen and progesterone to properly support the uterine lining.

6. If your doctor has any doubts as to whether your lining is absolutely appropriate, he will perform an endometrial biopsy, which should also be done seven to nine days after your LH surge. This will indicate whether the second half of your ovulatory cycle is still functioning normally and is timed properly, an essential part of maintaining a successful pregnancy.

Step Four:
Inspecting the Inside of Your
Reproductive Tract

Let's say you want to buy a house. You find a place with wonderful curb appeal, and quickly put down your money. Then you panic. Is it everything the sellers promise it will be? Do all the systems inside its walls—the wiring, the plumbing, the heating—connect and work properly? Your next call is to your local house inspector.

After examining the interior of the house, your inspector will be able

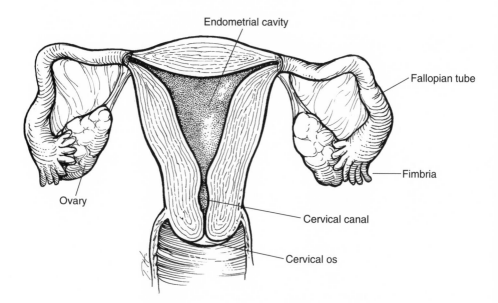

Figure 5-3: The Female Reproductive Tract

to tell you whether it is constructed properly and its systems are functioning correctly. Similarly, your doctor needs to inspect, as the next step in the basic workup, what's going on inside the female reproductive tract. He needs to see inside the uterine cavity to know whether it is normal. He needs to find out whether the fallopian tubes are open and healthy, and will allow passage of sperm, egg, and embryo. He has to find out whether your uterus can safely house an embryo, then a fetus, and finally a baby. He has to determine whether your ovaries, tubes, and uterus are positioned and connected properly, and whether your tubes move freely, as they should, or whether there are problems such as adhesions, scarring, endometriosis, and intestinal tract abnormalities that affect their ability to move and pick up an egg. (See Figure 5-3.) Just like the inspector who finds out what's really going on inside your new house, your doctor will determine the structure of your reproductive tract, and find possible tubal, uterine, and pelvic factor disorders. The five most common tests to help him do that are listed here.

THE HYSTEROSALPINGOGRAM

The first and most basic test is called the hysterosalpingogram (HSG). It is also the best and most accurate in most situations. HSG has been used for many years. It's a visualization study, which utilizes a dye that can be seen by X ray. The purpose of this test is to see whether your uterus is normal in shape, and whether your fallopian tubes are open (or patent). To have the test performed, you are sent to a facility with a large X-ray machine. The HSG is usually performed between the sixth and eleventh day of your cycle. You lie on your back under the X ray, in the same position as if you were getting a pap smear. The doctor performing the test, usually a radiologist, threads a catheter through your cervix and passes it into your uterine cavity. A dye, known as standard contrast solution, is then sent through the catheter into the uterine cavity, and allowed to flow back through the fallopian tubes. If your tubes are open, it will fill them; if there is a blockage, it will stop at that point. Your doctor will be able to see what has happened by looking at the shape the dye has produced on your X ray. (See Figures 5-4 and 5-5.)

Preparing for Your HSG

An HSG takes about an hour to perform. You may have heard that it is extremely painful, but if it is done by a physician who routinely performs the test, you should experience only minimum discomfort. And

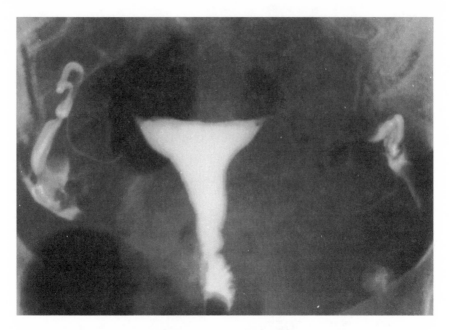

Figure 5-4: Normal HSG

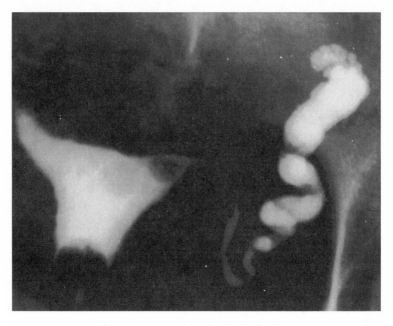

Figure 5-5: HSG with Blocked Tubes

since what the test will tell your doctor is extremely important, it is well worth doing.

Still, if you're very anxious about this test, or if you're one of those women who have a low threshold of pain, here are some helpful hints regarding medication that you should consider as you prepare for your HSG.

- First of all, it might help you to take one of the antiprostaglandin medications such as Motrin, Advil, Naprosyn, or Anaprox about 45 minutes prior to the test. They will help to minimize any possible pain that you might feel.

- In conjunction with an antiprostaglandin, Valium can be taken to relax your uterine and tubal muscles, and to help prevent the discomfort that can be caused by these muscles contracting and spasming.

- If you are extremely anxious, or are very prone to pain, a medication such as Darvocet, Tylenol with codeine, or Vicodin may help you feel more comfortable during the procedure.

Keep in mind that most women don't need these medications. We're just telling you about them to guarantee your comfort during the test.

One thing all women *will* need is a prescription for a broad spectrum antibiotic, such as Vibramycin. The sterile environment of the interior of the uterus and the fallopian tubes, which is normally protected against the bacteria that's in your cervix and vagina, will be compromised by the insertion of the tube and the dye. The antibiotic will protect against any bacteria that is passed this way from the vaginal-cervical area into the uterine environment and fallopian tubes. Without an antibiotic, you could get a bacterial infection or pelvic inflammation. If you have a history of pelvic inflammatory disease, or tubal disease as the result of a pelvic infection, you should have particularly close supervision during and following an HSG.

Sometimes, when a woman has a highly suspicious history of pelvic inflammatory disease, the test is not recommended because it carries with it a potential risk of further inflammation or infection. In such cases tubal patency testing and an internal check of the uterus can be done through a laparoscopy or a hysteroscopy, two tests that we will be telling you about later in this chapter. Another situation in which these alternative tests should be used is for a patient who is allergic to shellfish. Because the dye used in the HSG test contains iodine, it is not appropriate for these women.

━━━━━━━━━━━━━━━━ **IS HSG SAFE?** ━━━━━━━━━━━━━━━━

If you are concerned about X-ray exposure involved in a hysterosalpingogram, don't be. Having a hysterosalpingogram is equivalent to having a chest X ray. As you may know, you can have a chest X ray once a month for many years, and never receive enough radiation to be of any danger to you. The same is true of hysterosalpingograms. The amount of radiation that the ovaries receive from an HSG test is estimated to be between one and two rads. But the amount of radiation that is necessary to produce ovarian damage is somewhere between 1,500 and 3,000 rads. Having an HSG performed once, maybe twice, could never be considered dangerous to your health.

THE CARBON DIOXIDE TEST

While testing for patent fallopian tubes using carbon dioxide is an *outdated* procedure, it's still used by some doctors today. The doctor performing this test guides a catheter into the cervix, and then passes carbon dioxide through it and into the uterus and fallopian tubes. If the tubes are open, the carbon dioxide will flow through and then out of them, and will settle under the diaphragm. The doctor administering the test waits for you to complain of shoulder pain. If you complain of shoulder pain on both sides, the test is interpreted as having shown that both fallopian tubes are open. If you have pain on only one side, it indicates one open tube. This test has several shortcomings. First, it's extremely painful. Second, pain is totally subjective; the same amount of pain might be interpreted by some women as being extreme, and by others as being moderate. For example, a woman could complain of pain on both sides, even though only one of her tubes is blocked. Finally, because this test doesn't actually allow the doctor to view the uterine cavity or the fallopian tubes, the results aren't as accurate as those gotten from an HSG. Given these problems it's obvious that the only reliable way to determine the configuration of your uterine cavity and the patency of your fallopian tubes is by the visualization that an HSG offers.

ULTRASOUND HSG

An ultrasound HSG is often used after tubal surgery is performed to open the tubes, to confirm that it was successful. It is a more convenient, but less accurate, version of the standard HSG, which we previously described. Because in these circumstances the physician already has a fairly good idea of what he's looking for, ultrasound HSG is adequate to test tubal patency. It can be performed in the doctor's office, which saves you the time and expense of a visit to a specialized radiology facility.

An ultrasound HSG is given by placing saline in the uterine cavity, in exactly the same way that standard contrast solution is introduced for a standard HSG. The patient is then given an ultrasound procedure, which allows the physician to visually follow the progress of the saline as it moves through the uterus, the fallopian tubes, and the pelvic cavity. Though he can see the saline solution, the picture he gets is very poor compared to that which is produced in a standard HSG.

Since your doctor will be using a saline solution, instead of the dye that is used in a standard HSG, it is an option you might want to consider if there is a possibility that you are allergic to standard contrast solution. Also, some women prefer it because it involves absolutely no X-ray exposure.

COMPUTERIZED AXIAL TOMOGRAPHY AND MAGNETIC RESONANCE IMAGING

Computerized axial tomography (CAT) and magnetic resonance imaging (MRI) are two other possible means of imaging a woman's reproductive organs, but in general neither of these testing methods should be used during a basic infertility diagnosis. Both are more expensive than ultrasound and more inconvenient, as they must be done in a specialized facility outside your doctor's office. These two drawbacks make CAT scans and MRIs difficult to use as effectively as ultrasound. Ultrasound can be repeated at different stages throughout your cycle to track the changes in appearance of your ovaries and uterus that occur as a result of hormonal changes.

It *is* possible that your doctor will recommend a CAT scan or an MRI if your transvaginal ultrasound has shown an abnormal mass that he can't definitely identify. The use of these diagnostic methods should be limited to relatively rare situations, as they are relatively expensive to be used routinely, especially when imaging of the uterus and fallopian tubes can be better accomplished with a hysterosalpingogram or ultrasound HSG. And even in these cases, the usefulness of an MRI is limited, as it doesn't offer any kind of contrast enhancement to show the relative thickness or density of the suspicious tissue.

HYSTEROSCOPY

A hysteroscopy is a procedure that can take the place of a hystero-salpingogram for those women on whom an HSG cannot be performed—women who are allergic to iodine or to iodinated materials (the key ingredient in the solution used for the hysterosalpingogram), or women who have a history of severe pelvic inflammatory disease. If you fall within this group, you can be diagnosed with a greater degree of safety if your physician uses a hysteroscope to view the interior of your uterus and fallopian tubes.

During a hysteroscopy, a small telescopic instrument is inserted through your cervical opening, allowing your doctor to look inside the uterine cavity and see any type of abnormalities that may be there. He will also get a direct view of the uterine cavity's openings into the fallopian tubes, and can see whether they are blocked.

Your doctor might also use hysteroscopy if the results of your HSG are abnormal. Suspecting some growth within your reproductive organs, he would then use hysteroscopy to take a look at it, and perhaps remove it through hysteroscopic surgery.

Both of these are valid reasons for this procedure. But remember, if the results of your hysterosalpingogram were completely normal, a hysteroscopy won't offer any other advantage, and will only cost you more money.

Step Five:
Evaluation of the Pelvic Environment

If your doctor doesn't find anything wrong within the internal structure of your reproductive tract, he will next look to its exterior—to the landscaping that surrounds your house, so to speak. During the fifth and final step of the basic workup, he will examine the outside surfaces of your uterus and fallopian tubes, and check your entire pelvic environment.

LAPAROSCOPY

Laparoscopy was developed in the early seventies, and is now routinely used to view the pelvic cavity. In this procedure, a telescopelike instrument, called a laparoscope, is inserted into the abdominal cavity. It gives the physician an overall view of the pelvic area, as well as a look at the external reproductive tract.

Using laparoscopy, your doctor can both see and feel pelvic, tubal, or ovarian adhesions. These sometimes occur after surgery or infection, when the surfaces of the traumatized organs connect to each other (or adhere) during healing. These adhesions can cause a number of infertility problems. For example, if they interfere with the normal movement of the fallopian tubes, the tubes may not be able to move freely enough to pick up an egg once it ovulates from its follicle.

Laparoscopy can also diagnose endometriosis. Endometriosis occurs when pieces of the lining of your uterus (the endometrium) are shed into the abdominal cavity. They then stick to surfaces such as the ovaries, fallopian tubes, uterus, intestinal tract, and pelvic side walls. Once they find a home, these pieces of the endometrium start to grow under the influence of estrogen and progesterone, in just the same way that they would grow within the uterine cavity during a normal ovulatory cycle. Endometriosis can cause scarring and damage to the sensitive structures inside the pelvis—the fallopian tubes, ovaries, uterus, and intestinal tract. In addition to causing infertility, the resulting inflammation can be extremely painful.

The only way that endometriosis and adhesions can be definitely diagnosed is through laparoscopy. Your doctor has to actually see them to confirm that they are there. It's important that he does so, since either of these conditions can affect your ability to get pregnant.

What's It like to Have a Laparoscopy?

Laparoscopy means surgery. Some women draw the line at this point in their basic workup, and decide not to go on. If you're among those who feel that this procedure is too invasive, that's understandable. Other women, seeing this as the final step in their diagnostic workup, and hoping it will help solve their problem, resolve to go on. When making your decision about this, you should keep in mind that the results from a laparoscopy can be essential in helping your doctor make an accurate diagnosis.

Laparoscopy is performed in an operating room under a light but general anesthetic. Most often it is done in a hospital, but sometimes your doctor will have an operating room within his office suite that will accommodate this operation. During this procedure a slender telescope-like instrument, a laparoscope, is inserted into your pelvic cavity through a small cut just below the navel. Carbon dioxide is allowed to flow into the abdomen through a special needle. As it enters the abdomen, it pushes the abdominal wall and the bowel away from the other organs in the pelvic area, making it easier for your doctor to see your ovaries, uterus, fallopian tubes, and other nearby organs. His view is illuminated by a special attachment, which transmits light down through the tube and into the abdomen. If he needs to separate adhesions to see better, or sample tissue, surgical instruments are inserted through the laparoscope, or through another smaller incision lower down on your abdomen. Once the procedure is completed, the instruments are removed, the gas is released, the incisions are closed, and a small adhesive bandage is placed over them. You will be able to go home that day. Your doctor will probably tell you that you can resume normal activity as soon as you feel up to it, but you may feel some minor discomfort for the next day or two, so take it easy.

Beyond the Basic Workup

As you may recall, we explained when we started this chapter that the basic workup would be able to pinpoint approximately 85% of the abnormalities that infertile couples have. If, when your doctor has completed the five steps of the basic workup, he still has been unable to make a diagnosis and you are within the remaining 15%, he will probably move on to more sophisticated testing. First, men with normal semen profiles will be reexamined, using some of the more discriminating approaches that are normally reserved for men with abnormal profiles—the hamster test and the hemizona assay, for example. When this is done, 10% of them will be found to have subnormal sperm function that didn't show up in their basic semen analysis. Fortunately, most of these problems can be corrected, and the men they affect can still fertilize eggs using corrective procedures, which we will discuss in a later chapter.

Another way to narrow down the group of unexplained infertile couples is to do an endometrial biopsy, if one hasn't already been performed as part of the basic workup. As we pointed out, even a woman who has tested positively for ovulation can have a luteal phase abnormality. Such luteal phase defects are responsible for another 5% of the problems that remained unexplained after the basic workup.

If, after advanced testing, you end up in the small group that is still unexplained, you will be comforted to know that there are still certain advanced therapeutic approaches that you can take to help you increase your fertility potential. We will be discussing these later, in Chapter Twelve.

Think Positive!

The basic evaluation is essential to finding the cause of your infertility. No one says this diagnostic process will be easy. But it is necessary, and it needs to be completed before any therapeutic decisions can be made.

Don't let denial stop you from being tested; it will only hold you back. You'll find yourself wandering around, trying things hit or miss, only to further frustrate yourself emotionally and financially. Once tested, you may find your problem can easily be remedied. Perhaps it's a simple ovulation problem, which can be corrected with minimal medication. Or a difficulty with cervical mucus function, which can easily be overcome by an insemination procedure.

There are things you can do to alleviate some of the frustrations that are part of any basic workup. First, feel free to ask questions. Use the knowledge you've gained from this book and other sources to make sure you understand why your doctor has chosen each test he's giving you. He and the support staff within his office should be willing to provide you with a full explanation of each test, the thinking behind it, and the order in which your tests will be done. Be sure that each test is appropriate for your suspected condition. Also be sure that your doctor lets you know what to expect physically, before the various tests are performed.

As you approach the basic workup, remember that whatever plan your doctor chooses for you, he should offer examples of the way the process works, answer any questions you may have, project what you may expect with each step, and explain what and why certain things will be occurring over the course of time.

Once your physician knows what abnormalities, if any, are present within your systems, an appropriate treatment approach can be designed to correct them. Keep in mind that without the diagnosis, your therapeutic game plan will never be established.

Terms We Used in This Chapter

Asthenospermia: a term used to describe sperm that has poor mobility or progressive movement, i.e., low-motility sperm.

Basal body temperature chart (BBT):   a daily record of the body's temperature at rest. When ovulation occurs, the body's temperature will rise 0.6°F to 0.8°F above baseline.

Carbon dioxide test: an antiquated test used to determine whether there is any blockage of the fallopian tubes.

Computer-assisted semen analysis (CASA):   the measurement of sperm number, shape, and movement by computer technology.

Computerized axial tomography (CAT):   a diagnostic X-ray procedure that utilizes computers to project an image on film.

Electron microscopy: an instrument that can magnify structures 50,000 to 100,000 times.

Endometrial biopsy: sampling or removal of a piece of the uterine lining (or endometrium) for microscopic study.

Hamster penetration assay/Hamster test: see Sperm penetration assay.

Hemizona assay test: a test used to determine whether sperm binding or attachment to the zona membrane of the egg is normal.

Hysterosalpingogram (HSG):   an X-ray study in which a dye visible by fluoroscopy is injected into the uterine cavity to determine the shape of the uterus and patency of the fallopian tubes.

Hysteroscopy: a surgical procedure that uses a small telescope placed through the cervical canal to view the interior of the uterine cavity.

In vitro mucus penetration test: a test used to determine whether sperm/mucus interaction is normal; commonly done with bovine mucus and human sperm.

Laparoscopy: a surgical procedure in which a telescope is inserted through the abdominal wall to view the inner organs.

LH surge: the large release of LH from the anterior pituitary that causes the release of the mature egg from the follicle.

Luteal phase defect: inadequate production of hormone from the corpus luteum, or poor response of the endometrial lining to hormonal stimulation, which interferes with implantation.

Magnetic resonance imaging (MRI):   an imaging device that does not use X ray or ultrasound, yet gives a clear picture of our internal organ systems.

Oligozospermia: low sperm number.

Postcoital test (PCT):   a test used to determine whether sperm/mucus interaction is normal, i.e., whether the sperm can move properly through the cervical mucus.

Sperm penetration assay (SPA): a test utilizing hamster eggs to measure the ability of the human sperm to fertilize.

Teteratospermia: sperm that has an abnormal shape.

Ultrasound: an instrument that emits pulsed sound waves which are reflected off solid tissues to give an image of internal body structures without the use of X ray.

Varicocele: dilated veins around the testicle, most commonly on the left side, which can cause sperm abnormalities.

PART THREE

FINDING THE CAUSE
OF INFERTILITY AND
FIXING THE PROBLEM

6
Problems with Ovulation

You're probably eleven or twelve when it happens. You greet your first period with surprise, with fear, or with an incredible reluctance to suddenly leap into the unknown gulf of adolescence. And things get worse from there. Your period always seems to show up at the most inconvenient or embarrassing times, bringing along cramps as part of the package. Pretty soon you begin to call it "The Curse." Little did you know, during those early years, that the real curse is not having a regular ovulatory cycle. Some young women's bodies never mature sexually; they never have menstrual cycles and ovulation. And others—perhaps like you—have cycles that aren't normal enough to let them conceive a child.

What's Causing Your Ovulation Problem?

Ovulation problems, which account for approximately 40% of female infertility disorders, can be caused by any number of factors. Some of them are environmental, relating to lifestyle, diet, or medications. Others can be traced to physical sources, such as lesions within the brain, or to genetic disorders that have been present from birth. If your initial workup indicates an abnormal ovulatory pattern, which is commonly seen when menstrual bleeding patterns are irregular, all of these possibilities need to be considered. Before you work with your doctor to pinpoint the reason for your individual problem, you should try to remember when and how it started. This historical information will often lend clues to its cause, which can then be verified through medical testing.

Ovulatory dysfunctions normally fall into one of three main areas.

- Most commonly, an imbalance within the hypothalamic/pituitary/ovarian axis is the root of the problem.

- Less commonly, the ovary itself is the source of the ovulatory defect.

- And sometimes the problem occurs during the luteal phase of the cycle, affecting either the preparation of the uterine lining prior to ovulation or the proper timing of the lining's development.

Hypothalamic Pituitary Problems

As we discussed in Chapter Two, proper coordination and communication between the hypothalamus and the pituitary gland is essential as they work together to control the activities of your ovaries. This relationship between the central nervous system and the reproductive organs that it directs is the most common source of problems in women who aren't ovulating regularly. Such "hypothalamic pituitary problems" fall into two categories.

- Hypothalamic Pituitary Dysfunction
- Hypothalamic Pituitary Failure

Hypothalamic pituitary dysfunction refers to cases in which menstruation and ovulation are irregular. With *hypothalamic pituitary failure*, there is no ovulation or menstruation at all.

HYPOTHALAMIC PITUITARY DYSFUNCTION

The most frequent cause of ovulation problems—in fact, the reason for 90% of them—is hypothalamic pituitary dysfunction. Hypothalamic pituitary dysfunction is a broad, catchall term that is used to describe a number of different ovulation abnormalities. Typical examples are women who menstruate on a very irregular basis and ovulate only sporadically, or women who menstruate but don't ovulate. Hypothalamic pituitary dysfunction is by far the most common ovulation problem, and it is the most easily cured. Hypothalamic pituitary dysfunction is commonly associated with various environmental or medical conditions, such as inappropriate body weight, stress, drugs, or polycystic ovarian syndrome (PCOS).

Body Weight

Inappropriate body weight is a frequent reason for delayed menstruation in adolescent girls, and for abnormal ovulatory patterns in women of all ages. The precursors of estrogen change into this pivotal female hormone within fat, and without an appropriate amount of estrogen, sexual maturation and ovulation can't occur. Because of this, there is a critical body mass, or weight, that must be present before any woman can menstruate on a regular basis. There's no hard-and-fast rule as to what your critical body mass is. Since every woman's system has a different sensitivity to estrogen, women of identical height and build might have to achieve different weights and manufacture different amounts of this hormone in order to have a regular cycle.

Staying below their appropriate critical mass can delay the onset of ovulation and menstruation for adolescents. It can also lead to continuing irregular ovulation and menstrual periods for mature women for as long as their underweight condition persists. Classic examples include women who are active in competitive sports, and have a very low body fat ratio as a result of their constant exercise program—ice-skaters, tennis players, runners, and gymnasts. Keep in mind, if you are trying to get pregnant, that normal exercise may improve your chances of conceiving, but excessive exercise may negatively affect your ovulation. Women who are severely underweight for other reasons—those suffering from anorexia and bulimia—can also become anovulatory.

The same is true of women who are massively obese. A woman who has problems with obesity can ovulate irregularly, or not ovulate at all, because of an overproduction of estrogen in her excess fat. Some of these cases of obesity may be caused either by overfunctioning adrenal glands or by an underfunctioning thyroid. Each of these conditions has specific clinical signs, which help in its diagnosis, and each can be corrected through hormone therapy. Typically, women whose adrenal glands are overfunctioning gain weight in their chests, abdomens and upper hip areas, while their arms and legs remain thin. They also have high blood pressure and a rapid pulse rate. Women whose thyroids are underfunctioning have a generalized obesity, as well as a lethargy and slowing down of certain mental functions, such as concentration, and both their pulse and cardiac rhythm are slow. If you are overweight and have an irregular ovulatory cycle, these possibilities should be taken into consideration during your evaluation, and corrected with appropriate medication if they are found.

If you do not have a thyroid or adrenal gland problem, your weight can still be corrected, and normal ovulation restored, through appropriate diet, nutritional supplements, and in some cases through medication. But while making your weight adjustments, you should bear in mind that whenever there is a severe change in body mass or fat, hormonal blips may occur that can cause temporary changes in ovulatory function. These abnormalities are normally self-correcting once your body weight has stabilized.

Stress

If you want to get pregnant, you would be well-advised to steer clear of crisis situations. You may have noticed that during stressful times—office shake-ups, family problems, physical emergencies, or even the stress of competition—your menstrual period has been delayed or nonexistent. That's because your body reacts to these stressful states with surges in heart rate, respiration, and blood pressure, which are triggered by the same glands that produce the hormones you need to have a normal ovulatory cycle. And when your glands are occupied with dealing with emergencies, they tend to put aside less immediate concerns, like releasing pulses of GnRH, FSH, and LH, and producing estrogen.

ONCE IN A LIFETIME

Some situations are so stressful that they can cause a one-time problem with ovulation. A family trauma . . . the death of a parent, for example, can result in a skipped period if it happens at the time of ovulation. A situation such as this is totally self-correcting. Don't add it to your worries at an already stressful time.

If you are entering infertility treatment, you should be aware that tension can foster a vicious circle. The mere fact of not being able to conceive can bring on extreme levels of stress for many infertile women, which in turn can make it even harder for them to conceive. While there is very little hard scientific data as to the effects of stress on conception rates, there is a great deal of anecdotal information that tends to confirm its negative effects. The Infertility Program at Harvard's Deaconess Hospital in Boston, for example, put infertile women through stress management clinics during the period from 1989 through 1991 in an effort to help them overcome their depression, anger, and exhaustion. Most of these women had been suffering from infertility for more than three years. Once in the program, and managing their stress better, a third of them conceived within six months.

These results lead to an obvious conclusion. Women who are experiencing irregular ovulation may be contributing to their problem by subjecting themselves to persistent stressful situations. Women who are trying to juggle a family, a job, and school, for example, or women who are chronically depressed, should consider the fact that the relationship between stress and ovulatory difficulties is a very direct one. If you are in this "overly stressed" group, solving your underlying lifestyle problems may sometimes provide a solution to your infertility, as well.

Drugs

Most doctors will tell you that if you have decided to start a family, you would be well-advised to stop taking all nonessential drugs. This is good advice. A number of drugs work by raising various hormone levels. They can have the side effect of causing you to become anovulatory. Most antidepressants, for example, raise the level of the hormone prolactin. Prolactin is normally released by a woman's pituitary after she gives birth. It stimulates the breasts to make milk, and at the same time it interferes with ovulation. Certain medications, such as blood pressure medications, can have the same effect. If you are having ovulatory problems, you should be sure to give a complete list of the medications you're taking to your doctor, so he can evaluate their possible impact on your reproductive function.

One of the most common causes of drug-related effects on a woman's ovulatory pattern is the use of birth control pills. Whether a woman has been on the pill for six months or six years, her first few cycles after stopping it—one to three cycles is typical—may be irregular in length, or may have either irregular ovulation or none at all. Assuming that she had normal ovulatory cycles before using the pill, her cycles should then return to the same pattern.

However, those women who had irregular ovulatory cycles, or were anovulatory before pill use, will most often retain the same dysfunction after stopping the pills. The old wives' tale that the birth control pills can make you permanently infertile is false; they only make you infertile during the time you are actually taking them. Any ovulatory problem you have after their use was already present in your hypothalamic pituitary makeup before you took them. So while your prepill problems will resurface, this isn't something that the pills caused.

Polycystic Ovarian Syndrome (PCOS)

If your doctor diagnoses you with polycystic ovarian syndrome (PCOS), you are suffering from what is by far the most common cause of hypothalamic pituitary dysfunction. In fact, nearly 90% of hypothalamic pituitary dysfunction is the result of this condition and its several variants. A finding of PCOS is seldom a complete surprise. Since it usually starts sometime between a woman's first period and the age of twenty, an infertile patient who has PCOS will commonly have experienced years of either irregular, or anovulatory cycles. Women with PCOS tend to have a large number of eggs within their ovaries, ready to ovulate during each cycle. However, when it is time for a dominant follicle to grow and be selected, all of their follicles enlarge simultaneously and compete for the dominant follicle status, and none emerges as the winner. Because of this, no ovulation takes place. This process of multiple follicle development within the ovary is one of the diagnostic signs of PCOS. These multiple follicles look like a "ring of pearls" when viewed through ultrasound. This is a classic indicator of PCOS activity.

There is a great deal of controversy among reproductive endocrinologists as to the cause of PCOS. The majority feel that the problem lies within the ovaries themselves—that for some reason they are not responding to the hormonal signals that are being sent to them through the hypothalamic-pituitary feedback loop. However, some believe that the problem lies within the pituitary gland —that it is overproducing luteinizing hormone, which then sets up an ovarian condition that causes a chronic low level increase in estrogens (E_2) which can make follicle response erratic and irregular. Still others think that in a high percentage of PCOS patients, the adrenal glands are overproducing male hormones such as DHEAS, and that this causes PCOS. Practically speaking, it doesn't matter whether the source of the problem is the brain with a decreased production of dopamine, the ovary, or the adrenal gland. What matters is that the balance between them must be corrected to achieve normal ovulation. (See Figure 6-1.)

If you have PCOS, your physician should be able to diagnose it during your basic workup. Certain external signs will lead him to suspect this condition. Because one of the side effects of PCOS is an elevated level of certain male hormones (androgens), you may have some excess hair growth, and a weight gain in the trunk area of your body. And since your ovaries contain a large number of follicular cysts, they will feel enlarged during a pelvic exam. If he suspects that you have PCOS, your doctor can confirm your condition fairly easily. PCOS carries a number of hormonal markers that will show up on a blood test: overproduction of

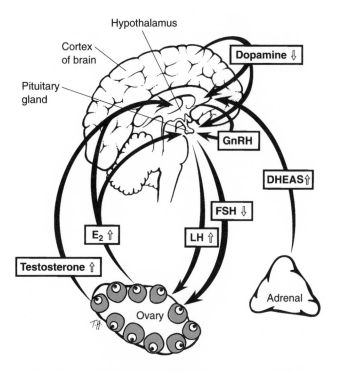

Figure 6-1:   Mechanisms of Polycystic Ovarian Syndrome

the male hormones testosterone and dehydroepiandrosterone sulfate (DHEAS), as well as of luteinizing hormone and prolactin. If he does suspect that you have PCOS, your physician should evaluate hormone production from your pituitary gland, your ovaries, and your adrenal system. The hormone levels of a patient with PCOS will differ from those of a normal woman. For example, when you have PCOS, your level of luteinizing hormone will be higher than normal when compared to your level of follicle-stimulating hormone. And your levels of testosterone and DHEAS also may be higher than expected.

Hormonal Markers of Polycystic Ovarian Syndrome

Luteinizing hormone (LH)	Elevated
Follicle-stimulating hormone (FSH)	Normal or Low
LH/FSH ratio	Greater than 3 to 1
Prolactin	Normal or Elevated
Estrogen	Normal or Elevated
Testosterone	Normal or Elevated
Dehydroepiandrosterone sulfate	Normal or Elevated

If his tests indicate that you do have PCOS, your doctor will have to carefully study your hormone levels before deciding on how a correct balance between them can best be achieved.

HYPOTHALAMIC PITUITARY FAILURE

Only a small percentage of the women who have infertility caused by ovulation defects—approximately 5% to 6%—have hypothalamic pituitary failure. If you fall into this category, you may have gone through puberty and started to menstruate at the regularly expected time, approximately 11½ to 12 years of age. Alternatively, your puberty and menarche may have been delayed until you were 15 or 16. In either case, your menstrual periods probably disappeared soon after their onset, and you haven't ovulated or menstruated from that point on. This loss of menstrual function can be due to a complete failure of your hypothalamus to send gonadotropin-releasing hormone (GnRH) to the pituitary at regular 60- to 90-minute intervals, or to a total failure of your pituitary gland to release luteinizing hormone (LH) and follicle-stimulating hormone (FSH) in response to the gonadotropin-releasing hormone that it receives from the hypothalamus. In either case, the ovaries never receive LH and FSH pulses, and follicle growth and ovulation is never stimulated.

While in *most* cases of hypothalamic pituitary failure, patients simply don't have the capability of producing the hormone release that is necessary to initiate ovarian cyclic activity on their own, others can be traced to an obvious physical cause—benign tumors in the hypothalamus or the pituitary.

Tumors of the brain, located either in the hypothalamus or the pituitary, can interfere with normal ovulation in any age group. The majority of these tumors are benign, but by throwing off the production of hormones coming from these areas of the brain, they upset the delicate balance between the central nervous system and the ovary. In most cases, other symptoms will show up well before a tumor interferes with ovulatory function. Symptoms such as headaches and visual problems are common. And, in some of the most extreme forms of tumors—larger tumors, such as pituitary macroadenomas—breast secretions and loss of vision due to pressure on the optic nerve will also occur. If you are experiencing symptoms such as these, you should report them to your doctor so that possible lesions can be diagnosed and properly treated. Don't let fear of treatment delay you. These days less than 1% of tumors of the pituitary are treated with surgery; the other 99% are reduced in size with medication.

OVARIAN FAILURE

Ovarian failure is caused by conditions that exist within the ovary itself, rather than by conditions within the central nervous system such as we have discussed in the prior pages. While every woman experiences ovarian failure when she reaches the age of menopause and her ovaries' production of follicles and eggs ceases, infertile women may experience it prematurely, during their reproductive years. Often, a woman with premature ovarian failure will initially have normal menstrual function, only to go through menopause at an abnormally early time. Such ovarian failure accounts for a low percentage of abnormalities in anovulatory women. It can happen for several reasons.

1. Autoimmune Conditions
2. Congenital Defects
3. Pelvic Infections

Autoimmune Conditions

Some woman don't ovulate because they have an autoimmune abnormality that causes their bodies to direct antibodies against their own ovarian tissue. Over time, this attack by their own immune systems destroys their ovarian cells, their egg cells, and their follicular apparatus, until they are rendered menopausal by all normal standards. Premature ovarian failure due to autoimmune disease can occur at any time—from the late teenage years through age 35. Happily, as there is no known treatment for it, this is a relatively rare condition.

Congenital Defects

Sexual development begins at the moment of fertilization, when the 23 chromosomes that are carried by the egg join together with the 23 chromosomes that are carried by the sperm. The female ovum always contributes an X chromosome to this mix. If the male sperm also contributes an X chromosome, the embryo becomes a female. When the sperm contributes a Y chromosome, the embryo becomes a male.

While this pattern is generally true, in some cases an abnormality in a single gene can be enough to change the sexual characteristics of an embryo. A Y chromosome with an abnormal gene can produce a fetus with a standard male XY combination of chromosomes, which will nevertheless develop as a female. And an X chromosome with an abnormal gene can result in a fetus with a standard female XX combination of chromosomes, which will never be able to develop a full range of female characteristics.

Congenital abnormalities such as these are rare and, unfortunately, incorrectable. Because, by their very nature, they produce not only a lack of ovulation but also abnormal sexual development, most are diagnosed at a very early age, usually before the affected individual gets to the point of attempting pregnancy. In cases of congenital abnormalities, a competent physician dealing with a woman who has never menstruated will encounter certain physical findings during his examination that will lead him to consider genetic testing. Several types of congenital conditions can be identified by this testing, including:

1. Turner's Syndrome

2. Ovarian Dysgenesis

3. Testicular Feminization

Turner's Syndrome   The most common congenital cause of ovarian failure is Turner's syndrome. Women with Turner's syndrome are born with one missing chromosome—the second X chromosome. Their chromosomal makeup is 46XO, instead of the normal female 46XX pattern.

Because they are missing the second X chromosome, which is necessary for the development of female sexual characteristics, these women do not have normal ovaries, or ovarian function. They don't produce estrogen or eggs, and can't be made to ovulate.

Ovarian Dysgenesis   A similar condition, called ovarian dysgenesis (or gonadal dysgenesis), results when a woman has a normal female chromosomal pattern (46XX), but an abnormal gene on the second X chromosome. Ovarian dysgenesis can be diagnosed through banding studies, which magnify the chromosomes to a point that it can be seen where pieces of the second X chromosome are missing.

Like all genetic abnormalities, ovarian dysgenesis exists from birth. Women who suffer from this condition have a uterus, but are born without eggs in their ovaries. Because of this they have a complete lack of ovarian function; they don't have normal follicle and egg production, and their bodies don't manufacture estrogen. Since they don't have eggs, they cannot have a child that is biologically theirs. However, they can carry a fertilized donor egg and give birth.

Testicular Feminization   Another condition that can be diagnosed through chromosomal studies is testicular feminization. This condition results when an individual is born with a male chromosome pattern (46XY), but with an abnormal gene on the Y chromosome.

A woman with testicular feminization appears to be normal externally. Yet when she's given a pelvic exam, she's found to have no uterus, and usually has a somewhat shortened vaginal canal. In addition, her "ovaries" will be made up of a mixture of ovarian tissue and testicular tissue. These gonads or "ovotestes," as they are called, produce both female and male hormones—estrogen, testosterone, and other androgens. Her condition may be identified during puberty because, since she lacks a uterus, she will never begin to menstruate.

Because these individuals both produce and respond to estrogen, they have normal female secondary sexual characteristics, such as breast development. Yet while they also produce androgens, they remain relatively insensitive to them, so the secondary sexual characteristics that these male hormones would normally produce—such as pubic, arm, and leg hair—remain sparse. As a result these patients have the appearance of being female, even though they are genetically male.

Women with testicular feminization can never be made to ovulate, because they have no normal ovarian tissue. Nor can they carry a donor egg, since they have no uterus. The condition must be treated by surgically removing the ovotestes, since in a very high percentage of cases they become cancerous.

Pelvic Infections

While they sound relatively benign, pelvic infections can actually be very harmful to your fertility. Severe infections, such as pelvic inflammatory disease—or chronic diseases, such as endometriosis—can attack and destroy your ovarian tissue over a period of time if they are allowed to progress. If you feel that you have a pelvic infection, or suspect that you might have endometriosis, don't hesitate. Go directly to your doctor. If you ignore these conditions, you run the risk of becoming prematurely menopausal due to the destruction of your ovarian tissue.

─────────── **SIGNS OF PELVIC INFECTION** ───────────

If you have the following warning signs of pelvic infection, it is important that you see your doctor: 1) fever and/or chills; 2) diffuse pelvic pain; 3) pain with walking; 4) nausea and/or diarrhea. The onset of these symptoms will often, but not always, follow your menses.

Another thing to consider is that if you have one of these conditions and it has been allowed to become chronic, you may need to be treated with a more aggressive therapy than would otherwise have been needed. While a pelvic infection can be cured with drugs in its early stages, one that is allowed to progress might require surgical intervention. Surgery can be a mixed blessing. It removes the pain and the problem—the infection or endometrial growths. But if done without consideration of your future ability to get pregnant, it can also remove your ability to conceive, and can push you into premature menopause in the process. You should be particularly alert to the possibility that the majority—even all—of your ovarian tissue could be removed if:

- Your surgeon is removing dermoid cysts from your ovary.

- Your surgeon is removing endometrial growths that have formed around your ovaries.

- Your surgeon is removing abscesses caused by pelvic inflammatory disease from your ovary or fallopian tubes.

If you are faced with conditions such as these, which may have long-term consequences for your ovarian function, you need to be sure that

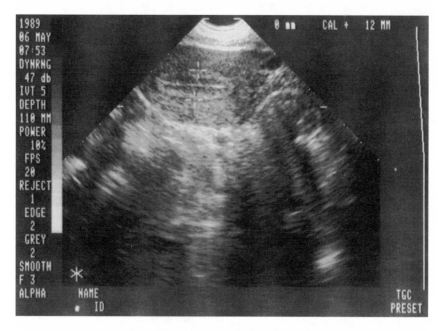

Figure 6-2:   Ultrasound of Endometrium

your surgeon is fully aware of your desire to have children. You should also question him very specifically as to the number of times he has successfully performed the operation he is about to attempt on you, to confirm his surgical expertise in dealing with your level of disease. Doing careful research prior to undergoing surgery can go a long way toward preserving your ability to have children.

Luteal Phase Problems

Problems with ovulation can manifest themselves as a lack of follicle growth or an absence of egg release, as we have already described. Or they can be related to the endometrial lining of the uterus. Such problems, which are known as "luteal phase abnormalities," can occur in two different ways. Either the endometrial lining can be poorly prepared prior to ovulation, or it can receive inadequate hormonal support after the egg is released from the follicle.

As ovulation takes place, the constant changes in follicle growth and hormone production that accompany it cause a matching, and just as precisely timed, set of daily changes to occur in the uterine lining. As estrogen increases, it stimulates the endometrial lining to grow, so that by the time of egg release, the lining has become thickened. Because this thickening of the lining can be easily observed through ultrasound by the time of ovulation, it is one of the markers that your doctor uses to determine whether you have a luteal phase abnormality relating to the preparation of the lining prior to egg release. To confirm such a problem, he would give you an ultrasound at the time of ovulation. In doing this, he would anticipate observing an endometrial thickness somewhere between 8 and 12 mm. He should also be able to make out what is called a trilinear pattern. This means that he should be able to see three distinct layers within the endometrial lining. If your endometrial lining passes both of these tests it is considered normal, and is optimally prepared to receive a fertilized egg. If it does not, your doctor will consider the possibility that there is some problem with the hormonal signals your ovary is receiving prior to ovulation, or with the ovary's ability to respond to them. (See Figure 6-2.)

After ovulation, your endometrial lining continues to grow and to change. This phase of its development is controlled by the corpus luteum, the structure that remains once the follicle has ovulated. It is not enough for your endometrial lining to achieve the appropriate thickness and structure; it must achieve them at exactly the correct time. By the seventh day following the LH surge, the endometrium should be prepared to nurture an embryo during implantation. Given this timing, an embryo will be able to implant between four and eight days after ovulation, the window within which most implantations take place. Whether this timing is achieved is largely dependent on the hormonal support that the endometrial lining receives from the corpus luteum. If the corpus luteum is not functioning correctly, development of the endometrial lining can take place out of synch with ovulation. The lining may be prepared either too early or too late to receive the fertilized egg.

If your doctor suspects that you have this type of problem, he will confirm it with a combination of two tests. The daily changes in your endometrial lining are controlled by two hormones that are secreted from the corpus luteum—primarily by progesterone, and secondarily by estradiol. To confirm that they are being secreted in adequate amounts, he will measure the estradiol and progesterone in your bloodstream. A progesterone reading of less than 10 nanograms per milliliter is abnormally low. If this is your test result, you have a luteal phase problem.

If your doctor finds adequate hormone levels, he will then look to the possibility that your endometrial lining isn't responding to them correctly, by performing an endometrial biopsy. A sample of the tissue from your endometrial lining will be sent to a pathologist, who will examine it, looking for the cellular changes that are typical of particular days in a normal cycle. Your doctor will then compare this result to the day of your cycle on which the sample was actually taken. You will be considered to have a luteal phase defect if your biopsy shows that the development of your endometrial lining is more than one day off from the point at which it should be, considering the day of your ovulation.

If he does find a luteal phase defect as a result of these tests, it can be easily treated. Unless there is a complicating structural problem, virtually all cases of luteal phase abnormalities can be corrected with drug therapy.

The Drugs That Treat Ovulation

Some ovulation problems, such as genetic abnormalities and ovarian failure, cannot be corrected. Those ovulation problems that *are* correctable—such as hypothalamic pituitary dysfunction and hypothalamic pituitary failure—are almost always treated with drugs, rather than surgically.

Today's drug treatments for infertility are an outgrowth of a 1958 decision by the Food and Drug Administration, which approved the use of two new medications that were specifically developed for the treatment of ovulation abnormalities. These two medications—clomiphene citrate (CC) and human menopausal gonadotropins (hMG)—have been marketed under a number of different brand names, some more expensive than others, and have been widely used ever since. In fact, forty years later they are still the most commonly employed fertility drugs.

These two basic drugs—CC and hMG—are supplemented by an ever-expanding arsenal of drugs, which go beyond ovulation stimulation to add various forms of support for both ovulation and pregnancy. Other new pharmaceutical alternatives can block the production of hormones, in cases where that is necessary, in order to achieve a better balance. Most recently a new generation of drugs, such as genetically engineered hormones, has been developed. Many of them are well along in their approval process by the FDA. They hold out the hope of doing even more to remedy ovulation problems in the future.

The first time you discuss fertility drugs with your doctor, you'll feel as if you've been dropped into a bowl of alphabet soup. Not only are a whole list of hormones involved in ovulation, there's an even longer inventory of drugs available to adjust them. These drugs have two things in common . . . almost all will be unfamiliar to you, and almost all will be unpronounceable. It will help you to get a clearer picture if you keep in mind that most fertility drugs do one of three things.

- Stimulate ovulation

- Block the production of competing hormones

- Support ovulation and/or pregnancy

Each category of fertility drugs has the ability to solve certain ovulation problems. It is important that you have some basic understanding of how each of them works. This will give you an idea of which conditions each is best at correcting, and help you understand why your physician chooses specific drugs for you. It is also important to educate yourself about the possible side effects that each of these drugs has, before taking it.

DRUGS THAT STIMULATE OVULATION

   1. Clomiphene citrate

   2. Human menopausal gonadotropin (hMG)

3. Urofollitropin (FSH)

4. Gonadotropin-releasing hormone (GnRH)

5. Human chorionic gonadotropin (hCG)

6. Genetically engineered hormones (FSH, LH)

Several types of drugs are used to stimulate various phases of ovulation. While each of them works toward the same end result—the development and release of eggs from the ovaries—each one does so in a slightly different way.

Clomiphene Citrate (Clomid, Serophene)

Of the drugs that are used to stimulate ovulation, clomiphene citrate is the most frequently used. There are several reasons for this. Clomiphene citrate is the least expensive choice, and since it is given in pill form, rather than injected, it is the least physically invasive and most convenient. Also, because it works indirectly to stimulate ovulation, rather than directly affecting the ovaries, it is less likely to cause overproduction of eggs when compared with the drugs that directly stimulate the ovaries, such as human menopausal gonadotropins (hMG).

How Does Clomiphene Citrate Work?

Normally, after a woman ovulates, her follicles form a corpus luteum. This corpus luteum releases estrogen and progesterone into her system for 12 to 14 days, at which point, if pregnancy does not occur, it stops releasing these hormones. As soon as the hypothalamus detects a lack of estrogen in the system, it starts to release gonadotropin-releasing hormone (GnRH), to start a new ovulatory cycle. This occurs even before the menstrual period begins. The presence of GnRH in a woman's system signals the pituitary gland that it is time to release follicle-stimulating hormone (FSH) and luteinizing hormone (LH). The FSH and LH then trigger the recruitment of the new ovarian follicles. As the follicles develop, they once again release estrogen into the bloodstream, correcting the lack of estrogen that the hypothalamus originally detected, and signaling it to decrease the amount of GnRH released.

When this new estrogen enters the hypothalamus, it links to estrogen receptors. The hypothalamus estimates how much estrogen is in the bloodstream by counting the number of receptors that are linked. When a large number of receptors are linked, the hypothalamus assumes

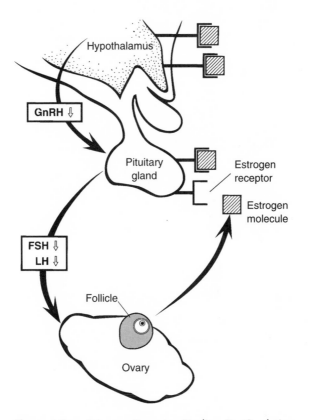

Figure 6-3a: Estrogen Receptor Binding Pre-Ovulation

there is a large amount of estrogen circulating. That tells it the follicles are in the process of developing. (See Figure 6-3a.)

If there are only a small number of linked receptors, the hypothalamus assumes that there is only a small amount of estrogen circulating. That tells it that the follicles are not developing, have already ovulated, or are no longer producing estrogen. When it gets these signals, the hypothalamus increases its releases of GnRH to initiate the next ovulatory cycle. (See Figure 6-3b.)

If a woman's estrogen levels do not vary appropriately for some reason, her hypothalamus won't get proper signals, and it won't function correctly—it will release too little, too much, or no GnRH. As a result, her follicles won't be given a signal to develop, and she won't ovulate.

Clomiphene citrate helps to correct this situation by working as false estrogen, or as an "antiestrogen" molecule. This means that it's the antithesis of estrogen, inhibiting processes that estrogen stimulates— such as the production of mucus and the growth of the endometrium.

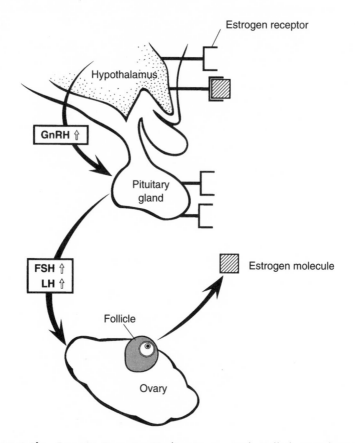

Figure 6-3b: Estrogen Receptor Binding During Early Follicle Development

When clomiphene citrate enters the bloodstream, it mimics estrogen and combines with the estrogen receptors in the hypothalamus. When the clomiphene citrate molecules bind with the estrogen receptors, they trick the hypothalamus into believing that there is no estrogen present, and the hypothalamus responds by releasing GnRH, which then starts a new cycle of ovarian follicle activity. (See Figure 6-3c.)

Who Should Use Clomiphene Citrate?:   If you aren't having menstrual periods, you aren't a candidate for clomiphene citrate therapy. That's because a lack of periods indicates a very low, or even menopausal, estrogen level. Under those conditions clomiphene citrate won't work to normalize your ovulatory system, because the binding of the clomiphene citrate molecules to the estrogen receptors won't produce a false low reading. Instead, it would simply be perceived by your system as the

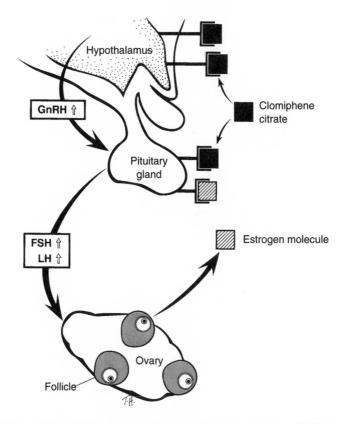

Figure 6-3c: Effect of Clomiphene Citrate on Estrogen Receptor Binding During Ovulation

normal state of affairs. That's why, in order for clomiphene citrate to work, you must already be manufacturing a somewhat normal level of estrogen, your ovaries must be able to function, and your hypothalamus and pituitary gland must be able to produce their respective hormones. Clomiphene simply balances this normal interaction between the brain and the ovaries. If you *are* having menstrual periods, but you are having them irregularly, clomiphene can help you to have more regular ovulatory cycles, which means that you will have more opportunities for eggs to become fertilized. And it can ensure that your follicles will mature before releasing their eggs. Clomiphene is also a good treatment possibility if your periods are overly long, or if you have a luteal phase defect. While clomiphene citrate is highly effective in patients that have hypothalamic pituitary dysfunction, it's a bad choice of medication for those with hypothalamic pituitary failure.

Patients whose conditions are appropriate for standard clomiphene therapy most often take one 50-mg tablet per day for five consecutive days. This regimen is usually started on the third, fourth, or fifth day after menstrual bleeding begins. If ovulation is still not normal, an increased dose of clomiphene is tried in an effort to correct it. Two tablets, or 100 mg, taken for five days is the maximum dose that should be used to normalize ovulation.

What Is Clomiphene Citrate's Success Rate?   Clomiphene citrate's success rate depends upon what your specific condition is. However, generally speaking, when women receive clomiphene citrate, around 80% of them ovulate approximately seven to ten days after completing their five-day regimen. Of those, approximately 50% become pregnant within six months of treatment.

What Side Effects Should You Expect?   A minimal number of side effects have been reported by women using clomiphene citrate. Changes in your brain's perception of your estradiol levels can cause hot flushes and, in about 10% of women, some ovarian enlargement or cysts. If your body is responding this way, you will probably experience symptoms such as abdominal discomfort or pain. Some other side effects reported frequently include mood swings, breast tenderness, headaches, nervousness, dizziness, nausea and vomiting, fatigue, and temporary visual disturbances. This all sounds reasonable on paper, but according to many women, nothing you can read will fully prepare you for the emotional and physical side effects of fertility drugs.

It's Not Fun!

On my way to getting pregnant, I took both Clomid and Pergonal. It's hard to control the emotional swings they bring on. It's as if you're standing on a beach and a large wave is building up behind you, but you don't see it coming. When it hits you, it's a total surprise. It's as if six months of anger and resentments suddenly well up and spill out all at once. How did I deal with it? I got in my closet and pulled the sliding mirror doors shut. When my husband came home and asked what was going on, I told him, "I'd highly recommend that you leave the room. I'm having a snit fit. I'll get over it." By the time he came home and found me standing in the freezer, he was used to my swings. Clomid brought on hot flushes. My makeup would melt, my hair would droop, my clothing would be soaked with sweat. The freezer was the only way I could cool down. So when I looked at him, said, "Don't even ask," he didn't. But when it came to the weight gain, he did speak up. "Where is it written we need to have a wardrobe allowance?" he asked our doctor. And believe me, we needed one. Because the sad fact is, you're bloated all times of the month, and you can't do anything about it.

—Sharon, age 40

————

Luckily, not everyone has the same extreme reaction to fertility drugs as Sharon did.

Human Menopausal Gonadotropin (Pergonal, Humegon, Metrodin)

Gonadotropins are substances that act on, or stimulate, the gonads— which, in the case of women, are the ovaries. Human menopausal gonadotropin (hMG) is second only to clomiphene citrate as a choice of treatment for encouraging the follicles to develop when a woman's pituitary doesn't release adequate FSH and LH, or when it releases these important hormones in an improper balance.

There are several reasons why human menopausal gonadotropin is in this runner-up position. It is much more expensive than clomiphene—a typical hMG cycle costs $800 to $1,000, compared to $50 to $100 for a typical cycle of clomiphene. And it is more difficult and inconvenient to use. Because hMG is a natural hormone that is a protein, it can't be taken orally in the form of a pill. If it entered the stomach, it would be broken down by the digestive system and inactivated. So human menopausal gonadotropin must be given by intramuscular injection, into the muscles of the buttocks or hip. This location presents some obvious logistical problems if you are trying to give injections to yourself. Treatments of hMG are usually initiated on the second, third, or fourth day of your menstrual bleeding. The drug comes in ampules, in the form of a powder, and must be mixed with saline to liquefy it before use.

————

You Always Hurt the One You Love!

Before you start thinking I'm some kind of wimp, you should know that I sailed through the army, and then the police academy, without missing a beat. Except when I was sick, of course. Show me a needle, and I go catatonic. So you can guess how I felt the morning our doctor looked across his desk at me and said, "Now you'll have to give your wife these shots once a day."

"She's much better at that kind of thing than I am," I told him. But short of being a candidate for a sideshow act, she wasn't going to be able to reach the right spot, so I was on.

"This is going to hurt me more than it hurts you," I told her the first time. After all, this was the woman I love. Later she told me I was wrong . . . it hurt her more. But as time went on, I got better at it, and she could begin to sit down again. My hard work and her patience paid off. We gave birth to twins a year and a half later.

—*Frank, age 36*

———

Finally, side effects from hMG are more difficult to regulate. Unlike clomiphene citrate, which is a manufactured chemical merely masquerading as the hormone estrogen, human menopausal gonadotropin is a distillation of the actual human hormones FSH and LH. They are harvested from the urine of postmenopausal women. Women who are postmenopausal excrete large amounts of FSH and LH from their pituitary gland on a daily basis, which is metabolized and concentrated in their urine. Their urine is collected, chemically separated, purified, made into powder, freeze-dried, and then sealed in sterile glass ampules, where it remains until it is administered by injection. It then travels through the bloodstream to the ovary, and directly stimulates the same follicular activity that would occur if it were actually released from the pituitary gland. Human menopausal gonadotropins work directly on the ovaries, rather than indirectly via the hypothalamus. Because of this direct push, there is a greater chance that they may overstimulate the ovaries.

Who Should Use hMG?   Human menopausal gonadotropin is usually used by the same women who use clomiphene. Its extra cost and inconvenience is justified when a woman's system is resistant to clomiphene. Sometimes, when a woman's pituitary is stimulated indirectly with clomiphene citrate, it doesn't respond with enough FSH and LH to produce ovulation. In those instances natural FSH and LH—in the form of hMG—can be injected. Their direct action on the ovaries will often bring a response where clomiphene was ineffective. HMG can also be used to produce multiple follicle growth for use in IVF, GIFT, and other assisted reproductive technologies.

HMG offers an additional advantage over clomiphene. Clomiphene acts by making a woman's body think it has inadequate estrogen, when it really doesn't. As we periodically discussed, estrogen triggers the production of cervical mucus. Clomiphene citrate, which has antiestrogen effects, will sometimes produce mucus that will not allow sperm migration to occur. HMG, which does not act as an antiestrogen, doesn't interfere with mucus production.

While human menopausal gonadotropin is available under a number of different brand names, these brands are not necessarily interchangeable. Each one contains different percentages of FSH and LH, and each one is best used when treating specific conditions.

Pergonal   is a combination of FSH and LH in equal amounts. It was the first type of human menopausal gonadotropin that was approved for medical use. Another brand name for this 50-50 combination of FSH and LH is Humegon.

Metrodin   is a purified form of hMG called urofollitropin. It contains only FSH and no LH. It increases follicle stimulation without elevating LH levels. It is a good choice for women who have too much LH compared to their FSH—women with polycystic ovarian syndrome, for example, who have an elevated LH level accompanied by a low to normal FSH level.

As you can see, there are a number of different options available, which must be fine-tuned for each patient. This is a process that requires both experience and intuition. For this reason it is important that your doctor has worked frequently with all of the human menopausal gonadotropins, so that he can expertly decide which is most suitable for you.

What Is hMG's Success Rate?   Studies show that if you take human menopausal gonadotropin, you have about a 95% chance of ovulating. If you do ovulate, you then have about a 25% chance of becoming pregnant each cycle, assuming your fallopian tubes are open and your partner's sperm count and function is adequate.

What Side Effects Should You Expect?   Like clomiphene citrate, human menopausal gonadotropin has some relatively mild side effects, which you might experience—things such as rashes, swelling, or irritation at the injection site. These are easy to deal with by simply alternating the area of your body where you are receiving injections. Also, if more than one of your follicles is stimulated, your estrogen level may be higher than in normal cycles, and the amount of cervical mucus you produce may be increased. Finally, you may experience fatigue, mood swings, headaches, bloating, and some weight gain.

Other possible side effects have the potential of being more serious, and should be monitored more closely. Because hMG bypasses your system's control centers—the hypothalamus and pituitary—and goes directly to your ovaries, there is a greater chance that the ovaries will be overstimulated. About 20% of women treated with hMG get a mild ovarian enlargement, sometimes accompanied by abdominal distension and pain. In uncomplicated cases this condition reverses itself without treatment within one to two weeks. If a more severe ovarian enlargement, known as hyperstimulation syndrome, develops, there can be both a sudden enlargement of the ovary and an accumulation of fluid in the abdomen. This fluid can also accumulate around the lungs, and if the ovary ruptures, blood can accumulate in the abdominal cavity as well. Fortunately, severe hyperstimulation occurs in only 1.3% of patients; it can almost always be avoided through a combination of blood tests, which check your serum estrogen levels, and ultrasound, which visually follows the development of your follicles and records how many of them are maturing.

If you are receiving hMG therapy, the amount of monitoring that you will need to gauge your response to the drug, to adjust dosage, and to prevent side effects, depends upon what your condition is and how the drug is administered. This is one place where your choice of physician can be very important in helping to contain the costs of your therapy. For example, patients with hypothalamic pituitary failure rarely hyperstimulate with gonadotropin therapy, or produce more than two or three follicles with standard doses of Pergonal or Metrodin. If you are in hypothalamic pituitary failure, and you go to a reproductive endocrinologist who is experienced in this therapy, he will only have to do minimal tests to monitor your condition. He will give you an ultrasound before you start your ovulation-induction cycle, another one about five days later, and a final ultrasound a couple of days after that. On the other hand, an obstetrician/gynecologist who has limited experience with ovulation induction would need to monitor you more closely, drawing blood for estrogen levels and doing ultrasounds daily, or every other day.

Beyond lowering the cost of your treatment, an experienced reproductive endocrinologist can also lower the risks. For example, if you are a patient with PCOS, there is a tendency among many obstetrician/gynecologists, and some reproductive endocrinologists, to go directly to the use of hMG alone if there is not a clear response to clomiphene. There are potential dangers to the patient inherent in this decision. Most of the time, with this form of ovulation induction, multiple follicles are produced, none mature properly, and follicle rupture doesn't take place. The ovaries can be overstimulated as a result, with hyperstimulation being quite common. An experienced reproductive endocrinologist will have developed enough finesse with fertility drugs to avoid these problems while still succeeding with ovulation induction. He might extend the period of time over which the drugs are administered, and administer them in very low doses. Or he might give them sequentially—first clomiphene citrate, and then hMG. These adjustments balance good results with a high margin of safety. While your ovulation may be delayed until Day 18 or 20 in your cycle, you'll be assured of having a manageable number of mature follicles—probably one, two, or three. The risk of hyperstimulation will be almost nonexistent, the risk of multiple pregnancy will be low, yet your chances to ovulate and become pregnant will still be excellent.

───────────── **CAN I RUIN MY CHANCES FOREVER?** ─────────────

Many patients are concerned about the possibility of ectopic pregnancies as a possible side effect of hMG ovulation induction. The results of studies regarding this possibility are mixed. There have been three major studies since 1970, two of which indicate the possibility of ectopic pregnancy. However, the most thorough study that has been done to date argues against this. It followed 1,200 women who experienced treatment with ovulation-inducing drugs, and found no elevated risk of ectopic pregnancy. It is normal in the general population for one half of 1% of all pregnancies to be ectopic. The percentage rises to 2% for women with any history of fertility problems, no matter what their problem might have been, or how it was treated. The sample group of hMG-stimulated women matched this 2% figure, and showed no apparent rise in ectopic pregnancy as a result of having had previous hMG induction of ovulation.

Gonadotropin-releasing Hormone (Factrel, Lutrepulse)

While clomiphene citrate and human menopausal gonadotropin are the most commonly used therapies, other drugs are also administered for ovulation control. For example, supplemental doses of gonadotropin-releasing hormone (GnRH) have been used over the last ten to fifteen years to help women whose hypothalamus fails to produce enough GnRH naturally, and whose pituitary isn't stimulated to release LH and FSH, as a result. However, since GnRH is both inconvenient and expensive to use, it is rarely prescribed unless other therapies have failed.

As we explained in Chapter Two, a woman's body normally releases pulses of GnRH every 60 to 90 minutes. If you are using supplemental GnRH, it has to be released into your body at the same frequent intervals. Since it is virtually impossible for you to give yourself shots every hour on the hour, 24 hours a day, a constant-infusion pump is normally used, which administers GnRH subcutaneously or on a continuous, intravenous basis. These infusion pumps are about the size of a credit card. They pump GnRH into your body through a needle that is worn inserted into your abdominal wall or into a vein in your arm. While these pumps are prohibitively expensive for most patients to buy—costing several thousand dollars—they can usually be rented through the physician who's treating you for several hundred dollars a month.

GnRH is rarely used for women who are having spontaneous periods, since clomiphene is much cheaper and easier to use, and in their cases can usually accomplish the same thing. For women who are suffering full hypothalamic pituitary failure, hMG is normally a better stimulant. However, in some severe cases of PCOS, GnRH has an advantage over hMG. Since GnRH is an *indirect* ovarian stimulus, working on the pituitary rather than on the ovaries themselves, it can correct difficult ovulatory problems without risking high rates of hyperstimulation.

On the plus side, therapy with GnRH has a high success rate. It usually produces ovulation within three to four weeks. And for those women who can tolerate having a needle in their vein continuously, two out of three become pregnant within four months, assuming they have no other infertility problems.

——— MULTIPLE BIRTHS WITH FERTILITY DRUGS: ——— DOCTOR, IS IT TWINS?

Maybe you're approaching the use of ovulation-induction drugs with visions of double and triple strollers dancing in your head. Are multiple births really more common under these circumstances? The answer is yes.

Ten percent of clomiphene citrate–induced pregnancies result in the delivery of twins, with slightly under 1% being triplets or more.

Of the pregnancies following therapy with human menopausal gonadotropin, around 20% are multiple births, with 5% of them being births of triplets or more.

If you don't see multiple strollers in your future, the possibility of multiple births can be minimized—though not entirely eliminated—if your physician monitors you closely with ultrasound to track the number of follicles that are developing.

Human Chorionic Gonadotropin (Profasi, Pregnyl, APL)

While the drugs we've described to this point are effective in helping your follicles to grow and mature correctly, yet another drug is necessary to create follicle rupture (ovulation). As we told you in a previous chapter, the rupture of the follicle, causing the actual release of the egg, is normally triggered by a surge of luteinizing hormone (LH). If you are not manufacturing enough LH to accomplish this, which is often the case if there is a problem in your hypothalamus or pituitary, the deficiency has to be corrected before you can ovulate. Human chorionic gonadotropin (hCG) is a hormone that is produced by the placenta during a normal pregnancy. Its structure is so similar to that of LH, it can be used to replace it. HCG is given when LH release is inadequate, or when hMG has been used to stimulate ovulation. In 99% of hMG cycles, hCG is used to correctly time the follicle rupture (egg release) for control of ovulation.

Genetically Engineered Hormones

The newest forms of hormones, which will soon be used for ovulation control, are made by genetic engineering. This method of manufacturing is producing purer forms of follicle-stimulating hormone, luteinizing hormone, and human chorionic gonadotropin than have ever been available before. In 1993 our clinic tested one such genetically engineered hormone—Gonal-F—which should be coming on the market as this book is published. With the development of such highly purified forms of FSH, LH, and hCG, ovulation correction should improve dramatically in the next decade.

DRUGS THAT BLOCK THE PRODUCTION OF HORMONES

As we've pointed out, different patients can have dramatically different reactions to an identical drug protocol. Because of this, the possibility always exists that a woman's system will receive too much stimulation, and that a new hormonal imbalance—an excess of hormones—will be created in the process of correcting a prior hormonal inadequacy. Medications known as "agonists" are used to prevent this.

Agonists

Agonists are synthetic versions of natural hormones, which are longer lasting and considerably more potent than the hormones they mimic. One form of agonist that is commonly used in ovulation control is gonadotropin-releasing hormone agonist. When natural GnRH is released from the hypothalamus into the bloodstream, it has a very short life. Normally it is active for just a couple of seconds to a minute. GnRH agonists, on the other hand, have an active life of anywhere from 90 minutes to 6 hours. Used correctly they can "level the playing field"— they can temporarily shut down your body's natural production of hormones so that only the controlled amounts, which are being given to you by your doctor, will be circulating in your system.

When a GnRH agonist reaches the pituitary, it stimulates the release of FSH and LH, just as natural GnRH would. But since its action continues for hours, rather than seconds, it eventually exhausts the pituitary, which then shuts down and stops producing these hormones. Once this is accomplished, your doctor knows that the only FSH and LH that will be circulating in your system is the amount he is putting there. This gives him an extra factor of control over ovulation, particularly in preventing hyperstimulation or premature ovulation, which can be caused by premature release of LH prior to follicle maturity.

Currently, the only GnRH agonists available in the United States for ovulation control are the injectable leuprolide acetate, which is marketed under the brand name Lupron, and a nasal spray, which is available under the brand name of Synarel. Lupron is administered subcutaneously, starting either on Day 2 of your cycle, or during your cycle's luteal phase—usually Days 22 to 24. It is then taken until the point at which you receive an hCG injection to stimulate follicle rupture (ovulation). Synarel is administered by nasal spray two or three times a day, beginning at the same cycle times as Lupron.

Bromocriptine mesylate, which is marketed under the brand name Parlodel, is another type of agonist. It is used to suppress the production of prolactin, the hormone that is released by the pituitary gland after the delivery of a baby to stimulate the breasts to make milk. Prolactin has a secondary effect as well: it can interfere with normal ovulation, or with the luteal phase, which is why women who are nursing rarely become pregnant.

In some cases, women who are not nursing also have an abnormally high level of prolactin. This excess of prolactin in women who aren't pregnant can be caused by a variety of things. Drugs—including antidepressants, blood pressure medications, or anesthetics—may be responsible. It can also be the result of stress, of excessive exercise, or of an underactive thyroid. But in most cases it is brought on by a benign growth (an adenoma) in the pituitary gland. No matter what causes it, an excess of prolactin can interfere with ovulation, either making it irregular, or stopping it altogether. Parlodel corrects this situation by imitating dopamine—a chemical compound that is naturally in your system.

Dopamine functions like a hormone, producing a response in a target organ in the same way that any hormone would. But since it is manufactured by cells in the cortex of the brain, rather than by cells in the endocrine glands, it is called a neurotransmitter. Dopamine suppresses the release of prolactin from the pituitary gland; a high level of dopamine in the bloodstream tells the pituitary to stop manufacturing prolactin. Once a pregnant woman gives birth, her dopamine level drops, and prolactin is sent into her bloodstream. Not only does prolactin stimulate the production of milk, but the decrease in dopamine can also cause a decrease in GnRH, which interferes with the manufacture of FSH and LH, thereby disrupting her menstruation and ovulation. If a woman who has not just given birth has an elevated level of prolactin, Parlodel—a manmade, longer-lived substitute for dopamine—can be used to suppress the release of prolactin from her pituitary gland.

Once their prolactin level is normalized, these woman may resume normal ovulation. Assuming they have no other fertility problems, 60% to 80% of them become pregnant after treatment with Parlodel.

GnRH Antagonists

GnRH antagonists are a new form of ovulation-induction drug that is now being developed. If all goes well with the Food and Drug Administration, they will be available for medical use in the United States sometime before the end of 1998. GnRH antagonists counteract, or block, the effect of gonadotropin-releasing hormone. They accomplish the same thing as the GnRH agonists that are currently in use, but they do it faster. They can produce a complete shutdown of the pituitary gland within hours. In certain patients, they will be used in conjunction with either human menopausal gonadotropin, or pure FSH, for ovulation control.

DRUGS THAT SUPPORT OVULATION AND PREGNANCY

Progesterone

As we discussed in Chapter Two, progesterone is normally released from the ovary after ovulation. It causes changes in the lining of the uterus to make it more receptive for implantation to occur. If the amount of this hormone, which is naturally present in your body, isn't adequate, your doctor will give you additional progesterone to stimulate more of your own progesterone to supplement it. This is done in an effort to make the lining of the uterus as receptive as possible to a fertilized egg.

Natural progesterone, when used as part of ovulation therapy, can be given by injection, suppository, or by mouth. Injectable progesterone is an oily fluid that is injected into the hip. Because it is so thick, it has a slow, even release into the bloodstream. For the same reason, you will have to take your time when you draw it up into the needle for injection. The time of day that injectable progesterone is administered is not crucial. It can be given at whatever time is most convenient for you, but this should be at approximately the same time each day. If vaginal suppositories or oral tablets are used, they must be administered three times a day in varying doses, depending upon the individual.

How These Drugs Are Used

All of the drugs we've discussed in this chapter can be used either alone or in combination with each other. Since there is such a variation in the way women respond to them, it is difficult for us to describe here exactly what your doctor should prescribe for you. However, there are some general therapy plans—or "egg production protocols"—that are commonly used, and should be considered as possible starting points for your treatment. The appropriate one for you will vary according to your condition—hypothalamic pituitary failure, hypothalamic pituitary dysfunction, or ovarian failure.

HYPOTHALAMIC PITUITARY FAILURE

Maintenance Therapy

As we explained earlier in this chapter, most women who have hypothalamic pituitary failure become aware of their problem well before the time at which they might want to become pregnant. If you happen to be among this group, you should begin estrogen/progesterone replacement therapy as soon as you learn of your condition, rather than waiting until the point at which you want a child. Because your estrogen levels are low, you share many symptoms with women who have gone through menopause. While you may not be having hot flashes, your skeletal structure will, over time, begin to show osteoporotic changes and lose bone mass. And since your cardiovascular system won't be receiving the beneficial effects that estrogen normally provides for premenopausal women, you will be more prone to develop heart disease.

All of these problems can be corrected with hormone replacement therapy (HRT), sometimes referred to as estrogen replacement therapy (ERT). Under this therapy you would receive both estrogen, to replace the female hormone that your system lacks, and progesterone, to help prevent possible side effects that can be caused by an excess of estrogen. These hormones would be given sequentially over a 25-day period. Estrogen replacement would be used for Days 1 through 25, with a progesterone replacement added for 10 days, from Days 16 through 25 of the cycle. Your estrogen supplement can be taken either orally (Premarin, Ogen, or Estrace) or worn as a skin patch (Estraderm or Climara). Your progesterone will be given orally (Provera). No matter which type of medication you and your doctor choose, the dosage of estrogen and progesterone must be carefully adjusted for your individual needs and responses.

Fertility Therapy

If you have hypothalamic pituitary failure and you decide you want to become pregnant, your ovulation will have to be medically induced. Unfortunately, the least expensive and most convenient fertility drug—clomiphene citrate—can't be used in your case. As we explained earlier, there has to be a minimum level of estradiol circulating in a woman's bloodstream—at least 40 pg per milliliter—in order for clomiphene citrate to be effective. Most hypothalamic pituitary failure patients have levels of estradiol that are virtually undetectable—usually less than 20 pg per milliliter.

HOW BIG IS A PICOGRAM?

There are 454 grams in a pound, 1,000 milligrams in a gram, 1,000 nanograms in a milligram, and 1,000 picograms in a nanogram. This should give you some idea of how delicate the measurements really are that must be made to adjust your ovulation.

Having eliminated clomiphene citrate as an appropriate therapy for you, your doctor will move on to human menopausal gonadotropins in one of three forms—Humegon, Pergonal, or Metrodin (purified FSH). Any one of the three will bypass your faulty hypothalamus or pituitary, and will directly stimulate your follicles' growth and maturity. However, once the follicle is mature, none of them will produce actual ovulation for you. Since a faulty pituitary gland doesn't produce LH—the hormone that initiates the rupture of the follicle and the release of the egg—

human chorionic gonadotropin (hCG) must be given to accomplish this final step.

The common protocol that I use in the first treatment cycle for women with hypothalamic pituitary failure is as follows:

Day 1: An ultrasound is performed to ensure that your ovaries have no preexisting cysts. If the scan is clear, two ampules of hMG are administered by injection.

Days 2–5: Two ampules of hMG are injected daily.

Day 6: Another ultrasound is performed, and blood is drawn and tested for serum estradiol levels, to determine whether your follicles are developing normally. If the estradiol level is lower than 100 pg per milliliter, the dosage of hMG is increased to three ampules daily.

Day 8 and on: A third ultrasound is performed. If your follicle(s) are developing normally, they will have reached at least 12 mm in diameter. Assuming they have, you will continue to receive the same dose of hMG, and to be scanned every 2 to 3 days, until your follicle is between 18 mm and 20 mm in diameter. As soon as this size is attained, you should receive a 10,000 IU injection of hCG, and 36 to 40 hours later you should ovulate.

──────────────── **TIMING IS EVERYTHING** ────────────────

HCG comes in powder form in vials that contain the normal dosage— 10,000 units. You will also receive a second vial, which contains fluid to dissolve the powder. If you are going to be receiving hCG as part of your treatment, your doctor will give you a time at which he wants you to administer it. It is important that you give yourself the injection at this time, particularly if your doctor is going to be doing an insemination procedure.

Seven days later: You should receive another 5,000 IU of hCG.

Ten days later: A pregnancy test is performed. If it's positive, you will continue to receive hCG every three to five days, until the pregnancy produces enough hCG on its own (in excess of 3,000 IU) to maintain estrogen and progesterone production adequate to support the implanted embryo.

On rare occasions, women with hypothalamic pituitary failure cannot be made to ovulate with normal doses of human menopausal gonadotropins. If this happens to you, your physician might first try considerably higher doses of hMG. If this still doesn't work, he might choose to try gonadotropin-releasing hormone (GnRH), which normally means wearing a pump. Your doctor will probably use the Lutrepulse system, which is readily available commercially. As inconvenient as this is, it seems to be effective. Once pulsatile GnRH is started, it usually produces ovulation within three to four weeks.

HYPOTHALAMIC PITUITARY DYSFUNCTION

As we explained earlier in this chapter, there are four frequent causes for hypothalamic pituitary dysfunction. These include stress, drugs, body weight problems, and polycystic ovarian syndrome (PCOS). The first two—stress and drugs—cannot be helped by therapy with fertility drugs. Eliminating the problems they produce can be accomplished only by eliminating the cause—by controlling the stress, or by stopping the drug intake. While the same is true of body weight problems, fertility drugs are sometimes called for to get ovulation started after the weight is normalized. PCOS, on the other hand, is almost exclusively treated through fertility drugs. Since it is a complex condition, with several possible variations, a number of drug protocols are used in its treatment.

Body Weight Problems

Only a small percentage of hypothalamic pituitary dysfunction is caused by abnormal body weight, or abnormal percentages of fat in the body. Whether the problem is excessive obesity or being severely underweight, nothing can be done to correct this type of ovulatory failure until a nutritionally balanced diet is adopted, with food intake adjusted to achieve a normal body mass. In addition to changing their eating habits, severely underweight women may also have to change their lifestyle by lessening their participation in competitive sports, or by reducing their training schedules. Women whose underweight condition is caused by psychological conditions, such as anorexia nervosa, should be aggressively treated by a team consisting of both a psychologist and a reproductive endocrinologist. Even after normalization of their body mass, some women will still need to have ovulation induced with clomiphene citrate, but will usually respond quite well and begin to ovulate normally once this drug therapy is completed.

Polycystic Ovarian Syndrome

While it can be fairly easy to control ovulation in women whose hypothalamic pituitary dysfunction is caused by abnormal body weight, overcoming the most common type of hypothalamic pituitary dysfunction—polycystic ovarian syndrome—can be even more difficult than dealing with hypothalamic pituitary failure. That's why, if you have irregular or nonexistent menstrual periods, you should be tested not only for PCOS but for several other unrelated conditions before you conclude that PCOS is your problem and begin treatment for it. These blood tests should be done on the second or third day of your cycle, and should include measurements of your FSH, estradiol, prolactin, DHEAS, and thyroid-stimulating hormone (TSH) levels.

If your thyroid panel shows overproduction of TSH, it can affect your prolactin levels, and that could be the reason you aren't ovulating. When this problem is detected, your thyroid balance can easily be restored. If your diagnosis is hypothyroidism, you would be given thyroid hormone replacement therapy—synthetic thyroid hormones administered to replace the hormone lacking from your underactive thyroid. Once this is done, your ovulation may become normal.

If your thyroid is functioning well, but your blood has an elevated FSH level, you have probably found the cause of your poor ovarian activity. Unfortunately, in the case of elevated FSH, no treatment to improve ovulation can be undertaken. An elevated FSH level indicates ovarian failure or decreased ovarian responsiveness, conditions in which normal ovulation may never be produced. There are other options, however, which we will discuss later in this chapter.

If your blood tests eliminate thyroid problems and ovarian failure as possibilities, your doctor should then consider the likelihood that your problem is PCOS, and look for certain telltale "markers." Elevated levels of prolactin, estradiol levels that remain steady during your cycle instead of varying, or an elevated level of DHEAS (one of your "male" hormones, or androgens) would all help to confirm this diagnosis. PCOS, which causes around 90% of hypothalamic pituitary dysfunction, comes in a number of variations, each one requiring a different type of medical therapy. As we stated earlier in this chapter, the various types of polycystic ovarian syndromes include those involving:

- Low estrogen production
- Prolactin overproduction from the pituitary
- Androgen overproduction from the adrenal gland

By analyzing your blood tests, your doctor can come closer to pinpointing the exact cause of your problem, before choosing an appropriate treatment and initiating a game plan for your medication. However, it is often quite difficult to determine precisely which treatment—or treatments—is appropriate in any particular case, even for the skilled physician. This is because a patient's PCOS may involve more than one of these complicating factors. As a result, medicating to correct PCOS is often a trial-and-error process, and you should be aware that you may experience some disappointments along the way.

Beyond the challenge of choosing appropriate medication, another word of caution should be given regarding PCOS. Using fertility drugs to treat PCOS poses more problems from a safety point of view than medicating complete hypothalamic pituitary failure. That's because when you are in hypothalamic pituitary failure, your physician knows that you are starting with a very low, or nonexistent, level of hormones in your blood. Given this, he can safely assume that for all practical purposes, the only hormones that will be affecting your system are those he adds to it. In hypothalamic pituitary dysfunction, however, your hypothalamus and pituitary are producing some hormones; their levels just aren't adequate for normal ovulation. Though your doctor can assume you are not producing the minimum level of hormones necessary, he cannot measure the amount you are producing. Therefore, he can't be sure what base level he's starting from when he begins supplementing, and because each woman's response to drugs can be quite different, your doctor will have to monitor you carefully to avoid overstimulating your ovaries while in the process of achieving regular ovulation.

Beginning PCOS Therapy   Since all the drug therapies that are used to help women with PCOS ovulate regularly are structured around the days of your menstrual cycle, the first thing your doctor will have to do is start you menstruating, if you aren't already. This will accomplish two things. It will help you to shed the endometrial lining of the uterus, which may have been building up for some time if you're not menstruating regularly. It will also give your doctor a starting point from which he can exactly time the events he is artificially inducing. In order to make you menstruate, your doctor will give you either progesterone or Provera, an artificial substitute for progesterone, for five to seven days. Assuming your estrogen levels are normal, you should menstruate within seven days after your withdrawal from the drugs. Once you menstruate, ovulation induction therapy can be started.

The most common therapy for women who menstruate irregularly, and the one that is usually tried first, is clomiphene citrate. Clomiphene citrate used on its own is a catchall therapy for women who do not appear to have any additional factors—such as overproduction of prolactin or of androgens—complicating their PCOS. Clomiphene citrate therapy is both simple and safe for hypothalamic pituitary dysfunction patients. If your doctor chooses this therapy for you, he will start giving you clomiphene on either the third, fourth, or fifth day of your Provera-induced menstrual period. He will initially try to produce ovulation using a very low dose—50 mg of clomiphene per day for five days. He will then have you confirm whether you have ovulated by using either basal body temperature graphs or an at-home LH surge monitoring kit.

If you don't achieve ovulation using 50 mg doses of clomiphene, your doctor will induce another period by giving you Provera, and will then repeat your clomiphene citrate treatment for five days using a higher, 100 mg dose. If you still fail to ovulate, and you are of normal weight and body stature, it would be rare for your reproductive endocrinologist to exceed this 100 mg dose. He might, however, try using 100 mg for a longer period—eight to ten days instead of five—to see if ovulation will occur. As we will be discussing in our chapter on cervical problems (Chapter Seven), clomiphene, especially when given at higher doses, has the potential of creating mucus problems that could interfere with sperm transport.

PCOS with Elevated Prolactin Levels   It is quite possible that your blood tests will indicate that you have a high level of the hormone prolactin in your system. If your test shows a level higher than 50 to 60 nanograms per milliliter, this prolactin could be significantly interfering with your ability to ovulate. Your doctor may have been led to suspect this possibility prior to your testing, particularly if your irregular menstrual periods are combined with galactorrhea—a milky discharge from your nipples. As we discussed earlier, prolactin is the hormone that the pituitary gland releases to stimulate the production of milk. If so, the high prolactin level that is indicated by your blood test will confirm his suspicions.

While an elevated prolactin level is most often caused by PCOS, in about 25% of cases it is brought on by a tumor (adenoma) within the pituitary. Adenomas in excess of 10 mm (known as macroadenomas) could require surgery. That is why the first thing your doctor should do if you have these symptoms is to perform a CAT scan or an MRI of your pituitary to see if you have a tumor, and determine its size. If a tumor in excess of 10 millimeters is found, an evaluation of your optic nerve function—called a "visual field examination"—should be done to determine whether it is putting pressure on your optic nerve, and whether surgery should be considered to remove the growth.

Twenty years ago, surgery was the first treatment of choice for tumors of all sizes. Today, surgery is rarely done for pituitary adenomas. These small tumors are now treated in the same way that a high prolactin level caused by PCOS is treated—with drug therapy. It doesn't matter whether you have a small tumor, or PCOS. Your doctor will give you Parlodel to bring your prolactin levels down to a normal level. This should then allow you to resume menstrual and ovulatory function. Once Parlodel has suppressed prolactin production, pituitary adenomas will begin to shrink. With long-term Parlodel treatment, they may even disappear.

PCOS with Elevated DHEAS Levels   Your blood test may have indicated another possibility—an elevated level of dehydroepiandrosterone sulfate (DHEAS). DHEAS is one of the male hormones, or androgens, that regularly circulates in your system. If it is found in excess, it indicates that your adrenal gland is producing so many androgens that the hormonal balance necessary to achieve ovulation is being interfered with. To correct this condition, your doctor will probably prescribe a combination of clomiphene with dexamethasone. Dexamethasone is a steroid medication that reduces the release of adrenocorticotropic hormone (ACTH) from the pituitary. Since it is ACTH that stimulates the adrenal gland to produce androgens, dexamethasone will reduce your body's production of male hormones.

Dexamethasone is normally given in a dose of 0.25 mg or 0.5 mg daily. Other than the suppression of excess androgens, minimal, if any, significant adrenal suppression occurs with a dose this size. Therefore, no adrenal side effects would be expected. In some cases of PCOS, the DHEAS level is normal, but the ovary produces increased amounts of testosterone (another male hormone). This overproduction doesn't affect ovulation, but it can cause severe side effects such as hair growth, acne, and weight gain.

Under this regimen you would take half a milligram of dexamethasone each day for at least two weeks, prior to starting clomiphene citrate. The dosage of clomiphene would be gradually increased if necessary, in the same way that it would in straight clomiphene therapy. If this still doesn't work, your doctor might try a regimen of 100 mg of clomiphene citrate used for five days, followed by two ampules of pure FSH every other day. Because the FSH will be working directly on your ovaries, this medication plan should be accompanied by ultrasound monitoring to determine whether follicle growth is occurring. Once follicle growth and maturity is reached, hCG will be administered to trigger the release of the follicle and ovulation.

Severe PCOS   If you are diagnosed with severe polycystic ovarian syndrome, and don't respond to standard doses of clomiphene citrate, or to clomiphene in combination with Parlodel or with dexamethasone, yours is the most difficult type of ovulation induction. Nevertheless, whether you are having ovulation control for insemination, for intercourse timing, or for in vitro fertilization or gamete intrafallopian transfer, there are a number of other drugs that might be tried. Keep in mind, as you step into this realm, that the decision as to which would be best for you, and the possible negative consequences each might cause, such as hyperstimulation, becomes more complicated.

If you make a decision to try therapies beyond clomiphene citrate, your condition cannot be adequately treated by an obstetrician/gynecologist. You should see a reproductive endocrinologist, and you should make sure that he has extensive experience in ovulation-induction therapies for patients such as yourself. There is no hard-and-fast rule as to which drug or drugs will work best. It's a patient-by-patient decision, which only an experienced reproductive endocrinologist can make, based on your prior history and your reaction to clomiphene.

Learning the Hard Way

I'm one of those women who gave up a lot of years and wasted a lot of time by staying with my ob/gyn for infertility treatment. She had a great reputation, and she was sure that she could help me. After three and a half years, she still hadn't. I really felt tortured . . . not only by the disappointment of not having a child, but physically tortured. I was using Pergonal— 40 to 50 ampules a month—and instead of diluting it with 1 cc of liquid, she had me mixing it with a full 10 cc's, all of which I then had to inject into myself. She took blood from me every morning while I was on Pergonal, and got results every afternoon. When she finally gave up and sent me on, telling me I was a candidate for GIFT, I discovered from my new reproductive endocrinologist that I'd spent years taking a multiple of the amount of Pergonal that I actually needed. In my case, no matter how much Pergonal I took, I was still only going to get one egg per cycle. When I meet people now who are considering infertility treatment, my immediate advice to them, especially if they're over 30, is to go directly to a reproductive endocrinologist.

—Karen, age 40

Your reproductive endocrinologist might use clomiphene citrate in combination with FSH, or he might use pure FSH or hMG alone. Since all of these more advanced ovulation-induction regimens leave severe PCOS patients at very high risk for hyperstimulation syndrome, you should discuss in detail with your physician how he intends to administer your drugs.

In those rare instances when human menopausal gonadotropins or FSH alone are used, your doctor should first use a GnRH agonist such as Lupron or Synarel to reduce the amount of hormones naturally being released. As we've noted before, pulsatile subcutaneous administration of GnRH, which is the most effective way to administer the drug on a 24-hour basis, is quite cumbersome. But since its use offers more control to your doctor, and reduces the chance you will hyperstimulate, in cases of PCOS where other options have failed, it is worth the inconvenience.

In some very severe cases of PCOS, where there is no response to treatment with drugs, surgery may be required. Previously, a surgery called an "ovarian wedge resection" was done in these cases. This procedure surgically removed a quarter to a third of the ovary, reducing both its size and its surface area. By reducing the amount of ovarian tissue that was there to respond, doctors also reduced the amount of out-of-balance hormone—most probably testosterone—that was produced. Unfortunately, while wedge resection could sometimes make a patient ovulate for a short time, it created tremendous long-term problems. The surgery produced adhesions between the fallopian tubes and the ovaries so frequently that it has generally been condemned by physicians for the last ten to fifteen years.

Today, the same results can be achieved with far fewer complications through a newer laser drilling procedure. In this current version of ovarian surgery, the physician gains access to the ovaries using a laparoscope. Once there, he punctures the surface of the ovary with a laser beam in a number of different places, drilling into the substance of the ovary. When he has finished, it resembles the uneven surface of a golf ball. By doing this he reduces and interrupts the surface area of the ovary—the same thing that was formerly accomplished through ovarian wedge resection—without actually cutting into it. In a high percentage of cases, once laser drilling is done, women begin to ovulate. However, this resumed ovulation is usually only temporary, lasting eight to twelve months. Laser drilling can be done on selected individuals without any long-term side effects.

OVARIAN FAILURE

Once a woman experiences ovarian failure—due to natural causes, surgical removal of the ovary, or destruction of ovarian tissue as part of an autoimmune response—nothing can be done to reverse it. These patients, just like patients who have experienced hypothalamic pituitary failure, should use long-term hormone replacement therapy to replace the estrogen and progesterone they are no longer manufacturing on their own. While it will not help them to get pregnant, this therapy will protect their cardiovascular and skeletal systems.

Since women with premature ovarian failure can never be given ovarian function or made to ovulate through any form of therapy, egg donation is their only option if they wish to carry a baby. And of course, adoption is another alternative for establishing a family.

LUTEAL PHASE DEFECTS

If your endometrial biopsy, and/or a reading of your progesterone level, indicate that you have a luteal phase defect, the first line of attack is usually clomiphene citrate. Clomiphene stimulates better follicle growth and improved estradiol production. It both increases hormone production prior to ovulation and improves the quality of the corpus luteum, which remains after the follicle has released the egg. As a consequence, the corpus luteum produces more estrogen and progesterone. Because it works both pre- and postovulation, clomiphene citrate is the most effective treatment for the majority of luteal phase problems. The standard dose of 50 or 100 mg for five days is still used in these cases.

If you have a luteal phase defect and you are undergoing ovulation induction—in which either hMG or clomiphene has been used to induce ovulation, followed by hCG to trigger egg release—supplemental doses of hCG may be given every three to five days during the luteal phase, to maintain estrogen and progesterone production from the corpus luteum, and thus correct the luteal phase abnormality.

While it is effective, hCG therapy for luteal phase problems does present one problem: it delays an accurate determination of whether you have become pregnant. As you will remember, your doctor assesses whether or not you are pregnant by measuring the level of hCG in your blood. The supplemental injections of hCG that are given for luteal phase defects will cause your level to rise, and will result in early pregnancy tests being falsely positive.

Alternatives to hCG therapy—after ovulation induction—for luteal phase defects include the use of supplemental progesterone in one of three forms: injectable, oral, or vaginal suppository. In some cases, additional estrogen may be used along with the progesterone. This would be appropriate if the reading of your hormone levels shows that your estradiol level is low.

A Quick Guide to Giving Injections

By this time you've noticed that many treatments involving fertility drugs require a large number of injections. One, Lupron, is given subcutaneously—injected into the fatty layer directly under your skin. Others, such as Pergonal, Metrodin, Humegon, hCG, and progesterone are given intramuscularly—injected below the level of the skin, into the muscles. Given the time problems and expense involved in going to your doctor's office for every shot, you'll probably decide to take your injections at home. It's a good idea to go to your doctor's office to have your first injection, so that a nurse can show you the proper way to administer it. Some offices even have videotapes to instruct you. Of course, by the time you get home, you will have forgotten at least part of what they told you. Here is an outline of some general rules you'll need to know.

SUBCUTANEOUS INJECTIONS

Subcutaneous injections can be given either on the front surface of your thighs or the back surface of your upper arms. You can protect your skin from irritation by changing the location you use for each shot. Before you start, you should wash your hands thoroughly, then you should prepare your syringe. First, clean the rubber top of the medicine vial with an alcohol wipe. Then take the syringe out of its package, and screw the needle down to the syringe. Check your doctor's instructions carefully, and draw air into the syringe corresponding with the amount of medication he told you to inject. Then push your needle through the center of the rubber stopper on the medicine bottle, and push the plunger all the way in. Keep your needle in the bottle as you turn it upside down, and holding the bottle straight up and down with the needle tip still in the liquid, pull back on the plunger to withdraw slightly more than the amount of medication you need. As you look at your syringe, you may see that there are tiny air bubbles in the medication it holds. If there are, tap them to the top of the syringe, then, leaving the needle in the vial, push down on the plunger to push them out. Remove the needle from the medicine vial, and if you are not going to give yourself the injection immediately, replace the protective cover on the needle to keep it clean.

Once your medication is prepared, you should clean the injection site you've chosen with an alcohol wipe, and let it dry. Then hold the syringe in one hand, and use your other hand to either hold the skin taut or pull up a little flesh. Hold the syringe alongside the skin at a 45-degree angle, and slide the needle quickly under the skin as far as it will go. Release the skin, and push the plunger in to inject your medication. Next, holding an alcohol wipe down on your skin where the needle is inserted, withdraw the needle at the same 45-degree angle you used while putting it in.

Congratulations . . . you did it!

INTRAMUSCULAR INJECTIONS

Many of the things we told you about subcutaneous injections hold true for intramuscular injections. However, since a number of the fertility drugs that are administered this way come in the form of a powder, your preparation will be somewhat different. Powdered medications—such as Pergonal or Metrodin—come in glass ampules. They are accompanied by additional ampules of liquid, such as sodium chloride (saline), which are used to dilute them. To prepare your medication, you should start by tapping any powder that's gathered in the top of the ampule back into its main body, so that it isn't lost when you open the ampule. After you assemble your syringe, you should break open your ampule at the thin neck portion by holding it with one hand, and using the other hand to apply pressure on the small dot found at the side of the ampule. Be sure to protect your fingers as you do this. The wrapper from your syringe or your alcohol wipe, or a paper towel, are handy for this purpose. Draw up 1 cc of liquid into your syringe, and inject it into the powder ampule. The medication will mix instantly. Once the mixing is complete, draw the solution into your syringe. Hold the needle upright, tap any air bubbles to the top of the syringe, and clear them out by pushing up slowly on the plunger.

Intramuscular injections are given in the upper quadrant of the buttock, into the gluteal muscle.

You should prepare the area where you are going to give the shot with an alcohol wipe and let it dry. Then, holding the syringe in one hand, push the flesh up, or gently squeeze it, with the other hand. Insert the needle straight in, pushing it down as far as it will go, then release the skin. Hold on to the syringe with one hand, while you pull up slightly on the plunger with the other hand. If the syringe remains clear, you can push the plunger down to inject your medication. If blood appears in the syringe, you should remove it, replace the needle, and attempt another injection in the opposite hip. Once the medication has been injected, you should hold an alcohol prep at the needle site, and pull the syringe out on the same straight angle you used to put it in. Hold the alcohol prep on the injection site for ten seconds, before covering it with a Band-Aid. Just as with subcutaneous injections, you can protect your skin from irritation by injecting each dose at a different site.

I Hate Needles

When I initially consulted with Dr. Marrs, he confirmed that I had end-stage tubal disease. This meant that in vitro fertilization (IVF) would be the only means through which I could become pregnant. He proceeded to explain that the IVF procedure would entail daily injections of hormonal medications, and frequent blood withdrawals. I panicked. The procedures didn't frighten me; the needles did. You see, I had a morbid fear of them. I knew I wouldn't be able to survive the treatment. But I also knew, deep in my heart, that the alternative was worse than my obsessive fear. For weeks I worked with a therapist and with one of the nurses in Dr. Marrs' office. I was finally able to survive a month of injections. Luckily, my hard work and determination resulted in my delivery of a healthy baby girl nine months later.

—Kimberly, age 30

Are Fertility Drugs Safe?

In most cases the treatment of choice for ovulation defects and failures involves the use of various forms of ovulation-inducing drugs, as we've discussed above. We can't leave the topic of ovulation induction without discussing the controversies that have surfaced in the last two to three years concerning these drugs. Numerous publications have raised questions about the long-term safety risks that they may pose, particularly in respect to ovarian cancer and birth defects. Some advocates have even warned of a cancer epidemic bursting forth in twenty years, when women who are now taking these drugs reach their sixties.

The fact is that, while these articles are suggesting theoretical risks, clomiphene citrate and human menopausal gonadotropin have been in use since the late fifties, and have been studied in over 400 scientific articles that have been published since the drugs were approved for use in humans. These articles have looked at side effects, adverse reactions, and long-term effects (greater than 20 years) related to their use. None of them—with the exception of two recent articles, which we will discuss—has found any adverse events that could be considered health threatening, either to the patient taking the drugs or to children produced after their use.

Of the hundreds of research articles that have been written on the effects of ovulation-induction drugs, one of the most comprehensive reviews to date was published in 1986 by a group of doctors in Israel. This group also wrote the first article ever published on the use of Pergonal in humans, in 1960. Their 1986 article was a follow-up study of over 2,000 women who had received multiple cycles of ovulation induction with Pergonal and hCG. They found no adverse effects on these women, a full 20 years after their treatment. This included no increased incidence of breast, ovarian, cervical, or uterine cancers. They also found no abnormalities in the children these women gave birth to after multiple cycles of ovulation induction. And because of the time span of this study, they were also able to examine the grandchildren of some of these women, and to pronounce them equally clear of any birth defects that might have been a result of the use of fertility drugs.

While both doctors and patients were reassured by this study, new concerns surfaced with the publication of a 1993 article by the Stanford University Ovarian Cancer Surveillance Group. The group was studying the relation of various environmental factors and medical treatments to an increased frequency of ovarian cancer. One aspect of their study was to look at women who were infertile, to determine the type of infertility treatment they received, and to analyze its relation to ovarian cancer. They found nine women who developed ovarian cancer after a history of fertility drug use. Using this data, the study concluded that an infertile woman who took ovulation-inducing drugs and did not have a baby had a 27 times greater chance of developing ovarian cancer than a woman who did not take ovulation-induction drugs. This statement created a huge controversy and an understandable panic in the infertile population using ovulation-inducing drugs. However, even before its publication, a group of investigators (several of us involved in ovulation-drug studies), had reviewed this study extensively and found many problems and flaws in its data design, which negated its findings. For example, the surveillance group studied just a small subset of patients, which they compared to inappropriately matched controls. They didn't have information about which fertility drugs were used, how long they were used, or what doses had been given. In fact, two of their nine cases of cancer occurred before clomiphene and Pergonal were even developed. Following the article's publication its senior author, Alice Whittemore, made a statement that their data on ovarian cancer in infertile women using ovulation-induction drugs could not be relied upon, refuting the authors' own published findings. Unfortunately, numerous consumer magazines and newspapers had already written articles based on this flawed data, creating massive amounts of fear and concern in the minds of the public.

A more recent article, which was published in 1994, looked for potential adverse health effects in individuals who had used clomiphene citrate. This article reviewed over 3,800 woman who had taken the drug for multiple cycles of ovulation induction. Eleven cases of ovarian tumors were found within this group. Of the eleven cases, seven were benign or borderline tumors of the ovary, and four were ovarian cancers. The overall incidence of cancer reported in this study was no different from what would be expected in the normal population, where about one in every 1,000 women has a risk of developing ovarian cancer. But the incidence of borderline tumors was higher than would be expected in a group of this size. A closer look at the data showed researchers that the seven women who developed benign, or borderline, tumors were patients who had taken at least 12 consecutive months of clomiphene citrate during their treatment. The authors rightfully concluded that prolonged use of clomiphene may increase the risk of ovarian tumors. Today, reproductive endocrinologists and gynecologists rarely use clomiphene for such an extended period of time. But looking at this data should make you aware, as a patient, that if clomiphene citrate has not been successful within your first six months of therapy, alternative methods of ovulation induction need to be found and utilized.

Overall, ovulation-induction drugs have not been shown to increase the incidence of ovarian cancer, or to have a demonstratable relationship to any long-term type of medical condition. But while scare articles are usually inaccurate, they can perform a service. They bring to the surface the fact that you need to discuss the potential long-term side effects of any medications that are prescribed for you, beyond just considering their more immediate relation to your success or failure in producing a pregnancy. Your doctor needs to constantly tailor his choice of drugs, the dosage given, and the number of continuous repetitive cycles that you receive, to your specific physical condition and ovulatory problem. Individual women have different responses to these fertility drugs, and this must be taken into consideration when deciding on the best therapeutic approach.

As an aware patient you need to be alert to any signs of trouble if you are using drugs for ovulation induction. If you are having difficulty with cyst formation or overstimulation, talk to your doctor. If he isn't responsive to your concerns, leave him and go to a doctor who has more expertise in ovulation-induction therapy, and who will work with you to protect you and your ovaries. Correcting ovulation problems is one of the most successful treatments for the infertile woman. But you should insist that it be done properly and safely.

The Layman's Guide
to Common Fertility Drugs

Substance	What It Is	Brand Names	Administered
Clomiphene citrate	Antiestrogen	Clomid, Serophene	Orally
Human menopausal gonadotropin (hMG)	Natural FSH and LH	Pergonal, Humegon	By injection
Urofollitropin	Natural FSH	Metrodin	By injection
Gonadotropin-releasing hormone (GnRH)	Natural GnRH	Factrel, Lutrepulse	Injection or pump
Bromocriptine mesylate	Dopamine agonist	Parlodel	Orally
Leuprolide acetate	GnRH agonist	Lupron, Synarel	By injection or nasal spray
Human chorionic gonadotropin (hCG)	Placental hormone used in place of LH	Profasi, Pregnyl, APL	By injection
GnRH antagonist		Not yet available	By injection

Terms We Used in This Chapter

Agonist: a drug or chemical designed to perform the same function as the natural, or parent, compound. For instance, Lupron is a synthetic preparation of gonadotropin-releasing hormone, but lasts longer and performs longer than the parent compound.

Androgens: male sex hormones produced by the testes and ovaries that give rise to male characteristics.

Anorexia: an aversion to food.

Anovulation: failure to ovulate.

Bulimia: a disorder involving binge eating and self-induced vomiting.

Chromosome: the structure in each cell's nucleus that holds the parent's genetic information in the form of DNA (deoxyribonucleic acid).

Congenital abnormality: a malformation that takes place during fetal development.

Corpus luteum: the cyst that forms after a follicle releases its egg. It produces estrogen and progesterone during the second half of the ovulatory cycle.

Dehydroepiandrosterone sulfate (DHEAS): a hormone made by the adrenal gland that has androgen (male hormone) effects.

Dermoid: a usually benign tumor of the ovary that can contain hair, teeth, and bone fragments—also known as teratoma or germ cell tumor.

Dysgenesis: faulty formation of any cell or organ.

Ectopic pregnancy: a pregnancy (embryo) that implants outside the uterine cavity. Most commonly this occurs in the fallopian tube, but can occur in the ovary or abdominal cavity.

Egg production protocol: the use of various combinations of drugs (i.e., clomiphene citrate, Metrodin, Humegon, etc.) to stimulate multiple eggs to ovulate.

Endometriosis: a disease in which normal endometrial cells get outside the uterus, stick to the surface of organs, and cause inflammation and tissue damage.

Endometrium: the lining of cells inside the uterus which is sensitive to estrogen and progesterone stimulation.

Estradiol: an estrogen formed and released by the ovarian follicle during ovulation.

Estrogen replacement therapy (ERT): the use of various types of estrogen to alleviate postmenopausal symptoms and diseases (i.e., osteoporosis).

Follicle-stimulating hormone (FSH):   a protein hormone produced and released by the anterior pituitary gland. FSH stimulates follicle growth in the female and sperm production in the male.

Galactorrhea: a milklike production from the breast of a woman who is either not nursing or has never been pregnant. Galactorrhea may indicate a benign tumor in the pituitary gland.

Gonadotropin-releasing hormone (GnRH):   a small protein hormone produced in the hypothalamus, responsible for controlling the production and release of FSH and LH.

Gonadotropins: the protein hormones FSH and LH; they stimulate ovarian function in the female and testicular function in the male.

Gonads: the glands that produce the male and female gametes (i.e., the egg and the sperm).

Hormone replacement therapy (HRT):   see Estrogen replacement therapy.

Hypothalamus: the midportion of the brain which produces GnRH and other hormones that control the pituitary gland.

Implantation: the attachment of the embryo to the endometrial lining of the uterus.

Luteal phase: the second half of the menstrual cycle; the luteal phase begins with ovulation, and is characterized by elevated levels of estrogen and progesterone.

Luteinizing hormone (LH):   protein produced and secreted from the anterior pituitary gland which is involved in ovulation.

Menarche: the onset of menstrual function.

Ovarian dysgenesis: a congenital condition caused by an abnormality in the second X chromosome, resulting in sterility in the female.

Ovarian failure: a condition in which the ovaries are either devoid of follicles and eggs, or they are nonresponsive to FSH stimulation.

Ovotestes: a congenital abnormality characterized by the presence of gonads that are a mixture of testicles and ovaries.

Ovulation induction: the stimulation of follicle growth and egg release through the use of fertility drugs.

Pelvic inflammatory disease (PID):   infection or inflammation of the female reproductive organs, usually caused by a sexually transmitted disease.

Pituitary: a small gland at the base of the brain that secretes hormones that control our endocrine organs.

Pituitary adenoma: a benign growth that causes the pituitary gland to be overproductive of certain hormones.

Pituitary macroadenoma: a benign growth in the pituitary gland that exceeds 10 mm in diameter.

Polycystic ovarian syndrome (PCOS):   the development of multiple ovarian cysts due to an imbalance of hormones in the ovary.

Progesterone: the hormone produced from the corpus luteum after ovulation. It is also the hormone responsible for maintenance of early pregnancy.

Prolactin: the hormone produced from the pituitary that prepares the breasts for lactation.

Puberty: the point in human development when sexual maturation occurs.

Receptor: the site on a cell surface where a hormone attaches to express its function.

Subcutaneous injection: the placement of medication immediately beneath the skin.

Testicular feminization: a syndrome in which the individual appears to be female, but her ovaries are testicular tissue.

Testosterone: the male hormone.

Turner's syndrome: a genetic abnormality in which the female has a missing chromosome and no ovarian function.

7

Cervical Problems

Wouldn't it be wonderful if you, too, could say, "Open, Sesame!" at just the right time in your ovulatory cycle, and have the door to your uterine cavity automatically unlock to let your partner's sperm flow easily in? You'd be one step closer to the riches *you* are seeking. Unfortunately, for those of you with cervical problems, it's not that easy. Your cervix is more than a door that connects your vaginal canal to your uterine cavity; it's also a mindful gatekeeper. A normal cervix will allow sperm to move from the vaginal canal into the uterine cavity on certain days of your cycle. But an abnormal cervix, much like the stone that blocked Ali Baba's cave, will stop all intruders until the day your doctor comes up with the magic to open it.

The cervix is an active structure, made up of fibrous tissue. During normal ovulation, sperm are transported through this opening and into the uterine environment by a clear, watery substance called mucus, which is produced by specialized cells in the interior walls of the cervix. (See Figure 7-1.) These cells are coaxed into action just prior to ovulation by the rising level of estrogen in your system. During your diagnos-

166

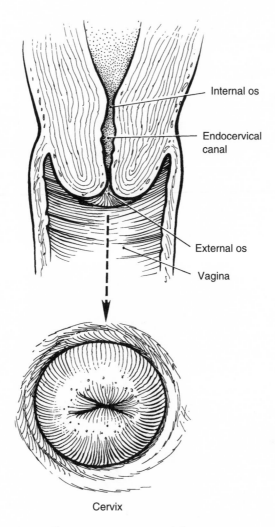

Internal os

Endocervical
canal

External os

Vagina

Cervix

Figure 7-1: Diagram of the Cervix

tic workup you learned how important the proper coordination of each
step of your monthly cycle is to conception, and the timing of this mucus
production is no exception.

   Unfortunately, there are a number of things that can go wrong with
this process; all of them fall under the general heading of cervical factor
infertility. If you are timing your intercourse correctly and you have
normal sperm, yet the sperm still don't make it into the uterine cavity,
you are probably among the approximately 15% of couples who fall
within this diagnosis.

What's Causing Your Cervical Problem?

Some cervical problems are caused by structural abnormalities in the cervix. These may be congenital, or they may have been caused by medical treatment. Structural abnormalities can cause the cervix to have too few mucus-producing cells, or to have a normal number of cells, which despite their abundance still don't produce enough mucus for good sperm transport. Other cervical abnormalities have a hormonal basis . . . your cervix just doesn't receive enough estrogen to stimulate the production of mucus. And despite testing, some causes of cervical problems remain unexplained. But don't let that diagnosis frighten you. There is treatment to help you get pregnant despite almost any cervical disorder, including those whose source isn't known. In some cases cervical problems can be corrected. In others, the cervix will simply be bypassed. And sometimes a combination of both methods will be used.

CONGENITAL ABNORMALITIES OF THE CERVIX

Congenital cervical abnormalities—those present at birth—are most often the result of drugs that were taken by a mother during pregnancy. The remaining cases are simply irregularities in the way the cervix forms during fetal development.

Drug Exposure

Each generation has its own unique infertility problems. One of the ones that is being faced by some women today is cervical abnormalities caused by their exposure to the drug diethylstilbestrol (DES) while they were still in their mothers' wombs. Starting in the mid-forties, DES was commonly prescribed for women who were having problems with miscarriage. By the mid-fifties the FDA recognized the damaging effects it was having on children born to these mothers, and quickly removed it from the market. Among the problems that frequently surfaced as these children matured were severe reproductive abnormalities. In fact, abnormalities related to DES exposure are probably the most common type of congenital cervical problems found in women today. These disorders can take several forms.

Vaginal adenosis is a DES abnormality in which a portion of the surface of the vaginal canal has been scooped out, leaving a raw, angry cavity of tissue. This is extremely rare. More commonly, DES changes the structure, and sometimes the shape, of the cervix and the uterine cavity. If your mother took DES during your fetal development and the drug altered your cervical structure, you can have abnormal mucus production, and because of that, poor sperm transport.

The severity of the changes caused by DES exposure depends on the stage of fetal development during which your mother took the drug, and the amount that was used. But in most cases, being told during your infertility evaluation that you have DES abnormalities won't come as a surprise to you. Since these structural changes are easily recognized by any gynecologist, most women become aware of their condition early on in their reproductive years.

As of now, no other drugs have been definitely proven to create a congenital abnormality of the cervix. There is, however, some surprising evidence that suggests other drugs may have the same effect. DES-type abnormalities have been discovered in women whose mothers definitely did not take DES during their pregnancies. One example is a woman who was born in 1965. Since DES had been removed from the market by then, her mother couldn't have taken it. Yet this woman's abnormalities are strikingly similar to those in women who are DES victims. This scenario opens up the possibility that the condition we refer to as "related to DES exposure" is not necessarily drug related, or that there are other drugs that can produce the same abnormality. Unfortunately, medical researchers are not yet aware of which drugs they may be.

Congenital Abnormalities Without Drug Exposure

Drug exposure does not cause all congenital abnormalities of the cervix. Others are simply due to a malformation during fetal development. Sometimes they involve just the cervical canal, but they can involve the uterus and vagina as well.

- The rarest and most extreme cervical abnormality is cervical canal atresia, a condition in which a woman is born with no cervical canal.

- A woman with a bicornuate uterus has a single cervical canal leading into a right and a left uterus, which are partially separated. (See Figure 7-2.)

- In cases of uterine didelphys, a woman has two complete uteri, a duplication of the cervix, and two vaginal canals. (See Figure 7-3.)

- In yet another variation, a woman's cervical canal, her uterus, and/or her vagina can be divided into two halves by a thin sheet of tissue called a septum. (See Figure 7-4.)

As you might imagine, any of these conditions can complicate cervical function, sperm transport, and uterine function, as we will discuss in Chapter Eight. While they sound severe, it's not necessarily hopeless if you are diagnosed with one of them. In most cases, there is treatment. We'll be discussing the various possibilities later.

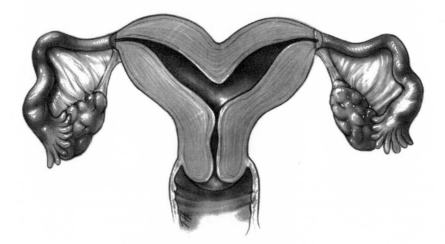

Figure 7-2: Bicornuate Uterus

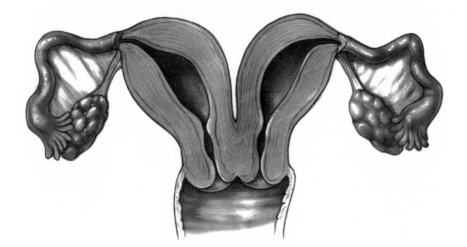

Figure 7-3: Uterine Didelphys

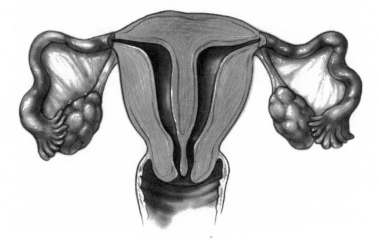

Figure 7-4: Uterus Divided by a Septum

MAN-MADE CERVICAL PROBLEMS

Ironically, the most common types of cervical factor problems seen today are those created by doctors. Many women have a medical procedure, or multiple procedures, that damage their cervix to a point where it no longer functions properly. This can take two different forms. An "incompetent" cervix won't stay closed during pregnancy, and the baby is delivered prematurely. Another variation occurs when the mucus-producing cells of the cervix are damaged. Either of these situations could occur after a woman has had multiple therapeutic abortions. Most therapeutic abortions are accomplished through a D&C dilatation and curettage: the cervix is dilated, and then suction curettage is used to remove the fetus and other tissue from the uterus. During the process of dilatation, as the cervix's fibrous tissue is expanded to allow the suction tube to enter the uterus, the bundles of fibers within its tissue may break. After dilatation, scar tissue forms at the site of these breaks, making the cervix more rigid. As a result it narrows and becomes what we call "stenotic." Dilatation can also damage the mucus-producing glands of the cervix, leaving you with a cervix that no longer produces mucus, despite the normal hormonal influence of estrogen during ovulation. Multiple cervical dilatations to treat repetitive miscarriages can have the same effect. In some cases of severe stenosis, sperm transport is virtually impossible because of poor mucus production and an almost complete closure of the canal.

Another danger point for the cervix occurs when mild abnormalities are found in a pap smear. Many doctors respond to this finding by removing the suspicious cells surgically. They may perform cryocautery, a freezing of the cervix; or they may use a laser to remove abnormal cells; or they may do a cervical conization—cut a cone-shaped slice of tissue out of the cervix where the abnormal cells were found. Each of these therapies can leave the cervix in a nonfunctional state. If this has already happened to you, you should take heart from the thought that this problem will not necessarily prevent you from getting pregnant. Today there are reproductive technologies that can help you succeed. Better yet, if you have not had surgery involving your cervix, you should be aware of the danger areas and of how you can avoid them.

How to Avoid Man-Made Cervical Problems

If you are notified that you've had an abnormal pap smear, especially if you are within your reproductive years and are interested in bearing children, you should ask your doctor to try to medicate, rather than operate. If he doesn't want to do this, preferring to proceed directly to surgery instead, you should seek a second opinion.

These days, the cytology laboratories that evaluate pap smears are painstaking in reading abnormalities and locating any inflammation in the cervical cells. If inflammatory cells are present, most often the pap smear will be reported as "having atypical cells" or "Class II." This type of reading often merely indicates that inflammation in the cells is preventing the laboratory from being able to see clearly whether they are dysplastic (abnormal) or premalignant. Since the abnormal reading that results may simply be due to the presence of inflammation, not disease, it should be treated, and a new pap smear done, before any more-invasive treatment is attempted. Despite this, some physicians respond to all Class II pap smears as serious, and as a result, they are overly aggressive in treating them.

Even today, many gynecologists immediately use cryocautery for the treatment of all Class II pap smears, though these infections usually do not require any type of surgical intervention, and can be cleared up with topical medications. As the patient, you should request a less aggressive treatment prior to agreeing to any type of surgery or cryocautery of the cervix. To treat your cervix topically, your doctor will give you a vaginal cream or suppositories, which you will use daily for seven to ten days. Once a possible infection has been eliminated, a second pap smear should be done to confirm that your cervical cells are now normal. If your pap smear still shows inflammation or abnormal cells after topical therapy, your doctor is then correct in assuming that you may have early premalignant changes of the cervix, known as dysplasia. While the treatment at this point should be very aggressive in removing these cells, some ways of accomplishing this are less risky to future pregnancies than others. If you are a woman of reproductive age and you wish to incur the least possible amount of trauma to your cervix, there are several approaches to take.

If dysplastic cells are affecting only the surface layer of your cervix, the most precise—but also the most expensive—way to remove them is with a carbon dioxide laser. A carbon dioxide laser can be adjusted so that it vaporizes tissue only to a specific depth, leaving the normal tissue that lies beneath virtually untouched. This type of laser is so precise that it can be adjusted to destroy only the top millimeter of tissue. If your problem lies deeper, and a portion of your cervix must be cut out, conization can be performed through a new procedure called LEEP, which uses a wire and electric current to cut through the cervical tissue. Using this electrosurgical cutting wire is probably the best way to preserve a functional cervix for women of reproductive age; LEEP is an improvement over standard surgical tools, in that it causes far less trauma to the tissue. If your goal is to minimize the chances of scarring and avoid the poor cervical function that it so often causes, you should insist on one of these procedures instead of conventional conization surgery. You can talk to your doctor to learn more about each of them, and how they might apply to your specific case. But keep in mind as you approach your surgery that even with these improved methods, a loss of cervical function can still result, which could cause you to have an infertility problem.

Perhaps you are reading this too late . . . your cervix has already been damaged in one of the ways we've described. If you find yourself in this position, there are other roads for you to travel. We will discuss these approaches in the treatment section of this chapter.

HORMONAL PROBLEMS THAT AFFECT THE CERVIX

If your postcoital test results are abnormal, and this can't be explained by any structural abnormalities or prior surgeries of the cervix, your problem may be hormonal. There are two ways in which this could happen. First, your mucus-producing glands, or the estrogen receptors within them, could be nonexistent or simply not functioning. Alternatively, your glands could be functional, but they could require a larger amount of estrogen than they're receiving to stimulate them. As we explained earlier, your cervix begins to produce mucus when your estrogen levels rise just prior to ovulation. A problem can arise if your cervical gland's estrogen "threshold" is set higher than the amount of hormone it receives at this important point in your cycle. In fact, your cervical gland's mucus production may never get turned on because of this high threshold. You can understand this more clearly by thinking of your pain threshold. You and another person might experience identical injuries, yet if you have a lower threshold for pain, you would feel it more. Similarly, if your mucus-producing glands have a high estrogen threshold, they may not respond to the same amount of estrogen that would stimulate mucus production in another woman. Happily, as we will explain later, cervical problems that have a hormonal basis are easily remedied.

UNEXPLAINED CERVICAL PROBLEMS

Perhaps, during your basic workup, you learned that you're ovulating normally, your hormones are signaling your cervix to produce mucus, and yet your postcoital test showed that your mucus doesn't have the correct properties to assist in sperm transport. If your problem isn't explained by any physical malformation of the cervix, or by any history of prior surgery, you fall into a group of approximately 15% of reproductive-age women who are in the same position, and are just as perplexed as you are. Don't be discouraged. There is treatment for unexplained cervical factor infertility. It usually involves improving the sperm transport—either through hormonal therapy or by bypassing the cervix—to increase your reproductive odds. We will examine the different ways of accomplishing this next.

Treating Your Cervical Problem

If you've been diagnosed with a cervical problem, the good news is that even if it takes a while, there's usually a course of action that will give you a healthy pregnancy. The treatment of cervical disorders generally falls into three basic categories:

- Surgery
- Hormonal therapy
- Intrauterine insemination

SURGERY

Some of the congenital infertility problems that stem from an abnormally shaped or abnormally structured cervix can be improved or corrected through surgical procedures. Specifically, if you have a septum dividing your cervix, if you have a narrowed or closed-down cervix, or if you have no cervix at all, your doctor will attempt to treat your problem through surgery. The type of surgery he uses, and the chances of its success, will depend on the exact nature of the problem you're facing.

Surgery to Remove a Septum

Picture a curtain running down the middle of a room. A septum is just like that—an extra curtain of fibrous tissue that divides the cervix, the vagina, or the uterus into two parts. If you have a split like this, your doctor can remove it and create a single structure through hysteroscopic surgery. During this procedure you will be under a general anesthetic. Your doctor will insert the hysteroscope—a small telescopic instrument that lets him view the interior of your uterus—through the opening in your cervix. Once he is able to see the septum, he will remove it, in most cases with a small cutting wire or microscissors. You can have this procedure done on an outpatient basis. It will leave you with only a minimal amount of discomfort, which should be gone after a one- or two-day recovery period.

Surgery to Repair a Narrowed or Closed-down Cervix

If you've been surgically damaged as a result of multiple abortions or cervical dilatations, you have a condition that is referred to as a stenotic cervix. What this means is that your cervix has become too narrowed and restricted for it to function properly. This is one situation in which there is good hope that your doctor will be able to help you regain proper cervical function. He will probably use a procedure that attempts to reopen your cervical canal gradually, in such a way that the fibers of your cervix won't be further broken or damaged in the process. He will time this to happen during your menstrual period, since that is the time when your cervix will have opened as much as it can on its own.

First your doctor will give you a light anesthetic. He will then mechanically dilate your cervix—opening it the smallest distance that will still allow him to insert a thin stick of dried seaweed, called a laminaria, into the opening of your cervical canal. Once in place, the dehydrated laminaria will begin to absorb natural fluids from your tissue, and to expand like a sponge, until it has reached a size approximately four times its original diameter. Yet as it grows over a period of about 12 hours, the laminaria will still remain rigid enough to slowly and safely dilate and soften your cervical tissues. In many cases, the opening that's created will be permanent, but in a few it will have to be repeated if the cervix closes up again. If the opening that results still isn't adequate in size, your doctor can gradually move up through progressively larger laminaria to establish a normal opening without further damaging your cervix.

When your doctor inserts a laminaria, he will most likely tell you to come back in 24 hours to have it removed. You should pay careful attention to this instruction, since you run the risk of developing an infection or other complications if it is left in place longer than that. Laminaria can be uncomfortable for some women; the feeling can be similar to having a menstrual cramp. If this happens to you, you'll want your doctor to prescribe a mild painkiller or muscle relaxant to help you through your 24 hours of treatment.

Using the laminaria, your doctor will be able to re-create a cervical opening for you, but he won't be able to restore the cells in the interior walls of your cervix if they have been severely damaged by your prior surgeries or as a result of a congenital condition. If this has happened, and your cells aren't manufacturing enough mucus for sperm transport, your doctor can give you the additional assistance of intrauterine insemination (IUI). We'll be discussing this procedure—which mechanically passes the sperm through the cervix and delivers it directly into the uterine cavity—later in this chapter.

Surgery to Build a Cervical Canal

If you were born with no cervix or cervical canal at all—a condition called cervical canal atresia—you suffer from an extremely rare condition. In fact, there have been fewer than twenty reported cases throughout the world's literature. Women with this condition become aware of it well before they decide to reproduce, because of the complications it presents. For example, when they begin to menstruate, the menstrual blood has no way to escape from the uterus. Their doctors must quickly stop their bleeding by suppressing their hormones, in order to prevent other complications. When women with cervical canal atresia decide they want to become pregnant, they face an obvious problem—there's no way for sperm to move into their uterine cavity.

Of the small number of cases of cervical atresia that have been reported, I have treated three. In all of these cases, the uterus and cervix were present, but no connecting canal ever formed through

the cervical tissue. As a result, there was no possible way for sperm to travel from the vaginal canal into the uterus.

While it was quite difficult, we were able to surgically reconstruct a cervical canal in all three women. In one of the cases, the woman was able to conceive after surgical correction and intrauterine insemination. Unfortunately, in the case of one of the women, such extensive problems existed as a result of her having had no cervical canal over an extended period of time, that despite several operations attempting to maintain a cervical canal, she eventually had a hysterectomy. The third patient was a twenty-two-year-old woman in whom we established a canal surgically, only to have it close again approximately eight months later. She is maintaining her uterus in hopes that future advancements in reproductive technologies will allow her to carry a pregnancy.

HORMONAL THERAPY

If you have an unexplained cervical problem, the first thing that your doctor should attempt is hormonal therapy. All hormonal therapy for cervical factor infertility involves increasing the amount of estrogen received by the mucus-producing cells in your cervix. This can be done in two different ways.

If your history leads your doctor to suspect that you aren't ovulating properly, he may try to remedy your mucus production problem in what you may think is a roundabout way, by improving your ovulation. Once your ovulatory cycle is improved through drug therapy, your follicles will produce additional estrogen, and your cervical mucus production may also improve as a result. As we discussed in the chapter on normal female function (Chapter Two), follicle growth and estrogen production are closely intertwined; in fact, it is increasing estrogen within your selected follicles that indicates their health and maturity. So it follows that if you have poor follicle growth, you may also have poor estrogen production. By giving you clomiphene citrate or FSH to stimulate your follicles, your doctor may also be able to increase your estrogen levels, and your cervical mucus production may improve itself to the point where your problem is fully corrected.

One possible negative side effect to this treatment is that your cervical mucus, while abundant, may become too thick for your partner's sperm to move through. In some cases, you can visually see that this is happening. Good mucus is runny, slippery, and transparent. Thick mucus, on the other hand, is opaque, and has a tacky, sticky feel. There's a very simple, nonprescription remedy that is commonly used to combat this: take one tablespoon of an expectorant cough medicine, such as Robitussin, every four hours beginning two days prior to your ovulation. In some cases, it will thin your cervical mucus in the same way that it thins mucus in your lungs. Since it's an easy preventative with no side effects, it's worth trying. If you are placed on clomiphene citrate, your doctor should perform an additional postcoital test, to confirm that your mucus is behaving properly. As we've told you, clomiphene acts as an antiestrogen and can interfere with mucus production.

If your doctor doesn't think that poor ovulation is the source of your problem, he will give you natural estrogens—Estrace (micronized estradiol) or Premarin (conjugated estrogens)—in very low doses. This would be a logical first step if your mucus glands are present and your mucus-producing cells are functional, but they may have a high threshold and require a greater than normal amount of estrogen in order to be stimulated. If Estrace is used, it is commonly given orally, in a dosage of 1 or 2 mg per day, beginning five to seven days before your expected ovulation. If your doctor chooses Premarin, it is given orally either in a 0.3 mg or a 0.625 mg daily dose, also beginning five to seven days before expected ovulation. Because these doses are physiologic levels—the same levels that would naturally be found in the body—they won't cause any side effects or interfere with ovulation. With either of these medications, 30% to 40% of patients will have normalization of their cervical mucus production. But you should be aware that if you receive larger doses of these medications—"pharmacologic" levels, which make your levels higher than they would naturally be—they can impede, or even shut down, ovulation.

Hopefully, with one of these hormonal treatments, your next postcoital test will show a normal result and you will be on your way to a pregnancy. But if your mucus-producing cells are damaged or nonexistent, or if they don't have estrogen receptors to tell them how much hormone they're receiving, your doctor will have to consider the more aggressive therapies that are involved in bypassing the cervix.

INTRAUTERINE INSEMINATION

If all else fails, and you are not able to get your cervix to function normally through surgery or hormonal therapy, your doctor can still help you to conceive by moving your partner's sperm through your cervix mechanically, and placing it directly into your uterine cavity. This procedure is called direct intrauterine insemination (IUI), and there are a number of instances when it is appropriate. Most commonly, IUIs are performed when an abnormal postcoital test indicates poor sperm/mucus transport. Another example is uterine didelphys. In this case, your doctor would first do an ultrasound during ovulation to determine whether you are ovulating from the right or left ovary. He would then move your partner's sperm through the cervical/vaginal opening, and place it in the uterine cavity on the side where your ovulation is going to take place. Since surgery can't improve cervical structure or function for women with problems related to DES exposure, they are also treated through IUI.

The History of IUI

Prior to the development of our current methods, intrauterine inseminations were attempted in various forms for decades, and produced both complications and extremely poor results. These early efforts at IUI were performed very simply. Semen was collected, and once it had fully liquefied after a waiting period of 20 to 30 minutes, it was placed directly into the uterus. This was both painful and somewhat dangerous for the women who received it. That's because seminal plasma—the liquid portion of the semen that is naturally left behind in the vaginal canal during normal intercourse—contains the hormone prostaglandin, which causes extreme uterine cramping when it comes in contact with the endometrial cavity. Since semen is made up of protein, there is also the possibility of dangerous allergic reactions. And because it can contain bacteria, there is a chance that once it is inserted into the sterile environment of the uterus, it can cause infection.

These concerns became less important in the early eighties, when the IUI method that is currently being used was developed. This improved method for doing intrauterine insemination used "washed" sperm instead of liquefied semen. Sperm washing, which was originally developed for use in the laboratory with in vitro fertilization techniques, both concentrates sperm and separates them from their seminal plasma. During this separation, both prostaglandin and bacteria are also left behind.

The use of sperm washing for insemination procedures other than in vitro fertilization was started by a medical group in Australia in their donor sperm program. They realized that by using "washed" sperm they could eliminate the source of cramping and allergic reactions that was making the IUI procedure difficult or impossible for many of their patients. It also improved pregnancy rates, despite the fact that the number of sperm hadn't increased. Their work proved to be successful, and the treatment was introduced into several clinics in the United States, including ours, in 1981. As we began performing intrauterine inseminations for various forms of infertility, we realized that washed sperm offered a great advantage in certain clinical situations. Because the washing process creates a concentration of the number of sperm per milliliter of fluid, it improves our ability to get large numbers of sperm into a woman's reproductive tract. This gives an important boost to the fertilization process, especially for a woman with abnormal cervical function, or a man with decreased sperm count.

——————— HOW DO YOU WASH A SPERM? ———————

Little brushes? Well . . . not really. Sperm washing "cleans" a semen sample by filtering out improperly formed and nonmotile sperm in the same way that cervical mucus does. In cervical mucus, sperm swim through a series of small channels as they make their way through the cervical canal. Abnormally formed sperm, or those that don't move well, aren't able to negotiate their way through these spaces and are left behind. The same thing is accomplished in sperm washing, by filtering liquefied semen through a solution called Percoll, which contains millions of tiny, microscopic balls. The Percoll solution can be concentrated to different degrees; depending on its density, it can be used to separate the motile sperm from those that don't move well, and can be used to weed out abnormally formed sperm. By centrifuging semen to separate the heavier sperm cells from the fluid in which they are suspended, and then filtering the sperm cells through a series of Percoll solutions in different densities, doctors are able to collect about 80% of an ejaculate's motile, normally shaped sperm. They place these sperm into a tissue culture solution such as Ham's F-10, and concentrate it into a very small volume. When this concentrated solution of highly motile sperm is placed directly into the uterine cavity, it dramatically increases the number of motile sperm that will reach the fallopian tubes and encounter the egg.

One thing to remember, if you are having an IUI procedure, is that while washing can remove almost all danger of infection, there is still a small possibility that one will develop. If you have lower abdominal pain, vaginal discharge, spotting, or fever after your IUI, you should let your doctor know immediately. If caught in a timely fashion these infections—known as endometritis—can be eliminated with oral antibiotics.

How Well Does IUI Work?

Since its introduction, the process of doing intrauterine inseminations with washed spermatozoa has become extremely widespread. Its popularity is explained by its high success rates, particularly in some categories of infertility. For women under the age of 40 with cervical factor infertility, IUI produces a pregnancy rate of 10% to 12% per cycle. If women of all ages are considered, including those over 40, the pregnancy rate drops to about 6% per cycle. If couples having cervical factor infertility have four to six cycles of IUI, about 60% will conceive, although age will decrease this percentage somewhat. While IUI's success rate in patients with unexplained infertility, or male factor infertility, is slightly lower, it is still a good place to start before moving on to more invasive and expensive assisted reproductive technologies. If you are considering IUI, you should ask your doctor what his IUI pregnancy rate is for patients with your condition. If they don't approach the figures we've given, you might want to try to find another physician who's had greater success with the procedure.

How IUI Works

If you are going to be undergoing an IUI procedure, your partner will have to give a semen sample to your doctor ahead of time. After his sperm is washed and prepared, it's placed into a catheter. This could be any small tube 20 cm in length; in our clinic we use a 5 french pediatric feeding tube. The catheter is then inserted into your vaginal canal, and worked past your cervix until it extends into the uterine cavity. The sperm is then pushed through the tube and into your uterus. You should expect the procedure to cause you even less discomfort than a pap smear. After the sperm is in place in your uterus, your doctor will ask you to remain lying down on the examination table for five to ten minutes. (See Figure 7-5.)

This method of insemination, which is guaranteed to get the sperm into your uterus, is complicated by one very important problem. When the sperm bypasses your cervix, it also bypasses your cervical mucus. Under normal circumstances your cervical mucus works both as a means of transport for sperm and as a reservoir in which they can wait for as long as two days before migrating up into the uterine cavity. As we explained in the chapter on male function (Chapter Three), different sperm take different amounts of time to work their way up into the uterine cavity. Assuming there are no complications, the cervical mucus keeps them viable during this 24- to 48-hour period. Because of the reservoir effect of

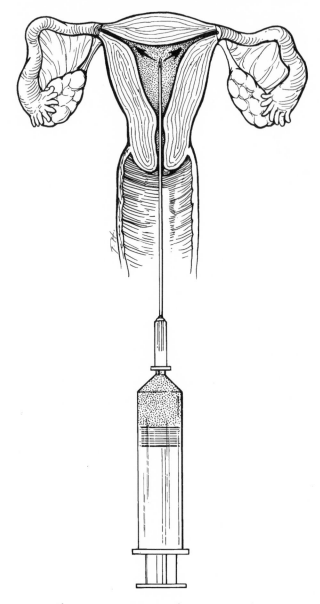

Figure 7-5:   Diagram of an IUI Procedure

the mucus, you and your partner don't have to have intercourse just before ovulation; it can occur up to two full days prior to ovulation, and you may still accomplish a pregnancy.

This advantage is lost when direct IUI is performed. By jumping past the mucus, the sperm lose their chance to wait in this natural reservoir. Once inserted into the uterine cavity by IUI, they very quickly migrate through the uterus and into the fallopian tubes. Because of this, if ovulation doesn't happen within several hours of a direct intrauterine insemination, fertilization probably won't occur. It's likely there won't be enough sperm remaining in the uterine environment or fallopian tube to accomplish the feat. But don't worry. Luckily, there are ways to compensate for this.

The Basic Protocol for IUI

One of the ways to do this is to perform IUI twice. Since it's impractical to know precisely to the hour when ovulation is going to occur, your doctor may "bracket" the time when he expects the egg to be released, inseminating you once at or before your anticipated time of ovulation, and inseminating you again 24 hours later. Because sperm can stay available in the fallopian tube for only ten to twelve hours after IUI, the egg has to be in the fallopian tube within ten to twelve hours of the insemination. This doubling up of the process should guarantee that some sperm will still be available when the egg arrives in the tube.

The goal of bracketing is for you to ovulate halfway between the time of the first insemination and the second one, which is performed the next day. Therefore, being able to precisely time ovulation is a key factor if IUI is to be successful.

Let's assume, for example, that you have a regular cycle—either because you're ovulating naturally or because you've been assisted by drug therapy. Two to three days prior to the midpoint of your cycle, you should begin testing your urine at home with an LH surge monitoring kit. When you get a positive reading, you should go into your doctor's office the following morning for an intrauterine insemination. Your partner should have provided a semen specimen enough ahead of time so that it can be properly washed and prepared. Before you are inseminated, an ultrasound should be performed to see whether you have already ovulated, or whether you are about to. If your follicle has already collapsed—indicating ovulation—you will receive a single direct intrauterine insemination. On the other hand, if your follicle is still present, indicating you haven't yet ovulated, your doctor should inseminate you, and then repeat the ultrasound and insemination the following day.

If you are not on a regular cycle, and are receiving the drug hCG to trigger ovulation, you will not need to monitor yourself with an LH surge kit in order to time insemination. Once an ultrasound determines that follicle maturity is reached, and hCG is given, your next ultrasound and your insemination will be timed to occur 36 to 40 hours after the hCG is administered. If, at that time, your ultrasound shows evidence that your follicle has ruptured, your doctor will perform a single insemination. If your follicle hasn't ruptured 36 hours following your hCG shot, a second insemination will be performed the following morning, or about 60 hours from the time your hCG was administered.

This method of using hCG to trigger ovulation for a single insemination can also be used if you are ovulating normally, assuming your doctor has ultrasound equipment that can accurately determine whether your follicle has collapsed. Some doctors still feel that two inseminations give you better insurance of achieving a pregnancy than a single insemination. But using the timing we've described above, and tracking the results of ten to twelve thousand cycles of intrauterine inseminations, we've found that pregnancy rates were the same, whether a single insemination or two inseminations were performed during a cycle, as long as one of the inseminations occurred when ovulation was visualized by ultrasound. This is particularly good to know if your partner has a low sperm count, making it more difficult to collect two good semen samples. But it is important to remember that for the single insemination technique to be this successful, your doctor will have to precisely time your ovulation/insemination synchrony. Timing is everything with IUI.

OTHER TREATMENTS FOR CERVICAL FACTOR INFERTILITY

Sometimes a difficult cervical problem doesn't respond to any of the therapies we've described. In the case of a severely traumatized or damaged cervix, for example, even IUI may not be able to help you establish a pregnancy. If you are among this small percentage of cases, don't despair. There are still alternatives for treatment, including in vitro fertilization and gamete intrafallopian transfer. The good news is that these assisted reproductive procedures are very successful for this condition. We will be talking about them in detail in Chapter Twelve.

Terms We Used in This Chapter

Bicornuate uterus: a malformation of the uterus resulting in two separate cavities, each with a connecting fallopian tube.

Cervical canal atresia: a congenital condition in which the opening or canal through the cervix does not form before birth.

Cervical mucus: a mucus secretion produced by glands in the cervical canal under the influence of estrogen.

Cervix: a narrow opening that connects the uterus to the vagina and produces mucus that allows the sperm to enter into the uterus.

Congenital abnormality: a malformation that takes place during fetal development.

Conization: the surgical removal of abnormal cells on the surface or within the cervical canal.

Cryocautery: the destruction of abnormal cervical cells by freezing.

Diethylstilbestrol (DES): a man-made estrogen originally used to prevent miscarriages. Is known to cause abnormalities of the cervix, vagina, and uterus of the unborn fetus.

Dilatation and curettage (D&C): opening the cervix and removing the contents of the uterine cavity by scraping or suction.

Dysplasia: abnormalities in the cell layers covering the cervix, vagina, or vulva.

Endometritis: infection or inflammation of the uterine lining (the endometrium).

Estrogen: a category of female hormone that is necessary for female characteristics.

Intrauterine insemination (IUI): placement of sperm into the uterine cavity.

Loop electrocautery excision procedure (LEEP): a procedure used to remove abnormal cells from the cervical area using an electric cutting wire; similar to a conization.

Pharmacologic: above natural physiologic levels.

Physiologic levels: hormonal levels that are identical to those produced naturally by a person's system.

Postcoital test (PCT): a test used to determine whether sperm/mucus interaction is normal, i.e., whether the sperm can move properly through the cervical mucus.

Prostaglandin: a hormone that is produced by the endometrium, which causes the uterine muscle to contract.

Septate uterus: a fibrous division of the uterine cavity.

Sperm washing: a technique used to separate sperm cells from seminal fluid.

Stenotic: a narrowed opening.

Uterine didelphys: duplication of the uterus; a double uterus.

8

Tubal and Uterine Problems

You're almost through with your basic workup when your doctor calls you and your partner into his office for a consultation. He tells you that he believes your uterus or your fallopian tubes may be the reason you aren't having a baby.

It's easy to understand why you wouldn't be getting pregnant if there are, in fact, complications with either of these organs. Your fallopian tubes are the pipeline between your ovaries and your uterus, as well as the meeting place where your egg and your partner's sperm come together. If they're not functioning properly, the ovulated egg may not be picked up from the surface of your ovary, thus the egg and sperm don't meet. Or, if your egg is picked up and fertilized, the embryo may not, in some cases, be transported safely to your uterus. If your fallopian tubes are functioning properly, and the egg has arrived in the uterus, the endometrial environment must be prepared to assume an equally important set of responsibilities—caring for the fertilized egg as it implants, grows, and develops.

While there are some instances in which a woman knows that her uterus or tubes have been damaged, other times she will have no idea that that's where her problem lies.

Even when a woman doesn't have any outward sign of her condition, clues can be picked up by her doctor during a series of diagnostic tests aimed specifically at examining the uterus and tubes. While the fallopian tube and the uterus are two different organs with two different functions, they do have some things in common when it comes to the diagnosis of their problems. The steps your doctor might go through in finding trouble spots in either of these organs include:

- Taking your *medical history*. This might lead him to suspect a uterine or tubal problem, particularly if you've had pelvic surgeries or infections in the past or have a family history of fibroids.

- Giving you a *physical exam*. In some cases this might help him to move toward a confirmation of his suspicions. For example, most uterine fibroids can actually be felt during a pelvic examination.

- Giving you a *hysterosalpingogram* (HSG). If your doctor thinks there might be some problem with the configuration of your uterine cavity, or with the opening through your fallopian tubes, an HSG is the most commonly used test to determine whether one really exists. If you'd like to review how a hysterosalpingogram is done, refer to our chapter on the basic workup (Chapter Five). By performing this test, your doctor can identify abnormalities within the uterine cavity, along with any obstructions that might exist inside your fallopian tubes.

- Confirming any abnormality or obstruction he finds, during your HSG, by doing an *endoscopic procedure*, in the hopes of visually seeing the problem.

Endoscopes are medical instruments that have been devised to let your doctor look into the interior of your body, or into certain organs. There are a number of different variations in these viewing tubes, each of which has its own distinct purpose. Some of them are so commonly used when diagnosing and treating problems with the uterus and fallopian tubes that we will be referring to them often, so you should be familiar with their names and purposes. A *hysteroscope* is used when your doctor wants to look inside your uterus. He inserts a thin fiber-optic telescope into your uterus through your cervical canal. We will be describing how this is done in greater detail later in this chapter. A *laparoscope* is used when he wants to see into your pelvic cavity and examine the area outside your uterus and tubes. The laparoscope is a larger telescope than the hysteroscope, and is inserted through the abdominal wall, just below the navel.

Endoscopes come in different sizes; some are large enough to allow your doctor to actually introduce surgical instruments into the cavity he's examining. Thus, once they've fulfilled their diagnostic purpose, they can also become the means of treating the problems that your doctor finds. By the end of this chapter you will, hopefully, understand how these, and other treatments, can help to restore your tubal and uterine function.

What's Causing Your Uterine Problem?

"Hope is the belief, more or less strong, that joy will come. . . ."

—*Sydney Smith,* Lady Holland's Memoir

Hope is the theme song of the normal uterus. No matter how many times it may have been disappointed in the past, it still prepares with each new cycle for the possibility that an embryo will implant, and will need to be housed and nurtured. It's a preheated oven, just waiting for a pan of batter to be put in so that it can bake it into a whole new size and shape. But when your oven isn't functioning normally, that cake never bakes. There are two reasons why this might happen. Either your uterus has a "physiologic problem"—a glitch in the way it functions—or there is something wrong with its structure, which is interfering with its ability to receive an embryo and carry it to term.

PHYSIOLOGIC ABNORMALITIES

The uterus is known to fall victim to only one type of physiologic problem: when its endometrium—the soft lining of the uterine cavity that's intended to protect and nourish the fetus as it grows—doesn't develop correctly, or at the proper time. This problem, known as a luteal phase defect, is the most common type of uterine difficulty, and happily it's one that can be treated fairly simply.

As you learned in the chapter on normal female reproduction (Chapter Two), the endometrium is a hormonally sensitive tissue. During the first phase of your ovulatory cycle, as estrogen production from the developing follicle is increasing, it influences the endometrium to grow and thicken. Once follicle rupture and egg release occur, the corpus luteum that is left behind begins to produce progesterone. It's the combination of these two hormones—estrogen and progesterone—that triggers the endometrium to become a receptive, spongy layer . . . one that will allow an embryo to attach, implant, and connect to the maternal bloodstream inside the uterus.

Sometimes this hormonal balance is off. When this happens, the endometrium either doesn't develop properly, or matures off schedule, usually too late to receive the fertilized egg. When the embryo enters a uterine cavity that isn't properly prepared for it, it doesn't implant, and the pregnancy that should have begun never progresses. This problem has been described in detail in Chapter Six.

STRUCTURAL ABNORMALITIES

It's a simple rule of biology—structure affects function. Your uterus is no exception. In order for it to carry a pregnancy to term, its shape must be appropriate. There are two reasons why it might not be. First, you might have a congenital defect—one that was present at birth. Or you may have developed problems during your reproductive years—things such as fibroids or tissue masses from surgical scarring. Either of these could affect the ability of your uterus to do its job.

Congenital Structural Abnormalities

Tracing the way your uterus took shape can help you to understand how flaws may have occurred as it was evolving. Both the uterus and fallopian tubes normally develop sometime between the tenth and sixteenth weeks of fetal life. The uterus is formed when two separate tubular systems called the "Müllerian ducts" turn into pouches, slowly move together, then fuse to become a unified single structure.

Several different types of abnormalities can occur if the Müllerian ducts don't fully fuse. Women whose uterine development was sidetracked before its completion can be left with a divided uterus, two duplicate uteri, or no uterus at all, as we explained in Chapter Seven. Whether these women can conceive and carry a pregnancy to term depends on the stage at which their fusion stopped.

Rokitansky Syndrome   Rokitansky syndrome is the most extreme type of congenital abnormality; it occurs when the Müllerian ducts don't fuse at all. When this happens the female child is born without a uterus, and usually without a complete vagina as well. While her ovaries are most often functional and will ovulate, she has no way to either conceive or carry a pregnancy.

Uterine Didelphys   A second type of congenital abnormality occurs when the Müllerian ducts fuse, but the wall between them doesn't disappear. The woman is left with two distinct uteri—a condition that is called uterine didelphys. If you have been diagnosed with this problem, you have a double cervix and duplicate uterine cavities. You probably also have a curtain of fibrous tissue called a septum dividing your vagina into two separate canals. This complete duplication or nonfusion of the Müllerian systems is rarely seen. (See Figure 7-3.)

Bicornuate or Septate Uterus   Incomplete fusion of the Müllerian ducts, in which a woman is left with a single uterus, a single cervix, and a single vaginal canal—but with a division that separates her single uterus into two cavities—is more commonly seen. If the division is made by fully formed muscular walls, she has what is called a bicornuate uterus. (See Figure 7-2.)

If it is divided into two compartments by a thin sheet of fibrous tissue, however, she has what is called a septate uterus. On a hysterosalpingo-gram a septate uterus can look like a heart-shaped cavity, or an upside-down triangle with a wall running through its middle. (See Figure 7-4.)

The septum can extend a third of the way, half of the way, or all of the way down, from the top of the uterine cavity to the cervical opening.

Congenital Abnormalities Caused by Drug Exposure   Yet another ab-normality of the uterus is found in women who were exposed to the drug diethylstilbestrol (DES) during the first twelve to sixteen weeks of their fetal development. DES contained large doses of synthetic estrogens—so large that they interfered with the fetal development of both the cervix and the uterus. If you have a congenital defect as a result of this exposure, the interior of your uterus may have formed in a distinctive shape. As your doctor looks at it via the hysterosalpingogram, he may see, for example, that it has the appearance of a *T*. This *T* is formed by a cervix that is very long in comparison to the shorter uterine cavity above it. (See Figures 8-1a and 8-1b.)

Because of this T-shaped configuration, the uterine cavity is left with a very small interior. That's why women with severe uterine abnor-malities as a result of exposure to DES have great difficulty getting pregnant, and even more difficulty carrying their pregnancies to term.

Developed Abnormalities

Most structural abnormalities that aren't congenital develop during the reproductive period of your life. Some, which are inherited disorders, occur naturally. You might develop uterine fibroids, or a condition called adenomyosis, in this way. Others, such as Asherman's syndrome, are the result of surgical procedures that created scarring and led to structural changes. Irrespective of the way your abnormalities were created, they can affect your uterus's ability to help an embryo implant and grow.

Uterine Fibroids   Uterine fibroids (or leiomyomas) are one of the most common structural abnormalities of the uterus. Fibroids inside the uter-ine cavity, or in the muscular wall of the uterus, can be diagnosed by

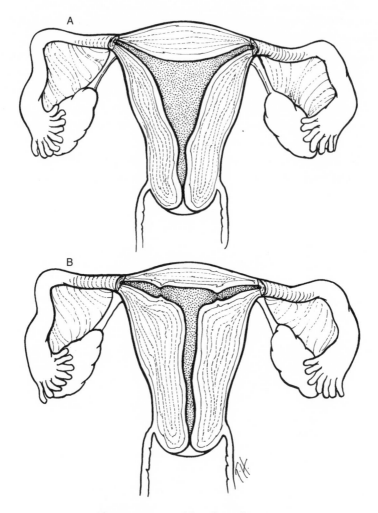

Figure 8-1a: Mild T-Shaped Uterus
Figure 8-1b: Severe T-Shaped Uterus

hysterosalpingogram and/or ultrasound. Those on the outer surface of the uterus can be seen by using an ultrasound or during a laparoscopic procedure.

If you have fibroids, don't blame yourself. There was nothing you did to create them; fibroids are an inherited disorder that was passed on to you from your mother. You may argue that your mother never had significant problems, and that may well be true. But the fact is, even if she never actually developed fibroids, the gene existed in her makeup, and she passed her genetic predisposition on to you.

Fibroids are rarely malignant, but as these benign fibrous tumors grow and develop, they can create significant problems with regard to your ability either to get pregnant or to carry a pregnancy to term. If you are one of those women who has fibroids, the two key elements you and your doctor will need to focus on in deciding how to treat them are their *size* and their *location*.

Fibroids are usually measured in centimeters. Your doctor may help you to understand how large yours are by referring to them using a recognizable analogy such as "golf ball size" or "grapefruit size." While size is an important factor, the location of your fibroids is the element that most affects your ability to get pregnant. (See Figure 8-2.)

- Fibroids that are growing inside the uterine cavity are called *submucosal*.

- Fibroids located within the muscular wall of the uterus are called *intramural*.

- Fibroids that protrude to the outside of the uterus, or are on the outer surface of the uterus, are call *subserosal*.

Submucosal fibroids are the most destructive to a potential pregnancy. Because they are found inside the uterine cavity, fibroids as small as one centimeter can cause your uterus to react as if it has a foreign body inside it. Just as an IUD's mere presence can interfere with the way the uterine

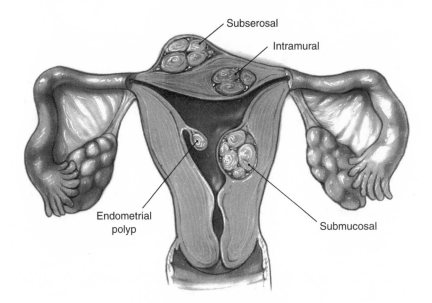

Figure 8-2:   Uterine Fibroids

lining responds to the hormonal changes that occur after ovulation, submucosal fibroids can disturb endometrial development, and stop the uterus from preparing itself for the embryo to implant.

While they are not technically fibroids, *endometrial polyps* are another type of lesion that can form inside the uterine cavity, where they can disturb endometrial development in the same way that submucosal fibroids do. A polyp is formed when a piece of endometrial tissue bulges out from its normal location and turns into a protruding stalk. Polyps are commonly seen in the nasal sinuses, the throat, and the large and small bowels, as well as in the uterine cavity. In very rare cases they can be malignant, but normally they are benign. However, when located in the uterus, these overgrown masses of endometrial tissue can interfere with endometrial development, and thus with the implantation of an embryo.

Intramural fibroids present less of a problem with respect to getting pregnant. Even the larger-size ones usually don't interfere with implantation, as long as they don't protrude to such a degree that they disrupt the endometrial cavity. They can, however, develop into a problem *during* pregnancy. Fibroids that are greater than four or five centimeters in diameter can push against blood vessels to such an extent that they create poor uterine blood flow. When this happens, it can interfere with the normal development of a fetus. Moreover, these fibroids can grow very rapidly during pregnancy, and interfere with normal uterine growth. Women with these large intramural fibroids often have premature labor and delivery.

Subserosal fibroids create less of a problem during a pregnancy, but when they're excessive in size they can affect your ability to get pregnant in the first place. Once a subserosal fibroid exceeds five to six centimeters in size, it may get in the way as your fallopian tube tries to pick up the egg after ovulation. The same can be true of an intramural fibroid that pushes against the outer wall of your uterus and protrudes into the pelvic cavity.

Adenomyosis   While adenomyosis is somewhat similar to fibroids, it develops in a different way. Adenomyosis occurs when endometrial tissue invades the muscle wall of the uterus and begins to grow.

Some women, particularly after several pregnancies, may have uterine enlargement or a thickening of the uterine wall. These are signs of significant adenomyosis. Instead of sloughing off and exiting through the cervix with the menstrual blood, some endometrial tissue invades the uterine muscle, where it thickens with the hormonal changes that occur during every ovulatory cycle.

Adenomyosis can begin as very small implants that create minor areas of fibrous scarring in the uterine muscle. Or they can be extensive, involving large portions of the uterine muscle and the endometrial cavity. Really invasive adenomyosis—extending from the endometrial cavity through the entire muscle wall of the uterus—can interfere with embryo implantation, or can hinder the ability of an implanted embryo to grow properly inside the uterus, resulting in a pregnancy that may not go full term.

Asherman's Syndrome   Of all the disorders that affect uterine function, the one that creates the largest number of problems is, ironically, created by physicians. Asherman's syndrome is caused by the formation of scar tissue within the uterine cavity after surgical procedures. While cases have been described in which it followed severe uterine infections, for the most part Asherman's is a condition that occurs after surgeries that manipulate and traumatize the endometrial environment. It's a commonly seen abnormality, probably due to the popularity of a minor surgical procedure called dilatation and curettage of the uterus, better known as a D&C.

In this country, D&Cs are done for a number of reasons. They're a frequent means of performing therapeutic abortions, and they're used to remove any remaining tissue from the uterine cavity after a pregnancy miscarries. A D&C is also performed when a woman has abnormal uterine bleeding that can be related to a pregnancy loss or hormonal abnormalities. No matter what the reason for the surgery, patients can be left with abnormal scarring if a surgeon who isn't well trained aggressively attacks the uterine cavity. Another operation that has been known to cause Asherman's is a cesarean section. If you are having a D&C or a cesarean birth, you should choose your surgeon carefully. The truth is, there's a potential for creating scars within the uterine cavity anytime these operations are performed.

Asherman's syndrome can be very mild—consisting of just a few scars in the uterine cavity—or it can be so severe that the entire uterine cavity is sealed shut with scarring. Even in its least severe forms, it can interfere with the uterine cavity's response to hormonal changes during ovulation. If you have Asherman's, you may be ovulating but not menstruating. This can happen when there's no endometrium left to be stimulated by the hormonal changes during your ovulatory cycle, and to slough off when it concludes. That's why the lack of menstrual bleeding after a D&C is a classic sign of Asherman's.

The most severe cases of Asherman's syndrome that I've treated resulted from cesarean sections in which the surgeons inadvertently

closed the uterine cavities of their patients by suturing their walls together. Unfortunately for them, because of their dense scarring, the surgery to reopen the walls of the uterus was extremely difficult.

Can Your Uterine Problem Be Fixed?

Most uterine problems, if correctable, are fixed surgically. In some cases, when problems can't be fixed, doctors are able to either bypass the uterus or produce a pregnancy despite it. While hormones and drugs may often be used prior to surgery—to shrink the size of the growths that are being surgically removed—only luteal phase defects, the one physiologic abnormality that affects uterine function, can actually be corrected with various drug regimens. The way in which this is done is discussed in detail in Chapter Six.

TREATING CONGENITAL ABNORMALITIES

Many congenital abnormalities of the uterus are not correctable either with drugs or any surgical approach. If you are born with uterine didelphys, bicornuate uterus, Rokitansky syndrome, or DES changes, you will carry them throughout your lifetime. But depending on the type and severity of the abnormality, you may still be able to carry a pregnancy to term.

Selective Insemination

If you have either a bicornuate uterus—two completely separated uterine cavities—or uterine didelphys—complete duplication of the cervical canal, which leads into two completely separated uterine cavities—you have great hope of getting pregnant and, with careful treatment, carrying your baby for a full nine months.

In either of these cases, your doctor will look at your ovaries by ultrasound, to determine which one—the right or the left—is ovulating during any given cycle. Once he determines which follicle is ovulating, he will perform intrauterine insemination; this process is explained in the chapter on cervical factor infertility, Chapter Seven. As he does this, he will maneuver the catheter into the uterine cavity next to the ovary that's releasing the egg. This process is called selective insemination. It puts the sperm as close as it can be placed, nonsurgically, to the place

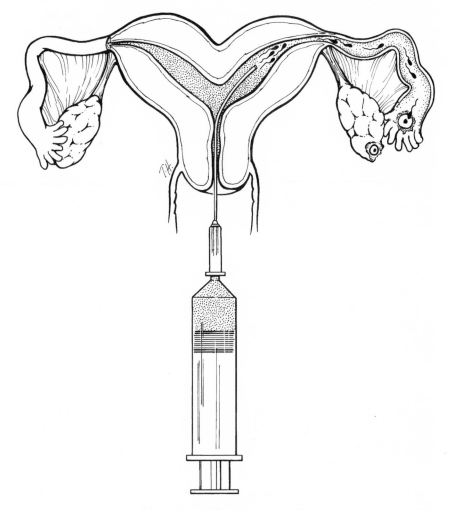

Figure 8-3: Selective Insemination

where it will meet the egg and fertilize it. The embryo will then, hopefully, implant on the correct side of the uterus—the portion where ovulation took place.

If all of this works, and you do get pregnant, your doctor will have to
follow your progress very closely.

Remember, your pregnancy will be growing in a uterine cavity that is
half normal size. Because of this, the baby will quickly begin pressing
against your uterine walls and cervix. Eventually the cervix could give
way, and the baby could be born prematurely.

Your doctor will probably try to counteract this by performing a cervical cerclage. He will place a suture in your cervix, and pull it tight around the cervix, like a drawstring closing a purse. Then he'll tie it in place to close the opening to the uterus. A cerclage is usually performed between the fourteenth and eighteenth weeks of pregnancy, and it remains in place, holding the baby inside the uterus until it has fully matured.

Once your pregnancy has reached its twenty-eighth week, your doctor will usually tell you that strict bed rest is required for its duration. Often, drugs are also used to keep the uterus from beginning premature labor. When the pregnancy does reach full term, your doctor simply removes the cerclage, which allows the baby to be born.

Because these pregnancies are high-risk and can present a great number of practical problems in their daily lives, women with uterine didelphys or a bicornuate uterus should spend extra time talking to their doctors before they elect to go into a pregnancy. It's especially important that they be fully counseled as to the potential risks and complications of miscarriage, premature labor, and delivery.

While women who suffer from DES exposure in utero, resulting in an abnormal, T-shaped uterus, do not undergo selective insemination, the same techniques for maintaining a pregnancy, once it's established, apply to them. Even though there is no known surgical correction for this condition, a cerclage and supporting therapies can help women who are lucky enough to become pregnant, despite having a T-shaped uterus, to safely carry their pregnancies to term.

A Surrogate Situation

While vaginal reconstruction is often done for women with Rokitansky syndrome (absence of a uterus) to facilitate their ability to have sex, there is no corrective surgery for this condition that will allow a woman who suffers from it to carry a baby. Nevertheless, if you are diagnosed with Rokitansky, you can still have a child that is genetically your own. Your eggs and your partner's sperm can be combined in a laboratory using in vitro fertilization, then another woman—known as a surrogate gestational carrier—can carry the pregnancy to term. We will be discussing both the physical and psychological aspects of surrogacy in more detail in Chapter Twelve.

Surgical Solutions

If your hysterosalpingogram shows that your uterine cavity has a congenital division, your doctor will need to determine whether it is bicornuate or septate before deciding how to treat it. Sometimes this will be suggested from the image on your hysterosalpingogram. However, the hysterosalpingogram cannot demonstrate whether the division is muscular or fibrous. The next diagnostic step he will go to is ultrasound. Sometimes ultrasound clearly shows a separate muscular division. But in most cases, it will still not be clear whether the division is a wall of muscle or a fibrous septum. At that point your doctor will use a laparoscope to view the exterior of your uterus. If the exterior of your uterus shows a clear muscular division, he will have discovered that you have a bicornuate uterus. If this is the case, your doctor will not operate. Attempting to remove the muscular wall that divides a bicornuate uterus into two halves not only can be dangerous but is often unsuccessful. The only alternative is to hope that you become pregnant, and that your doctor can use a cerclage to maintain the pregnancy once it's initiated. If your uterus appears to be a single muscular organ, your doctor will know that its division is formed by a fibrous septum. Because this type of septum isn't muscular and doesn't have a blood supply or nerves, it can easily be removed through a hysteroscope, without excessive bleeding or pain.

Hysteroscopy   Hysteroscopy is a relatively new surgical procedure, developed during the eighties. It enables a surgeon to see inside the uterine cavity, and in many cases to correct the structural abnormalities that he might find there, without making an abdominal incision or cutting through the uterine walls. This minimally invasive surgery is done by inserting a small, thin telescope called a hysteroscope through the vagina and the cervical opening, and on into the uterus. Inside the hysteroscope, there's a fiber-optic light. Using an eyepiece at its exterior end, your doctor can see the interior of your uterus, which will look like the inside of a cavern or a blown-up balloon. If your doctor finds an abnormality, he can usually correct it during the same procedure, by inserting micro-operating tools through the hysteroscope. (See Figure 8-4.)

For example, if you have a septate uterus, once the septum is viewed, your surgeon would then use hysteroscopic cutting instruments such as laser, electrosurgical fiber, or simple cutting scissors to remove the fibrous wall.

Hysteroscopy from the Patient's Point of View   Before you have a hysteroscopy, you will be asked to empty your bladder. Then your vaginal area will be cleaned with an antiseptic solution. Either a local or general anesthetic will be used for this minor surgery. Just before the procedure

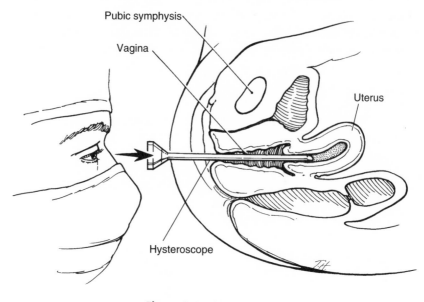

Figure 8-4: Hysteroscopy

your cervix may need to be dilated, or made wider, with special instruments. The hysteroscope is then inserted through the vagina, the cervix, and into the uterus. A fiber-optic light is shone through the scope to illuminate the uterus and the openings of the fallopian tubes, and a liquid or gas (such as CO_2) is usually released through the scope, to expand the cavity so that your surgeon can have a clearer look at its interior.

Recovery from hysteroscopic surgery is relatively simple. With either type of anesthetic, hysteroscopy is almost always performed as an outpatient procedure. If your doctor uses a local anesthetic, you will go home in a short time, usually one to two hours. If you have a general, you may feel groggy for a few hours, and won't go home for two to four hours. If your doctor corrects an abnormality during your procedure, you may have some menstrual cramping the day of the surgery, and some minor bleeding for a few more days. But serious complications are very rare, occurring only 1% to 3% of the time when hysteroscopic procedures are performed by an experienced surgeon.

One area of concern to me is the too frequent use of laparoscopy and hysteroscopy by undertrained and inexperienced gynecologic surgeons. If the surgeon you have chosen is not well trained, considerable damage to your uterus, its endometrial lining, and to your large

and small bowel can result. You must find out about the experience and reputation of your surgeon before, not after, your procedure.

TREATING DEVELOPED ABNORMALITIES

Treating Fibroids

The type of lesions that are known as fibroids are probably the most common uterine abnormality. These growths of fibrous connective tissue can develop at varying depths and locations in the uterine wall. They usually don't have any symptoms, but your physician may be able to feel them during a pelvic examination. If he does, he will then go on to determine their size and exact position in much the same way that he would diagnose congenital abnormalities—by using ultrasound, hystero-salpingogram, laparoscopy, and/or hysteroscopy.

Depending on what he finds, your doctor will then choose between two different types of surgical treatment. Because he will be removing a tumor from the muscular tissue of your uterus, which is known as the *myometrium*, either type of surgery will be known as a *myomectomy*. Fibroids that are located on the inside of the uterine cavity are most often removed through *hysteroscopic myomectomy*. But fibroids that are located either on the exterior of your uterus or within its muscular wall must be reached through an abdominal incision, a procedure is called a *laparotomy myomectomy*. (See Figure 8-5.)

Treating Submucosal and Subserosal Fibroids

Submucosal fibroids—those located on the inside of the uterine cavity—are a definite factor in infertility, since they can disrupt endometrial development and interrupt the normal implantation of an embryo. When they intrude into the uterine cavity, they can usually be detected by ultrasound. They can most often be removed through hysteroscopic myomectomy.

Hysteroscopic myomectomy was a great step forward in the removal of these sorts of fibroids. Previously, in order to remove them, a doctor would make an abdominal incision, enter the pelvic cavity, and open the uterus. Since the advent of hysteroscopic myomectomy, there is no longer any reason, in most cases, to do this, or to risk all of the complications that can be associated with this sort of procedure.

In order to do a hysteroscopic myomectomy, your fibroid is first

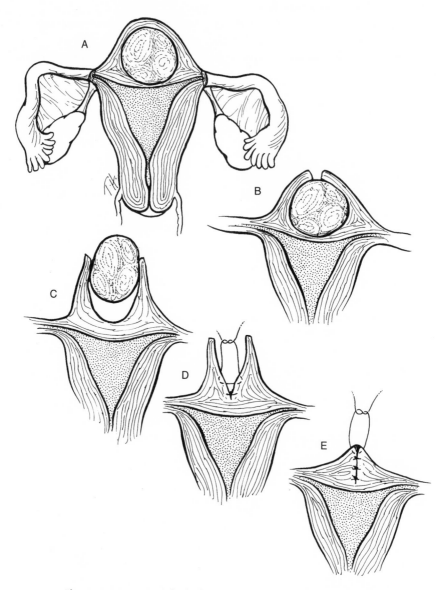

Figure 8-5:   Removal of Fibroid Tissues from the Uterine Wall

diagnosed through a hysteroscope, and your surgeon then uses a different type of scope, the resectoscope, to completely remove it. Even fibroids that are partially implanted within the uterine wall can be removed through the cervical canal via the resectoscope. For the patient, a hysteroscopic myomectomy is very much like having a simple diagnostic hysteroscopy. The only difference is that you may experience some menstrual cramping and bleeding following the procedure, due to the removal of the fibroid.

If your doctor discovers that you have an endometrial polyp, either through a hysterosalpingogram or by using ultrasound, he will most often operate in a similar fashion. He would first look at, then remove, the polyp through the hysteroscope.

Unfortunately, subserosal fibroids—fibroids on the outside of the uterus—or intramural fibroids—those that are in its wall—can't be reached via the hysteroscope, or even the laparoscope in the majority of cases. If you have either of these types of fibroid, and it needs to be removed, this will have to be done through laparotomy myomectomy. Since this is a more invasive surgical procedure, you should be sure, before embarking on it, that you really need to have it done. There are several things that you and your doctor should consider.

If your are trying to get pregnant, the location of fibroids that are on the exterior of your uterus is one important factor in making your decision. As we stated earlier, some of these fibroids are positioned in such a way that they interfere with the fallopian tube when it tries to retrieve the egg. This is particularly true when they exceed four centimeters in size. Fibroids such as these require surgical removal. But others of the same size, if they don't interfere with the tube, may not. (See Figure 8-6.)

Even if you are not trying to get pregnant, there may also be good general health reasons for you to have your fibroids removed. Some women with fibroids over four or five centimeters in size experience

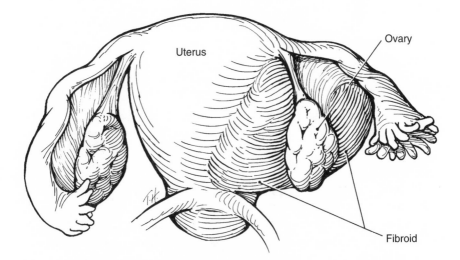

Figure 8-6: Subserosal Fibroid with Tubal Interference

heavy and prolonged menstrual periods, which can leave them anemic. If this is happening to you, it's a definite argument in favor of surgery.

Laparotomy Myomectomy from the Patient's Point of View   When you have a laparotomy myomectomy, your doctor accesses the uterus by cutting through the abdominal wall, either with a side-to-side "bikini" cut, or an up-and-down incision. These are the same type of cuts that are used to deliver a baby through cesarean section.

A laparotomy is considered to be major surgery. You will be operated on under either an epidural or general anesthetic, and your surgery will take anywhere from two to four hours. Afterward, you'll probably have to endure some pain and discomfort, mainly from the incision that has been made into your abdominal cavity. Your hospital stay following surgery will be several days, and during the first day you will be receiving fluids through an IV. After you leave the hospital, you will have a recovery period of four to six weeks before you'll be able to resume full physical activities.

The most common fear that women have when they are told they need an abdominal myomectomy is that their uterus will be removed along with the fibroids. This fear is not unfounded. The majority of gynecologists tell patients that a hysterectomy is advised—maybe even necessary—when they see large fibroids. These doctors believe that due to the fibroids' large size, it will be extremely difficult to maintain uterine function after they are removed. This is simply not true. In almost 100% of cases, an experienced surgeon can preserve your reproductive function, or even reestablish the functional ability of your uterus, despite large fibroids. If you're told otherwise, it's always worthwhile to get a second opinion before deciding that the recommended procedure is the correct treatment for you.

In the past 15 years I've performed hundreds of myomectomies in women who had been told by other physicians that they needed their uterus removed. They were told that their fibroids were too big or too many, and that their uterine function could not be maintained. This couldn't be further from the truth. In all of my cases, with the exception of one, I have never removed a uterus. And that exception was a case where I discovered that the patient's fibroid had a malignant change that necessitated its removal. I've removed fibroids up to 15 and 20 centimeters in size, while maintaining the uterus. Then I've watched those uteri heal properly and carry a pregnancy to term. Before you consider this type of surgery, I highly recommend you

research your surgeon's attitude toward hysterectomy. Then get a second opinion.

Because a laparotomy is major surgery, you should make sure before you consider undergoing it that:

1. the size of your fibroid exceeds four to five centimeters, and it needs to be removed either for fertility or general health purposes,

2. the position of your fibroids (e.g., submucosal—located inside the uterine cavity) makes their removal mandatory, and

3. you choose an experienced reproductive surgeon to do the procedure.

Given the invasive nature of abdominal myomectomy, you may be wondering whether drug therapy is a possible fibroid treatment. The answer is yes and no. Fibroids can be reduced by drug therapy, but only temporarily. Lupron is the drug that is most commonly used to suppress the size of a fibroid, but it can only shrink it by 50%. And as soon as you are taken off the drug, your fibroid returns to its pretreatment size.

While drug therapy isn't a cure for fibroids, it might be used if you have a fibroid that's greater than ten centimeters in diameter—about the size of a grapefruit—and your surgeon wants to reduce its mass in order to make its removal easier.

Treating Adenomyosis

While fibroids are treatable through surgery, the other type of growth that can invade your uterus—adenomyosis (invasive endometrial tissue)—is much more difficult to control. Because this type of misplaced endometrial tissue is often spread across multiple areas within the uterine wall, surgical removal is usually impossible. For the most part, adenomyosis can only be temporarily reduced in size by using GnRH agonists such as Lupron to suppress estrogen production. We will be describing this type of treatment in more detail when we discuss endometriosis in our chapter on pelvic factor disorders (Chapter Ten).

Treating Asherman's Syndrome

Solving the problems caused by Asherman's syndrome (postsurgical scar tissue) is a difficult challenge. The only way to try to restore uterine function is by removing all the scars within your uterus. Depending upon how severe your Asherman's is, this will be done either by hysteroscope or with a full laparotomy.

If you are lucky enough to have a relatively mild case of Asherman's, your surgeon will operate using the hysteroscope. Looking through it, he will be able to see inside your uterus and identify the scars. He will then use microscissors to remove each scar individually. Depending on the number of scars you have, this can be a lengthy process, lasting as long as one to two hours. After your surgery, your doctor will place you on a high dose of estrogen for 30 days. He'll do this in hopes of stimulating your endometrial tissue to regrow to a point at which it is once again functional.

In more severe cases of Asherman's—those in which the uterine cavity is completely closed by scarring—your surgeon's job becomes more complicated. Because the two sides of the uterine cavity are completely fused together, he won't be able to tell through the hysteroscope where the separation between its walls used to be, or whether he is moving his cutting tools in the right direction to re-create the cavity that was previously there. If he moves in the wrong direction, instead of opening the cavity he may cut through the muscle of the uterine walls and go into the pelvic cavity. To solve this problem, another surgeon assists him by watching the outside of the uterus through a laparoscope while he tries to separate the walls inside. If he goes off track and begins cutting in the wrong direction—through one of the walls and toward the outside of the uterus, instead of between them—the assisting surgeon will see the wall begin to bulge outward, and will direct him back in the proper direction.

Hysteroscopic correction of severe Asherman's may require two or more separate surgeries to completely normalize the uterine cavity. This is an extremely difficult surgery, which requires a surgeon with the utmost skills. Even with this approach, some cases are too severe to correct with the hysteroscope, or they continue to scar again after each procedure, which means that correction is never accomplished. In these cases one last procedure is sometimes attempted. Your doctor could perform a laparotomy to expose your uterus, then open it top to bottom. Next he would remove the scar tissue that wasn't removed during the prior hysteroscopic procedures. This is hardly a routine approach for treating Asherman's; it's used only in the most severe cases. The unfortunate part of Asherman's is that even after the scarring is removed, or the uterine cavity is opened, your doctor may discover that the damage to your endometrial lining was so traumatic that it won't regenerate or function. And once endometrial function is lost, no corrective therapy is possible.

What's Causing the Problem with Your Fallopian Tubes?

Like the uterus, the fallopian tubes have an important job to perform. So important, some doctors consider the tubes' responsibilities to be the most vital part of the reproductive process. They're the place where your embryo's life begins. They're responsible for its survival and development during its initial, delicate days. And they're in charge of delivering it safely to its next home, the uterus.

The fallopian tubes are well designed to accomplish this. They evolve during fetal development from a pair of structures known as the Wolffian ducts, in much the same way that the uterus evolves from the Müllerian ducts.

The normal fallopian tube is about 10 centimeters in length. Its distinctive appearance—like branches sprouting off the sides of the uterus—was first described by an Italian anatomist, Gabriello Fallopius, in the sixteenth century. While it may look delicate, a fallopian tube is a highly muscular organ.

As you travel from one end to the other, you can see that it has four parts:

- the interstitial
- the isthmus
- the ampullary portion, and
- the fimbrial segment.

The portion of the tube that travels through the thick wall of the uterus—the part that extends from the inside of the uterus to its exterior, where the tube becomes visible—is called the *intramural section*. The internal diameter of the tube at this point of connection is approximately 1 mm, about the size of a human hair. As the tube emerges from the uterus into the pelvic cavity, it enlarges and starts to widen, but not by much. This section is called the *isthmus*. Then, as it travels farther from this point, it begins to open up like a funnel. This funnellike portion of the tube—called its *ampullary portion*—is its widest part, with an interior

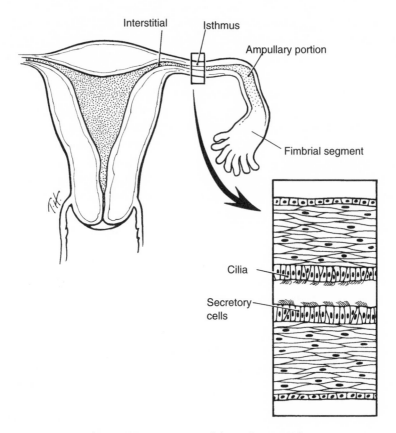

Figure 8-7: Anatomy of the Fallopian Tube

measurement of about 10 mm. At this point, the interior of the tube is about half an inch wide. The final portion of the tube, the section where it ends in fingerlike projections, is called the *fimbrial segment*. Each of these areas has its own distinct function. (See Figure 8-7.)

The first part of the tube to come into play during the reproductive process is the fimbriated portion. Before fertilization can take place, the fallopian tube has to move to where the egg is being released from the follicle, and pick it up. As we said before, when the follicle opens, the egg slowly oozes out and then rests on the surface of the ovary. If the fallopian tube is functioning normally, its muscular motion will move its fimbriated end into contact with the egg, and the fimbria will retrieve it. If sperm have already moved up through the uterus, they will be waiting in the tube's ampullary portion. That's where they will meet up with the egg so that fertilization can take place.

The fallopian tube does more than provide the perfect conditions for the egg and sperm's rendezvous. It serves as a nourishing environment, as well as a transportation system, for the developing embryo during its first and most crucial stage of life. The inside of the fallopian tube is lined with a sensitive layer of cells called *secretory cells*. These cells produce a protein substance that nourishes the sperm, the egg, and the developing embryo. Each tube is also lined with cells that have little hairlike projections called *cilia*. After embryo development begins, the cilia, by beating in one direction, move the embryo toward the uterine cavity. (See Figure 8-7.)

Because of the tube's distinctive structure, infections can cause great difficulties. The tube's narrow internal diameter, particularly in its intramural section, has just enough room for a developing embryo to pass through. Since there's no room to spare, the most minimal inflammation or bit of debris can stop the embryo from moving on to the uterus, squelching any hopes for a successful pregnancy. Also, if the fimbria are destroyed by inflammation, they won't be able to pick up the egg. And since damaged fimbria don't regenerate, this can make conception a permanent impossibility. While most tubal failures occur because of developed problems such as infections, one problem is congenital.

CONGENITAL TUBAL ABNORMALITIES

It is extremely rare to be born with an abnormality of the fallopian tubes; they almost always develop correctly from the Wolffian ducts. Even if you're born with a congenital abnormality of the uterus, it almost never affects tubal development.

This generally holds true for women with DES syndrome changes, as well. Even when their uterus develops abnormally, their tubes still develop normally. If you were born with abnormal tubes as a result of DES exposure, you are among the rarest of cases. And even for you, the only change in your tubes would probably be in their length; they would be longer than normal. This is one DES-related change that does not cause great concern. There is no hard scientific data to support the possibility that longer tubes function any differently than those of normal length.

NONCONGENITAL ABNORMALITIES

Most tubal abnormalities are noncongenital. Some form during a woman's reproductive years. This can happen either as a result of an intentional surgery, or following a random infection.

Surgically Caused Abnormalities

It is not uncommon for a woman, after delivering a baby, to have a tubal ligation performed. Tubal ligation is a sterilization procedure. When performing a tubal ligation, a doctor normally removes the middle section of a patient's tubes. He then ties the tubes off, blocking the sperm and egg from meeting. A tubal ligation is a type of man-made tubal obstruction.

Abnormalities Caused by Infection

While a tubal ligation is created deliberately, most tubal abnormalities are the result of some sort of tubal infection that occurs during a woman's reproductive years. Many types of bacteria (such as streptococcus, enterococcus, and staphylococcus) are harmless when they are in your vaginal canal, where they are neutralized by the acidity of their environment. But they can become destructive if they are taken out of the vaginal canal and introduced into the sterile environment of your pelvic cavity.

There are a number of ways in which these bacteria might enter the pelvic cavity. They can travel into it with semen, after intercourse. They can move up into the uterus during menstruation, using menstrual flow as a pathway. Or they can move from one area to another as a side effect of procedures in which a medical instrument is passed through the cervix and into the uterus.

Often when bacteria enter the pelvic cavity, they move into one or both of the fallopian tubes. Because of the delicate nature of a tube's tiny structure, it's very hard for the body to send infection-fighting white blood cells to the infected area. That makes the inside of the fallopian tube a perfect environment for these bacteria to multiply and spread. As they do, they release toxins that have the potential to destroy tissue. Once bacteria have a foothold, they can cause the fimbrial segment of the tube to close up, or they can break down the inner lining of the tube. Fallopian tubes can become permanently damaged after a single bout of infection.

While this sort of pelvic infection might be caused by any number of things, it most often involves at least one of the following two factors:

- Intrauterine devices (IUDs)

- Sexually transmitted diseases (STDs)

Intrauterine Devices (IUDs)   For years women who had never conceived, as well as women who had gone through previous pregnancies and deliveries, used the IUD as a birth control device. Unfortunately, many of these women were never told that the IUD could also provide a foolproof pathway for bacteria to move up into the sterile environment of the uterus. From there they would spread into the vulnerable tubes, where infections can create serious damage.

Once believed by most physicians to be a safe form of contraception, today the IUD is considered potentially dangerous. As a result, IUDs are not as frequently used as they were in the seventies, and problems relating to them are also being seen less frequently. However, they still do exist.

Chances are, the IUDs themselves were not the source of the infections that caused these problems; they were merely the conduit that transported bacteria. This can happen when an IUD is inserted—it can pick up bacteria in the cervix, and these bacteria can be carried into the sterile environment of the uterus. Or bacteria can ascend during the removal of an IUD, which can be particularly dangerous because removal often traumatizes the cervical canal or uterine cavity. The sites that have been traumatized are perfect places for infection to take hold.

One type of IUD was, and is, a particular offender in the transport of bacteria. The Dalkon Shield was the most damaging IUD ever developed. After it had been in use for several years, it became obvious that a large group of women who were using it suffered severe infections and loss of fertility. Doctors soon realized that this happened because the Dalkon Shield had a multistranded string which passed out of the uterus, through the cervix and into the vaginal canal. Bacteria moved up along this string and into the uterine cavity, just as oil travels up the wick of an oil lamp.

As you can see, the role IUDs play as the transporters of bacteria make them accessories to many tubal problems. These include problems that are created by the most prevalent source of pelvic infections, sexually transmitted diseases.

Infections Caused by Sexually Transmitted Diseases   IUDs are particularly hazardous when used by women who have multiple sexual partners. This points out the underlying problem these women face. The larger the number of partners a woman has, the greater the chance that she will be exposed to a sexually transmitted disease. And once she is, the greater the chance that she will get a pelvic infection.

The combination of STDs and IUDs did its greatest damage during the sixties and seventies. During this period both the frequency of sexual activity, and the number of partners women had, increased. This coincided with the time when IUDs were most widely in use. One of the STDs that was most frequently seen during that period was gonorrhea. It is still among the most common STDs today.

While it is not pleasant to have gonorrhea, it is less likely to cause fertility problems than some other sexually transmitted diseases. That's because gonorrhea makes itself known early on, giving you the opportunity to deal with it before it has a chance to permanently damage your reproductive potential. Keep in mind that a single pelvic infection can damage tubal function, and that the longer an infection is doing its damage, the less likely some of your tube's sensitive structures (such as the cilia) will return. With this in mind, it's fortunate that in most cases a woman with gonorrhea will have some symptoms within three to five days. And within seven to ten days she will usually have developed symptoms that are painful enough to send her to her doctor for treatment.

Since early treatment is the key to preserving your fertility, you should learn to recognize these symptoms, and if they occur, you should go to your doctor immediately. They may include cervical discharge, painful urination, abdominal pain, and high fever. Some women with the most severe cases even have difficulty walking.

Severe cases of infection can produce a condition known as *pelvic inflammatory disease (PID)*. Pelvic inflammatory disease is an inflammation of any or all of the organs in a woman's pelvic cavity. It can involve the uterus, the ovaries, or the fallopian tubes. Or the entire pelvic cavity can become inflamed. PID involves the fallopian tubes almost half the time that it occurs. If left untreated, pelvic inflammatory disease can cause scar tissue to build up around the fallopian tube, blocking it from picking up the ovulated egg. It can also invade the interior of the tubes.

Women who have suffered from PID at some time in their lives should not be overly surprised to find, when they try to get pregnant, that there is some problem with their tubal function. But often women who have never, to their knowledge, suffered from PID receive the same diagnosis. It is obviously confusing to discover that tubal function has been damaged when no known infection was ever present. Faced with this quandary, doctors have come up with a theory that attempts to explain it. They point to another type of STD—chlamydia.

Chlamydia is a cross between a bacteria and a virus. Unlike gonorrhea, chlamydia is usually a "silent infection." It can be harbored and passed back and forth between sexual partners without their ever knowing they have it. And it can be present in a woman's pelvic area without causing pain. A woman who has chlamydia might have no evident signs of an inflammation, or have symptoms that are so mild, she thinks she merely has a stomach virus or a cold. A woman with these minimal symptoms may simply take a painkiller and try to rest, instead of going for diagnosis and treatment.

Many times when tubal function has been damaged, doctors can connect the problem to a prior episode of PID that the patient reported in their medical history. When they can't, and when the patient can't remember any episode of pelvic infection, doctors tend to point to chlamydia as the culprit. They theorize that it lurked in the fallopian tubes, slowly scarring them, without ever causing any obvious symptoms of a pelvic infection. It's only later, when the tubes are visually examined because of a fertility problem, that the damage becomes evident. By this time, the infection is no longer active. Just the damage remains.

There is some basis for this theory. Chlamydia is found in 10% to 12% of women who have PID that has been treated ineffectively or not at all. But a careful reading of medical literature should lessen patients' fears somewhat. While chlamydia is often found as a secondary infection in partially treated PID, there is little or no proof that it can actually *cause* PID. In fact, it is very rare for an active case of chlamydia to infect the reproductive tract so significantly that it actually damages it enough to affect a woman's reproductive potential.

Because our understanding of chlamydia—and its possible effects on female reproductive potential—is incomplete, most reproductive endocrinologists now do screening cultures for it. If the results are positive, a 10- to 14-day regimen of doxycycline (Vibramycin), taken by both partners, clears up the problem. Because this treatment is so simple and inexpensive, your doctor may even proceed directly to it if you have unexplained infertility, without spending the time and expense involved in culturing.

DIAGNOSING INFERTILITY CAUSED BY PID

In most cases—whether your pelvic inflammatory disease was caused by gonorrhea, chlamydia, or some other bacterial infection—your physician probably just treated the infection at the time it was discovered, without going any farther. He didn't diagnose what damage, if any, had been done to your reproductive organs. It is only now, when you want to get pregnant, that your fertility specialist will do this. Irrespective of the cause of your pelvic inflammatory disease, tubal damage can be very difficult to treat. The first step in trying to correct it is finding out exactly where and how bad your damage is.

Assessing the Damage

Damage within the fallopian tube can take many forms. It can be in any portion of the tube, and is particularly common in the tube's sensitive fimbrial end. It can actually block the tube, or it can damage either the muscular wall of the tube or its sensitive inner lining, the place where the secretory cells and the cilia are located.

The first step in assessing the amount of damage you have is to determine whether you have a blockage, and if so, where it's located. Your doctor will try to do that by performing a hysterosalpingogram. If there has been damage caused by inflammation of the tube—a condition known as *salpingitis*—he will be able to see a change in the tube's shape. And if there is an obstruction in your tubes, the dye he injects will stop once it meets up with it.

If the dye stops at the intramural or interstitial segment of your tube—the very narrow portion that connects the tube with the uterus—and it does not move into the tube, you have what is called a proximal or corneal block. A block like this can be associated with a very distinctive change in your tubal architecture. The tube's damaged muscular wall develops a series of blind canals that begin to bulge out and block the passage of sperm, and prevent fertilized eggs from returning to the uterus. This condition, which also involves the sensitive inner lining of the tube, is called *salpingitis isthmica nodosa* (commonly referred to as SIN). In some cases SIN can cause a complete obstruction of the tube. And in other cases, while the tube remains open, SIN can interfere with the passage of the sperm, egg, and embryo, and pregnancy will not occur. (See Figure 8-8.)

If the dye passes through the interstitial segment of your tube, but is stopped in the ampullary (or distal) portion of your tube, the tube will look like a sausage-shaped structure. This happens when inflamed fimbria at the end of the tube bond together and close the tube, preventing fluid from escaping. Keep in mind that the fallopian tube's secretory cells are continuously releasing different nutrients. If the end of the tube becomes fused, these nutrients begin to fill this now-closed sack. Over time, the tube fills up like a balloon filling with water. This condition is called hydrosalpinx, which means a fluid-filled tube. (See Figure 5-5, Chapter 5.)

This buildup of fluid causes increased pressure inside the fallopian tube, which negatively affects the muscle layer and causes the cells that line the tube to die. If a hydrosalpinx exists over a long period of time and becomes very large, the entire tubal musculature, as well as the tube's sensitive endothelial lining, is usually destroyed.

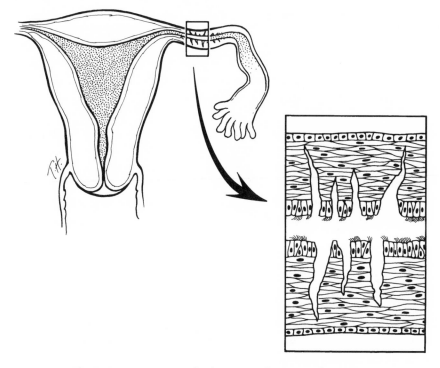

Figure 8-8:   Diagram of Salpingitis Isthmica Nodosa (SIN)

Hydrosalpinx are easily seen on a hysterosalpingogram, and can be graded as "mild," "moderate," or "severe." Their description depends on their size, and on whether the tubal lining can still be seen. If your doctor does still see some endothelial lining, this is good news. It means that the cells aren't completely destroyed, and there may be a chance for their regeneration.

Can Your Tubal Problem Be Fixed?

Women with infertility due to tubal factors once had a poor prognosis. Today, many of these women have a good chance of becoming pregnant. The treatment for tubal obstruction—in those cases where it *can* be treated—is usually surgery. The exact type of surgery that your doctor will do depends on what the problem is and where the problem is located.

- A *salpingostomy* is a procedure during which the fallopian tube is cut open at its fimbrial end to remove blockages or damaged tissue.

- A *fimbrioplasty* corrects damaged fimbria.
- A *reanastomosis* reattaches two sections of a tube that has been cut apart.
- A *tubal reimplantation* detaches the tube from the uterus and then re-inserts it through the uterine wall.

There is one exception to the rule of surgery to correct tubal problems. If you are fortunate enough to have your blockage within the proximal portion of your tube, a nonsurgical procedure called a tubal catheterization may clear away certain types of these obstructions.

As you and your doctor discuss your possible surgery, there are several things you should keep in mind. You should discuss the possibility of serious complications—such as tubal (or ectopic) pregnancy—occurring after your surgery, particularly if your tubes are badly damaged (we'll go into this in greater detail later in the chapter). You should also keep in mind that your surgery's chance for success depends on the extent of your tubal damage, the type of surgery you are having, and the talents and experience of your surgeon. And finally, you should be aware that if tubal surgery is recommended, your choice of procedure and of surgeon is of the utmost importance. *Tubal surgeries are tried only once.* Pregnancy rates are so low for repeated surgical repairs, they are rarely performed a second time.

During your discussions with your doctor, he may tell you that in your case, surgical repair isn't recommended. This could happen if your tubal disease has caused too much damage, or if your risk of ectopic pregnancy following surgery would be too high. Don't despair; you haven't necessarily reached a dead end. In some cases, a procedure can be performed that produces successful pregnancies through totally by-passing tubal function.

TREATING A PROXIMAL OBSTRUCTION

If during the HSG your doctor identifies a tubal blockage in the proximal area (the section where the tube connects to the uterus), he will first confirm that it truly is an obstruction, not just a muscular spasm of the uterine wall. Sometimes a laparoscopy is the only way to make this differentiation.

As we said before, if you are lucky enough to have your blockage in the proximal portion of your tube, there is a new nonsurgical technique that might possibly correct it. Tubal catheterization has come of age since the early nineties. It has proven itself to be a successful treatment for certain types of proximal obstruction—those in which the blockage is formed by protein building up and clogging the tube's small opening, rather than by actual tissue destruction.

A tubal catheterization is done at the same time the radiologist gives you your HSG. Using a series of small guide wires, he moves catheters up through your uterine cavity and into your fallopian tube. He then flushes fluid through the catheters into the blocked portion of the tube, in hopes of pushing the blockage out. If the tube is closed because of severe scarring, this catheterization will be of no benefit. But for 40% to 50% of women with proximal obstruction, the use of this type of catheterization—also known as *transcervical cannulation*—corrects the problem. If it doesn't, a surgical alternative may then be attempted.

Whether or not it will be, depends on the next step in your diagnosis. If you have a proximal blockage and the dye in your HSG stops before it enters your tubes, your doctor has no way to tell from this test what your tubes look like. Because of this, if a catheterization fails to open the tube, your doctor will then perform a laparoscopy and look at the exterior of the tube before he decides how to proceed. Sometimes he will see that the rest of the tube appears normal, and he will attempt to correct your proximal block surgically, with an operation called a proximal tubal resection and reanastomosis. But if your tube also appears to be blocked at its fimbrial end or ampullary portion, that option won't be available.

PROXIMAL TUBAL RESECTION AND REANASTOMOSIS

If your proximal block isn't caused by protein buildup, you most likely have salpingitis isthmica nodosa. Because SIN does such a good job of destroying tubal tissue, your doctor will have to correct it by first cutting out the affected tissue, and then reattaching what remains of the tube to your uterus. The portion of the operation during which he removes a part of your tube is called a "resection." The portion during which he reconnects it to the uterus is known as a "direct reanastomosis." (See Figure 8-9.)

In some cases of proximal obstruction a reconnection (reanastomosis) cannot be performed because the tube, on the uterine side, is destroyed. In this situation, a reimplantation or reinsertion of the tube through a different part of the uterine wall is done. (See Figure 8-10.)

Tubal resection and reanastomosis is relatively successful, averaging about 50% pregnancy rate, with less than a 10% risk that the pregnancy will be ectopic. But since it can be done only through a surgical incision, you should anticipate that you will experience the same postoperative events that you would have with a laparotomy myomectomy. As with any

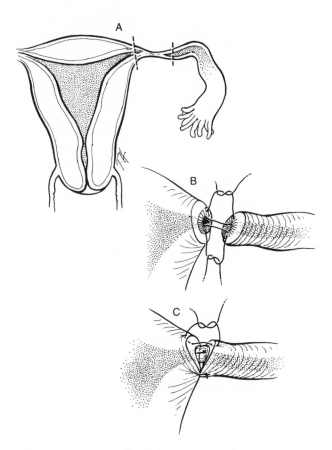

Figure 8-9:   Proximal Tubal Resection and Reanastomosis

type of abdominal surgery, you will achieve your best results if your doctor is an experienced microsurgeon who has worked on a number of similar cases.

In some cases, reanastomosis won't be successful. If the damaged area in the tube is extensive, there may not be enough tube remaining after it is removed for your doctor to be able to reattach it. In these cases, in vitro fertilization becomes the treatment of choice. It's the least invasive approach, and offers the highest pregnancy rate. We will be discussing it in detail in our chapter on assisted reproduction (Chapter Twelve).

TREATING BIPOLAR DISEASE

When your doctor performs your laparoscopy, and he sees that your fallopian tube is blocked at both ends, you have a condition that is

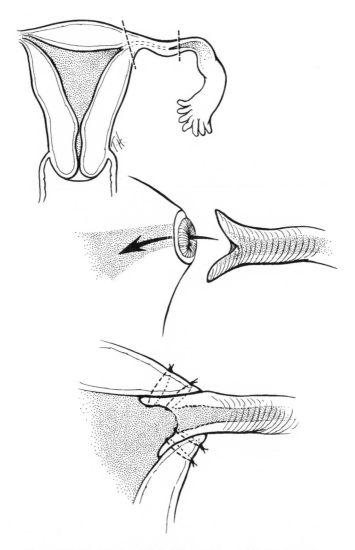

Figure 8-10: Proximal Tubal Resection and Reimplantation

known as bipolar disease. Prior to the advent of in vitro fertilization, doctors tried to correct bipolar disease surgically. This proved very difficult to do. Because so much of a tube is damaged when it has problems at both ends, corrective tubal surgery offered only a 5% chance that a pregnancy would result. In addition, there was a high probability that the pregnancy would prove to be ectopic.

Today, if your tube is blocked at both ends, your doctor will move in the direction of in vitro fertilization, rather than operating on your tube.

Because IVF bypasses the tube, it offers a true alternative for fertility enhancement in these cases.

TREATING DISTAL TUBAL BLOCKAGES

If, during your laparoscopy, your doctor sees a blockage in the distal portion of your tube—the widened portion that leads toward its fimbrial end—you may be facing a difficult decision. For the most part, if you have a distal tubal obstruction, but your hydrosalpinx is less than two centimeters in diameter and your endothelium (tubal lining) is still present, your surgeon will try to reconstruct your fallopian tube surgically. He should perform this surgery as part of the same laparoscopic procedure.

But if your doctor sees during your exploratory laparoscopy that your hydrosalpinx is greater than two centimeters, and if there is no evidence that your endothelial lining is still present, he will probably tell you that in vitro fertilization would offer you a better chance of success. Once this becomes obvious, many women have to make a choice. Most couples facing extensive tubal damage have insurance coverage for tubal surgery, but none for in vitro fertilization. Unfortunately, while surgical correction is covered by their medical insurance, it may not offer them their highest chance for a successful pregnancy. Yet often they can't afford IVF, so surgical correction is chosen, even though it may not be the better medical alternative. The rational behind this is that even if it's probably going to be ineffective, surgery is the only hope these couples have for increasing their chances, so they might as well try it. Because such financial concerns can, unfortunately, outweigh the best medical principles, you should make sure you're familiar with the limitations of your health insurance policy *before* you embark on your diagnostic procedures.

If you do opt for surgery—either because your hydrosalpinx is a correctable size, or because it's the only option financially available to you, your doctor will normally attempt only one surgical repair. This is because, like other tubal surgeries, repeated operations to correct distal obstructions have very low success rates. The surgical method your doctor should use is laparoscopy. He'll introduce microsurgical tools, probably a laser, through the laparoscope and use them to open the hydrosalpinx. (See Figure 8-11.)

This approach has been standard since the mid-eighties. Prior to the use of laser laparoscopy, doctors performed abdominal surgery to correct distal tubal correction. But since that is a more invasive procedure, and one that can create new scarring problems as a consequence, it is no longer chosen.

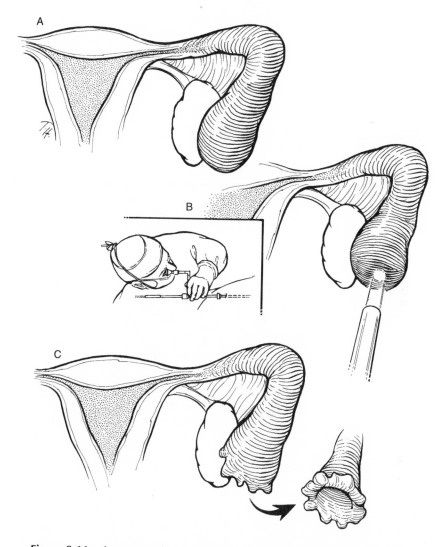

Figure 8-11: Laparoscopic Laser Surgery for Correction of Hydrosalpinx

The expected outcome for surgical correction of distal tubal obstruction can be very positive, but the possibility of complications is also high.
After surgery, you will have approximately a 25% chance of conceiving
safely. But depending on the size and severity of the damage to your
fallopian tube, and effectiveness of its correction, you will also face a risk
of ectopic pregnancy running anywhere from 15% to 50%. That is why in
women with extensive tubal damage who have a low chance of becoming
pregnant, and a high risk of it being ectopic once they do, surgical attempts to correct the fallopian tubes are not performed. They would

yield only a bad outcome—either a naturally occurring reclosure of the tubes, or an ectopic pregnancy. If you wish to go forward with infertility treatment, this is another case where in vitro fertilization becomes the only option. If the fimbria are stuck together, but the tube is not closed as in a hydrosalpinx, a fimbrioplasty is performed. Using the laparoscope, the surgeon merely separates the fimbria. The success rate with this procedure is normally very good, running 60% to 70%.

REVERSING A TUBAL STERILIZATION

About 10% of women who've asked for a tubal sterilization later change their minds. When they do, a microsurgical tubal reanastomosis is performed to reconnect their fallopian tubes. This type of tubal surgery is extremely successful in the hands of an experienced reproductive surgeon who does the procedure regularly. It can produce good results no matter which part of your tube was cut—close to the uterus, in the midportion of the tube, or toward the end of the tube. The critical factor is the overall length of fallopian tube that remains after the surgical correction is completed. In many cases, the previous surgeon removed more of the tube than is actually necessary to prevent pregnancy. This is the biggest problem a surgeon encounters in reestablishing fertility.

If only a moderate amount of the tube was removed, and the resulting fallopian tube after reanastomosis is at least five centimeters in total length, the surgical outcome is optimal, with an approximate pregnancy rate of 80%. This is especially true if the sterilization was performed in the middle portion of the tube, which is the most common situation. (See Figure 8-12A.) If, on the other hand, the fallopian tube has to be reconnected to the uterus, then the success rate drops to 50% to 60%. (See Figure 8-12B.) If the tubal ligation was done near the fimbrial end of the tube, the approximate pregnancy rate after surgery drops to 40%. (See Figure 8-12C.) In cases where the length of the tube would be less than five centimeters when reanastomosis is complete, in vitro fertilization offers a better pregnancy chance than surgery.

You may feel these percentages are rather high, but in fact they are accurate representations of your chances for pregnancy if you chose the right reproductive microsurgeon. The Society for Reproductive Surgeons, which can be found through the American Society for Reproductive Medicine, is one way to locate and check references when making your choice. Once you are in the hands of a skilled physician, you should be extremely hopeful.

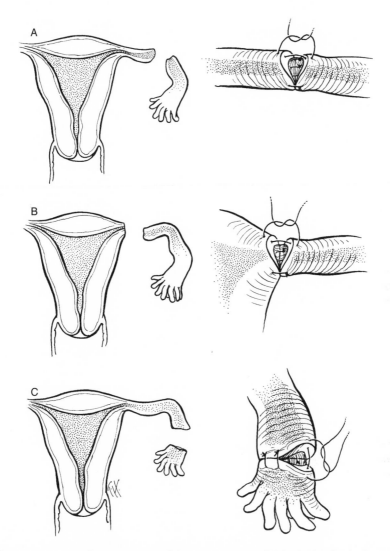

Figure 8-12:   Sterilization Reversal (Reanastomosis of Tubes) A) Isthmic Reversal
B) Corneal Reversal C) Ampullary Reversal

Complications with Tubal Surgery

One thing that you need to keep in mind, if you're having tubal surgery, is that even if your surgery is successful, your chances of having an ectopic pregnancy will increase. An ectopic pregnancy is one in which the egg is fertilized, but instead of traveling into the uterus to implant, it gets caught at some point within the fallopian tube and begins to grow and develop there.

Ectopic pregnancies occur in 0.5% of pregnancies for *all* woman of reproductive age. Woman who are infertile, even those who have nothing obviously wrong with their fallopian tubes, have a 2% risk of an ectopic pregnancy. And women who have a history of tubal damage caused by pelvic inflammatory disease, tubal surgery, or pelvic surgery have the highest risk—a 5% to 40% chance of ectopic pregnancy—depending on the cause and on the extent of damage to their tubes. Women with a history of DES exposure form another subgroup. Abnormalities in their uterine cavity, or in the length of their tubes, can affect the functioning of the tubes to such an extent that they have a 5% to 10% risk of ectopic pregnancy.

As high as these percentages seem, the risk of ectopic pregnancies used to be even greater before microsurgical techniques began to be commonly used. Large instruments and standard suturing material could create obstacles in tubes whose interior is sometimes no bigger than a pinpoint. Microsurgery, in which cutting is done more specifically, and suture material may be as thin as a hair, has helped to reduce the possibilities of that sort of blockage to some degree. Still, the increased risk of an ectopic pregnancy is one thing you should take into consideration if you are asked to make a decision between tubal surgery and simply bypassing the tubes by using in vitro fertilization.

Ectopic pregnancies can be very confusing from a clinical standpoint. A woman can become pregnant and have no apparent difficulty during the first six weeks of her pregnancy. It's not until she begins having either abnormal bleeding or pain that she seeks the advice of her obstetrician. The unfortunate aspect of this is that ectopic pregnancies, when diagnosed early, can easily be removed with a laparoscope. But when they are not detected, ectopic pregnancies can be life threatening. As the tubal pregnancy grows, it eventually causes the tube to rupture, and bleeding begins internally. Woman still die every year in this country because tubal pregnancies are not diagnosed properly. And since any woman who is an infertility patient is at a higher risk for an ectopic pregnancy, we advise that if you are in this category, you have early pregnancy testing for this condition.

Early testing means that your doctor should begin checking your hCG levels through blood tests during the first four weeks of pregnancy. Early testing of hCG levels will sometimes indicate an abnormal pattern, which will give your doctor his first clue that there is something wrong with your pregnancy. In a normal pregnancy hCG will start out at a level of anywhere from 25 to 100 mIU, per milliliter, and will begin to double every two to two and a half days throughout the first six to eight weeks of pregnancy.

If this doubling pattern falls off, your doctor will interpret this as an indication that your pregnancy may be abnormal. One possibility is that the fetus is developing in the fallopian tube, instead of in the uterus. If he suspects this, your doctor will try to confirm it by doing a transvaginal ultrasound. Once your hCG level has reached 1,800 to 2,000 mIU per milliliter, a pregnancy sac should be visible inside the uterine cavity during an ultrasound. If there's no sac inside the uterine cavity, and your hCG continues to rise, your doctor will then examine your fallopian tubes with ultrasound to see if he can find a sac in one of them. In cases where he locates a sac within one of the tubes—as well as in cases where none is visible, yet hCG continues to rise—he will terminate the pregnancy in one of two ways.

Tubal pregnancies that are diagnosed early enough—before the fetus is three centimeters in diameter, or before a woman's hCG level exceeds 7,500 mIU per milliliter—can be terminated with a drug called methotrexate. Methotrexate is a form of chemotherapy that attacks placental cells and causes a pregnancy to be reabsorbed. If it is given early enough, termination by methotrexate is usually successful. Methotrexate is administered through a single injection, and usually has no significant side effects.

In cases where the ectopic pregnancy is too large to be treated by methotrexate, a physician will most often choose to remove the pregnancy through laparoscopic surgery. Using the laparoscope, he will simply open the fallopian tube and remove the ectopic pregnancy. This allows the fallopian tube to remain intact. If the tube has not been severely damaged, it will heal itself once the tubal pregnancy is removed. But if the fallopian tube has been significantly damaged, or if the ectopic pregnancy has ruptured the tube, it will have to be surgically removed during the laparoscopic procedure. (See Figure 8-13.)

Surprisingly, whether the fallopian tube is left intact and heals properly, or whether it is removed, doesn't seem to matter. With either scenario—assuming a woman's remaining fallopian tube appears normal, if she does have one tube removed—the overall chance that she will become pregnant again is about 40%. And her risk of having another ectopic pregnancy ranges between 15% and 18%, whether she has one tube remaining or two. Since removing a tube doesn't seem to change a woman's risks or benefits, the decision whether or not to do so should be based solely on how damaged the tube appears to be.

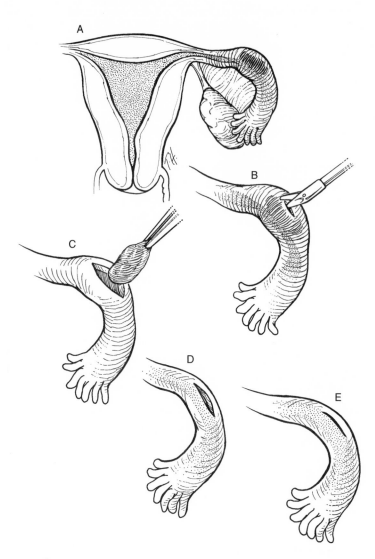

Figure 8-13: Laparoscopic Removal of Ectopic Pregnancy

Getting Ready for Surgery

Since abnormalities of the uterus and the fallopian tubes can be so detrimental to conception and to carrying a pregnancy normally, it's reassuring to know that so many of them can be corrected. But if you're facing a problem that falls into this area, you're probably also facing surgery. We've discussed in other chapters, as well as in this one, how important your choice of a surgeon can be. But even when you do choose carefully, and even if you have taken the time to understand what your doctor's findings mean and how they impact your options, a moment may still arrive when you feel that you are losing control of your situation.

Even the most levelheaded among us can grow anxious as we drive toward a hospital on our way toward inpatient surgery, a trip you may have to face if you have a tubal or uterine problem. So it's nice to know that there are some things you can do to ease your fears.

1. Be sure that your doctor has fully explained your surgical procedure to you ahead of time. He should have told you exactly what he will be doing, how long it will take, and when you will be released from the hospital.

2. Find out when your doctor will be there, and who you should direct your questions to when he isn't.

3. Find out ahead of time what medications you will be taking, and what side effects you can expect. And if something gets changed in your medication or treatment, don't hesitate to ask nurses or doctors why.

4. Call ahead of time to see if the hospital you're going to has a patient representative who is there to answer questions and resolve complaints. If so, have that person's name with you.

5. Ask your hospital if they adhere to the "Patient's Bill of Rights," which was drawn up by the American Hospital Association. If so, get a copy and read it.

Above all, remember that unlike some types of surgery, yours is a positive thing . . . a passing step along the road to what you want most in the world.

A Layman's Guide
to Uterine and Tubal Surgery

Endoscopic procedures	Endoscopic procedures use a telescope to allow the surgeon to enter the body without cutting through the skin. They can be used either for diagnosis or for correcting problems that are found.
Laparoscopy	The telescope is inserted through a small incision in the abdomen at the umbilicus.
Hysteroscopy	The telescope is inserted through the vagina and cervix into the uterus.
Resectoscopy	Like hysteroscopy, but is used to remove tissue (fibroids, etc.).
Laparotomy	Any surgery in which the doctor cuts through the abdominal wall.
Microsurgery	A technique in which very small cutting instruments and very small suturing materials are used. Can be applied to almost any type of surgery.
Uterine Surgeries	
Myomectomy	Removal of fibrous growths from the uterine walls. Depending on the location, can be done either as hysteroscopy or as laparotomy.
D&C	Dilatation and curettage. A surgery in which the inner walls of the uterus are scraped clean.
Cerclage	An operation in which the cervix is temporarily surgically closed in order to delay the onset of labor.
Tubal surgeries	
Tubal ligation	When a surgeon cuts and ties the tubes and ties the sections closed to prevent pregnancy.
Tubal resection	Cuts out a portion of a tube to remove blockages or damaged portions.
Tubal reanastomosis	Reconnects cut sections of a tube.
Salpingostomy	Removes blockages or areas of damaged tissue from the tubes.
Fimbrioplasty	Corrects damaged fimbria at the end of a tube.
Transcervical cannulization	Another term for a tubal catheterization.

Tubal catheterization	A nonsurgical procedure that tries to remove blockages from the proximal segment of a tube by flushing it with fluid.
Proximal tubal resection	Cuts out damaged portion of a tube that connects to the uterus, then reattaches the remaining tube.

Terms We Used in This Chapter

Adenomyosis: a condition in which the cells of the uterine lining (endometrium) invade the muscle of the uterine wall. This is similar to endometriosis, which is found on surfaces of the pelvic organs.

Ampullary: the outer or distal end of the fallopian tube. It is also the widest part of the fallopian tube.

Asherman's syndrome: a condition where scar tissue forms in the uterine cavity which interferes with normal uterine lining development. Usually this is associated with the loss of the menstrual period following a D&C.

Bicornuate uterus: a malformation of the uterus resulting in two separate cavities, each with a connecting fallopian tube.

Bipolar disease: blockage at both ends of the fallopian tube.

Chlamydia: a bacteria that is considered to be sexually transmitted, which may be an underlying cause of infertility.

Cilia: the hairlike projections inside the fallopian tubes that move the egg and/or embryo toward the uterus.

Congenital abnormality: a malformation that takes place during fetal development.

Diethylstilbestrol (DES):   a man-made estrogen originally used to prevent miscarriages. Is known to cause abnormalities of the cervix, vagina, and uterus of the unborn fetus.

Dilatation and curettage (D&C):   opening the cervix and removing the contents of the uterine cavity by scraping or suction.

Ectopic pregnancy: a pregnancy (embryo) that implants outside the uterine cavity. Most commonly this occurs in the fallopian tube, but can occur in the ovary or abdominal cavity.

Endometrial polyps: an overgrowth of normal endometrial tissue, forming a protrusion into the uterine cavity.

Endometrium: the lining of cells inside the uterus that is sensitive to estrogen and progesterone stimulation.

Endoscopic procedure: procedures such as laparoscopy or hysteroscopy in which a lighted telescope is used to see inside an organ (i.e., uterus) or body cavity (i.e., pelvis).

Estrogen: a category of female hormone that is necessary for female characteristics.

Fibroids: a benign tumor made up of fibrous tissues found in the uterus.

Fimbria: fingerlike projections on the end of the fallopian tube that pick up the egg after ovulation.

Fimbrioplasty: a surgical procedure to reconstruct the fingerlike projections on the end of the fallopian tube.

Follicle: a small fluid-filled sac contained within the ovary that prepares the egg for ovulation. The follicle is also the estrogen production factory in the female.

Gonorrhea: a sexually transmitted bacterial infection that can cause tubal damage in the male and the female.

Hydrosalpinx: closure of the fallopian tube at the fimbriated end, which results in a fluid-filled saclike structure.

Hysteroscopy: a surgical procedure that uses a small telescope placed through the cervical canal to view the interior of the uterine cavity.

Hysterosalpingogram (HSG): an X-ray study in which a dye visible by fluoroscopy is injected into the uterine cavity to determine the shape of the uterus and patency of the fallopian tubes.

Interstitial: the portion of the fallopian tube that travels through the muscular wall of the uterus to connect the endometrial cavity to the fallopian tube.

Intramural: any structure within the wall of another structure, i.e., intramural fibroids.

Intrauterine device (IUD): a small, inert, usually plastic device placed in the uterine cavity to block implantation of an embryo.

Isthmus: the most muscular part of the fallopian tube; the isthmus is connected directly to the uterus.

Laparoscopy: a surgical procedure in which a telescope is inserted through the abdominal wall to view the inner organs.

Laparotomy: a surgical procedure in which an incision is made through the abdominal wall in order to view the inner organs.

Luteal phase: the second half of the menstrual cycle; the luteal phase begins with ovulation, and is characterized by elevated levels of estrogen and progesterone.

Luteal phase defect: inadequate production of hormone from the corpus luteum, or poor response of the endometrial lining to hormonal stimulation, which interferes with implantation.

Methotrexate: a chemotherapy agent that destroys placental cells. Commonly used for the treatment of early ectopic pregnancies.

Müllerian ducts: the fetal structures that fuse to form the uterus.

Myomectomy: the surgical removal of fibroids (myomas) from the uterine body.

Myometrium: the muscular wall of the uterus.

Pelvic inflammatory disease (PID): infection or inflammation of the female reproductive organs, usually caused by a sexually transmitted disease.

Physiologic levels: hormonal levels that are identical to those produced naturally by a person's system.

Proximal (or corneal) block: obstruction of the fallopian tube at the junction of the tube and the uterus.

Reanastomosis: reconnection of a tubular structure such as the fallopian tube.

Rokitansky syndrome: the congenital absence of the uterus.

Salpingitis: inflammation of the fallopian tubes.

Salpingostomy: a surgical procedure where an opening is made in the fallopian tube either to alleviate an obstruction or remove a tubal pregnancy.

Septate uterus: a fibrous division of the uterine cavity.

Sexually transmitted disease (STD): a disease or organism that can be transmitted by sexual contact.

Submucosal: immediately beneath the endometrial layer of the uterus.

Subserosal: immediately below the silky outer lining of the uterus or other pelvic structures.

Ultrasound: an instrument that emits pulsed sound waves, which are reflected off solid tissues, to give an image of internal body structures without the use of X ray.

Uterine didelphys: duplication of the uterus; a double uterus.

Uterine fibroid: a benign tumor commonly found in the uterine muscle.

Wolffian ducts: the embryonic structure that forms into the fallopian tubes during fetal development.

9

Male Factor Problems and Solutions

Many men are disappointed when they find that a lifetime's supply of condoms was wasted. If you're among this disillusioned throng, you should take heart from the fact that progress in finding solutions to male infertility problems is being made at an incredible rate. Years ago, not much could be done for infertile men, other than bringing sperm closer to the egg through artificial insemination procedures. Today, men who can't even ejaculate, or who manufacture as few as fifty sperm, are able to fertilize their partner's eggs—with the help of laboratory technology—and father their own biological children. So if your doctor has told you that you have a male factor problem, don't despair. Instead, spend your energy locating a sophisticated practitioner who can accurately diagnose your problem, and help you to work around it.

━━━━━ MOST OFTEN ASKED QUESTIONS ━━━━━

Q: Does it matter what kind of underwear I wear?
A: *Probably not. But why not wear boxers just in case?*
Q: Does masturbation affect fertility?
A: *Only if it's done prior to intercourse or insemination, and it decreases sperm count.*
Q: What about lubrication with intercourse?
A: *No problem, as long as you don't use petroleum-based lubricants.*
Q: How frequently should I have intercourse?
A: *Daily, around ovulation.*

Finding Your Problem

As you know from reading our chapter on the basic workup, about 40% of infertile couples have problems related to sperm abnormalities. Since most of these problems can be detected by a routine semen analysis, they are normally identified early on in the diagnostic process. If your semen analysis demonstrated abnormalities in your sperm number, movement, or structure, you'll need to move on to a more extensive evaluation, which will locate the underlying cause of those abnormalities.

"I stood accused of manufacturing a brat pack of lazy sperm, layabout lads with minimalist tendencies and a lethargic bio-attitude. Disciplinary action was prescribed: I must sacrifice my beloved hot baths to the elusive future, wear boxer shorts like television dads do, ingest large doses of vitamins B and C to compensate for smoking. After ten days of ball-coddling and three more of restless chastity, I was ordered to have at it again with another peanut-butter jar."

Domesticity *by Bob Shacochis*
Copyright © 1994 by Bob Shacochis
Excerpt reprinted by permission of
Brandt and Brandt Literary Agents, Inc.

Normally, this means going to another doctor. For the most part, reproductive endocrinologists aren't well-enough versed in male disorders to be able to perform a complete diagnosis, or to treat the abnormalities that render some men infertile. So your reproductive endocrinologist will usually refer you to a urologic specialist. Be advised that this is not just any urologist. Just as most gynecologists don't have the necessary training to perform sophisticated infertility testing and treatment, most urologists don't have specific knowledge and experience in the diagnosis and treatment of male infertility. Your reproductive endocrinologist should be able to refer you to a subspecialist who has the required detailed knowledge in this urologic subspecialty.

Once you've interviewed specialists and decided on the one with whom you feel most comfortable, the two of you will go to work to find the source of your problem. The doctor will:

1. Take a medical history. In particular, he will be looking for a history of undescended testicle, postpubertal mumps, venereal

disease or other infections, illnesses with high fever, diabetes, liver disease, testicular trauma, or testicular surgery.

2. Do a physical examination, to rule out testicular or prostatic abnormalities and presence of a varicocele.

3. Do the types of sperm testing that we described in the basic workup chapter, for example: CASA, hamster test, in vitro mucus penetration test, electron microscopy, and hemizona assay test. This part of the urologic workup is similar to what a reproductive endocrinologist does when exploring male factor problems.

4. Do a testicular biopsy, if your sperm numbers are extremely low. A biopsy can determine whether you have a blockage, a maturation arrest pattern, hypospermatogenesis, or germinal cell aplasia. A testicular biopsy can be done under either a general or local anesthetic, and is considered to be minor surgery.

5. Do a routine test of hormonal levels: LH, FSH, prolactin, and testosterone.

By the time you've finished these tests, your urologist should have a very definite idea of what's causing your infertility problem. It will probably fall into one of three areas:

• Hormonal abnormalities

• Structural abnormalities

• Unexplained—or "idiopathic"—abnormalities

HORMONAL ABNORMALITIES

Although hormonal abnormalities are rarely the primary factor in male infertility—affecting only about 5% of men with problems—they cannot be entirely ignored. Hormonal abnormalities are detected both in men and women by looking at how their endocrine axis—the interchange of signals and responses between their hypothalamus, pituitary gland, and gonads—is functioning. For a woman this means testing the levels of the various hormones that are produced by her hypothalamus and pituitary, and then seeing how her ovaries respond to them. For a man it means analyzing the same factors as they relate to his hypothalamus, pituitary, and testicles.

In men and women both, a blood test will sometimes reveal that the level of a particular reproductive hormone is too high or too low. In a woman, this can cause problems with ovulation or implantation. In a man, it can interfere with his ability to manufacture sperm.

How Male Hormones Work

The hypothalamus and the pituitary gland control male gonadal function, just as they control ovarian function in the female. When pulses of GnRH are released from the hypothalamus, they trigger the production of FSH and LH in the pituitary. This FSH and LH, in turn, stimulates cells in the testes called the Leydig cells and the Sertoli cells, each of which influences sperm production and development in different ways.

The Leydig cells are the structures within a man's testes that produce testosterone. Without testosterone male physical and secondary sexual characteristics would be absent. The Leydig cells manufacture testosterone whenever they are stimulated by a release of LH. This testosterone is partially involved in normal sperm production. However, in order for the Leydig cells to receive these LH signals, they must first have developed mature "receptors." The formation of these LH receptors is regulated by the release of FSH from the pituitary.

FSH also influences the Sertoli cells, which line the seminiferous tubules. Each Sertoli cell is intended to support and nurture a single sperm as it grows. FSH stimulates the Sertoli cells to manufacture the raw materials that are necessary for the sperm cells to mature. Absent this cue from FSH, the sperm cells wouldn't receive nutrients, and would wither and die.

As you can see, it is the correctly timed release of FSH and LH, as well as the appropriate balance between them, that leads to good sperm development. That's why a full evaluation of your FSH and LH levels should be done if you have a male factor problem. Your doctor should also test the levels of some of your other hormones—thyroid hormone and prolactin, for example—both of which can influence the production and effectiveness of FSH and LH. He'll know that your hormonal balance is off if your blood test indicates:

- an abnormally high or low level of FSH and/or LH.
- an abnormally low level of testosterone.
- an abnormally high level of prolactin.

Fixing Hormonal Problems

A number of urologists and reproductive endocrinologists routinely try to correct male problems using the same drugs—clomiphene citrate, human menopausal gonadotropin, and FSH—that have proved to be so successful in regulating ovulation in infertile women. But while nearly all of the studies that have been performed over the years evaluating the efficacy of these hormonal treatments in the male have shown anecdotal improvement, *controlled studies have shown no significant benefit.* One explanation for this discrepancy may be the fact that sperm levels can show great variation naturally. When patients are studied for a short time, these natural changes in sperm levels can be misinterpreted by doctors as attributable to hormone therapy. But when long-range studies are done, the temporary nature of these increases is revealed. Since hormone treatments involve both expense and some side effects, such as weight gain and aggressive behavior, you should question your doctor carefully if he wants to use them. He should be able to give you a good explanation of why he's recommending drug therapy: some doctors routinely use it on men with low sperm counts, even when endocrine parameters are normal. He should also give you a projection of exactly what he thinks their effects will be. This dialogue can be very helpful to you in making your decision. There *are* a few situations in which drug therapy has been shown to be helpful, and you might fall into one of them.

For example, a patient who is deficient in FSH or LH can often benefit from therapy to increase their levels of these hormones. This may take any one of several forms:

- Men with mildly reduced levels of FSH and LH may be suffering from an abnormality in pituitary function. Taking 25 to 50 mg of clomiphene citrate on a constant basis can sometimes improve pituitary release of LH and FSH, and in turn produce higher sperm production. Clomiphene citrate will be prescribed on either a daily or an alternate day basis.

- More severe deficiencies of FSH, or of FSH and LH, can be treated either with 150 IU of Metrodin taken three times a week, or with 150 IU of Pergonal taken three times a week. If this is continued for three to six months, in some cases it will reestablish normal testicular function and sperm production.

- Occasionally, the use of hCG injected on a twice-weekly basis will help to elevate Leydig cell production of testosterone, which in turn may increase production of sperm from the testicles. Since hCG is a long-acting form of LH, it gives tonic stimulation to the Leydig cells.

Another situation in which drug therapy can prove effective occurs when a man has hypothyroidism, or a pituitary tumor. These conditions can cause his level of the hormone prolactin to become elevated. In women, excess prolactin interferes with ovulation. In men, it can interfere with LH activity in the Leydig cells, which in turn slows the production of testosterone and interferes with sperm production. If you have this problem, your doctor may find the use of Parlodel to reduce your prolactin level to be beneficial.

While some men who have abnormally low FSH or LH production may benefit from these replacement therapies, treatment with gonadotropins or clomiphene is fruitless for patients who have elevated FSH and LH. High levels of these hormones indicate testicular failure, in the same way that they indicate ovarian failure when found in a woman. The high levels come about because the man's pituitary never detects any testosterone or inhibin in his system. Testosterone is the male hormone produced by the testes, while inhibin is a protein made by testicular cells and regulates pituitary FSH release. Thus his pituitary continues to pump out FSH and LH in the hopes of triggering the production of these missing hormones. No amount of gonadotropin stimulation will cause resumption of ovulation in the female with ovarian failure, nor will it stimulate sperm production in men who have testicular failure due to trauma or to end-stage infection.

While we've spelled out some exceptions to the rule, you should keep in mind that for the most part, your doctor's ability to improve your semen parameters by using hormones is very limited, if not nonexistent. If your hormone levels seem to be normal, and your doctor is recommending hormone treatment on an experimental basis, you're better off avoiding it.

STRUCTURAL ABNORMALITIES

When your urologist gives you a physical examination, he will be looking for both congenital structural abnormalities and abnormalities that might have developed subsequent to birth. Since there are a number of physical abnormalities that can contribute to male infertility, this physical examination is extremely important.

For the most part, men with anatomic abnormalities of any type can now produce pregnancies. In some cases their conditions can be corrected surgically, to make sperm production and ejaculation normal. Failing that, sperm that are produced within the testicles can be removed from their storage area in the epididymis, and used either for in vitro fertilization or intrauterine insemination.

Congenital Structural Abnormalities

The abnormalities a man can be born with include:

- Hypospadia
- Congenital absence of the vas deferens
- Cryptorchidism (undescended testicles)
- Kallmann's syndrome
- Klinefelter's syndrome

Hypospadia   Hypospadia is a condition in which the opening of the urethra is on the underside of the penis, instead of on its end. While it is occasionally the cause of infertility, it is a relatively rare condition, affecting just 5% to 10% of men with fertility problems. Hypospadia can sometimes go unnoticed by the layman, but it is easily detected by a urologist when he does a thorough inspection of the external genitalia. In fact, if a man has hypospadia, it may well have been discovered during routine physical exams before he reached adolescence.

Because the opening of the urethra is farther up on the shaft of the penis in a man with hypospadia, he can't deposit his sperm as high in the vagina as he would if he had a normal urethral opening. This can make the migration of the sperm through the cervical mucus and into the uterine cavity and fallopian tubes longer and more difficult, and sometimes even impossible.

Mild or moderate hypospadias can usually be corrected surgically. In more severe cases of hypospadia, surgery is not an option. In these cases, intrauterine insemination is the clinical alternative. (See Figure 9-1.)

Congenital Absence of the Vas Deferens   Another relatively rare condition that is sometimes found in infertility situations is a congenital absence of the ejaculatory duct, or vas deferens. In this very small percentage of males, approximately 1% to 2% of men with reproductive problems, testicular function is normal, but since the vas deferens didn't form during the development of the reproductive system, it is as if these men have had a complete vasectomy.

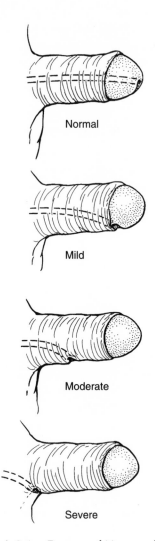

Figure 9-1:   Degrees of Hypospadia

If you have this condition, your doctor can still help you to produce a pregnancy by collecting sperm from your epididymis, and then using these sperm cells for in vitro fertilization. This process will be described in our chapter on assisted reproductive technologies (Chapter Twelve).

Other Congenital Conditions   A variety of other congenital conditions can also affect normal testicular function. Cryptorchidism (or undescended testicles), Kallmann's syndrome, and Klinefelter's syndrome are just a few. Some of these congenital abnormalities can be corrected, others cannot.

For example, Klinefelter's syndrome is a genetic abnormality in which a man is born with an extra X chromosome. Instead of the typical male 46XY karyotype, the man with Klinefelter's has a 47XXY karyotype. The extra X chromosome makes him sterile, and no treatment can correct his condition.

Unlike the genetic abnormality described above, some congenital problems are potentially correctable. In cryptorchidism, a condition in which a male infant is born with undescended testicles, timely correction is of the essence. If the testicles stay inside the abdomen for too long, the higher interior body temperature can damage the seminiferous tubules and other testicular tissues. Because of that, surgical treatment should be done as soon as this condition is discovered. And even if prompt surgical placement of the testicles into the scrotal sac is performed, many times enough damage has already been done that infertility is still present later in life.

Hormonal abnormalities, such as Kallmann's syndrome, are another type of congenital problem that can cause male infertility. In Kallmann's, a man's hypothalamus doesn't produce and release gonadotropin-releasing hormone (GnRH). The resulting condition is similar to hypothalamic pituitary failure in a woman. Hypothalamic pituitary failure can halt a woman's ovulation, even though her ovaries are normal. When GnRH is lacking in men, they don't manufacture sperm, and they have poor development of secondary sexual characteristics due to a lack of testosterone. Happily, Kallmann's is correctable with drugs. HCG can stimulate testicular production of testosterone, which will give the patient normal secondary sexual characteristics. And in order for sperm production to take place, treatment with FSH, or with FSH/LH (Pergonal) will be given. Using this two-pronged approach, men with Kallmann's can become fertile and have children.

Structural, or Functional, Abnormalities

During your examination, your doctor may also find that you have developed some structural abnormalities. These might include:

- Retrograde ejaculation

- Varicocele

- Blockages

- Vasectomy

Retrograde Ejaculation   While a small number of congenital conditions can affect ejaculation, physically based ejaculation problems are much more commonly found in males with neurologic difficulties, or with a history of diabetes or prostate surgery. Because these medical conditions sometimes weaken the nerves that close down the bladder's sphincter, they can cause men to have retrograde ejaculation. Retrograde ejaculation occurs when seminal fluid comes down through the ejaculatory duct normally, but instead of flowing forward through the urethra and then out the end of the penis, it flows backward into the bladder. Men with retrograde ejaculation can produce adequate seminal fluid and can have an orgasm, but little or no ejaculatory fluid will actually leave the penis.

There are several physical signs that can lead the doctor to suspect that a man experiences retrograde ejaculation. He will look at it as a possibility if there is a very small amount of semen, but a good sperm count. Or if there's a milky look to the urine when the man voids after an orgasm. Once the physician suspects retrograde ejaculation, he can easily confirm his diagnosis by testing the urine after an ejaculation for the presence of sperm.

Happily, if a man does experience retrograde ejaculation, the treatment is relatively simple. The urologist will place the individual on oral alkaline agents for three to four days prior to sperm collection. These agents will cause the urine to become less acidic. Once this is accomplished, the sperm cells will find themselves in a balanced acid/base solution when they enter the urine in the bladder. Because the urine is less acidic, it won't destroy them. The doctor will then be able to remove the urine after an orgasm—either through a tiny, lubricated catheter, or by asking the patient to void—and separate out the sperm for use in direct intrauterine insemination.

Retrograde ejaculation is also found in some men with spinal cord injuries. While these men have normal sperm production, their neurologic damage keeps them from ejaculating normally. These individuals can be helped with the use of electro-ejaculation, a procedure in which a probe is placed into the rectal area, above the prostatic urethra. Pulses of electrical current in the probe are then used to stimulate the nerves of the urethra and produce ejaculation. The sperm that is obtained can be used either for direct intrauterine insemination or for in vitro fertilization procedures.

Varicoceles   One of the most commonly found anatomic defects thought to relate to male infertility is the varicocele (dilated vein). This is suspected when an increased number of abnormally shaped sperm are seen in a routine semen analysis, or when sperm motility is markedly reduced.

A varicocele occurs when varicose veins form around the testicle. There are several ways to detect it. Some varicoceles are prominent enough to be diagnosed by touch when a urologist palpates the testicle. Other, smaller, varicoceles can be detected through ultrasound, or with the use of a Doppler stethoscope, which allows the urologist to hear the blood flow changes that are consistent with a varicocele.

Theoretically, varicoceles cause sperm problems by slowing the flow of blood around the testicle. This then causes the temperature of the testicle to rise, which can create problems in sperm formation such as abnormally shaped sperm, or a decrease in sperm motility. In severe cases, a varicocele can even cause a decreased sperm count.

While the possibility of these things occurring does exist, the varicocele is probably the most overtreated male infertility condition. If they were examined, literally 10% to 15% of the male population would probably be found to have a varicocele. Yet only a very small number of these affected men would have a problem with sperm production. Despite this, patients who have varicoceles are routinely told during evaluation by their urologists that they need surgical correction to enhance their fertility potential.

Some of these recommendations are given with the honest belief that repair will improve fertility. But a high percentage of these surgical corrections are more beneficial to the surgeon than to the patient. Just as general surgeons have been known to do appendectomies, and gynecologists have been known to do hysterectomies, more for their own financial gain than for the benefit of the patient, some urologists look to varicoceles to improve their income flow. As a result, varicoceles are often ligated, even in cases when it is an unnecessary and clinically nonindicated surgery.

How can you ensure that this doesn't happen to you? When men come into my office with a prior diagnosis of varicocele and question the need for surgery, I use a very simple approach. There are three common-sense rules I follow when separating men who truly need repair, from those who don't.

1) If the varicocele is large enough to create a change in testicular size or consistency—indicating the possibility of testicular atrophy—surgical correction is necessary. If there is no change in testicular size or consistency, and sperm parameters are only marginally abnormal, surgery should not be done.

2) If a varicocele isn't evident during a physical exam, and is found only through imaging or ultrasound, surgical repair *may not* be indicated.

3) If the changes in the appearance, motility, and number of the patient's sperm are marginal, and sperm function tests are normal, surgical repair is not indicated.

In these cases, not only is there no need for surgical correction, I recommend against it. There are several reasons for this. First, the question of whether surgically repairing a varicocele actually improves a man's fertility is still controversial. Several studies have attempted to show differences in pregnancy outcome after varicocele repair. But few, if any, controlled trials have actually shown improvement after surgical repair, when compared to varicoceles that were left untreated. In what is probably the best study to date, over 650 men with varicoceles were randomly assigned surgical correction or left untreated. While there was a minimal increase in sperm motility in the group that had surgical repair, the pregnancy outcome for the two groups was the same.

Next, the surgical correction of a varicocele is both expensive and somewhat painful. The operation is performed as an outpatient procedure, under a general anesthetic. Incisions are made above the groin area, and the large veins that drain blood from the testes are tied off. The area is painful for about a week after the operation, and is similar to a hernia repair from the pain standpoint. The cost may take longer to recover from, since charges for varicocele repair range from $8,000 to $12,000.

While there are a large number of reasons to forego surgery, there is one thing to keep in mind. When there is a varicocele that doesn't require surgery, the man needs to be checked on an annual basis to confirm that no change in its size or effect has taken place. These periodic examinations will assure him that testicular atrophy hasn't begun, and that his semen parameters haven't changed significantly.

Blockages   Blockages that prevent sperm from leaving the penis can occur in a number of places in the male reproductive tract. Some, such as vasectomy, are man-made. Some are the aftereffects of infections. And still others, such as congenital absence of the vas deferens, are present from birth.

In some cases, such as congenital absence of the vas deferens, blockages can be diagnosed by palpation. Others, such as those resulting from infections, require testicular biopsy to confirm their presence. Once a blockage is diagnosed, the same treatment is used regardless of its cause. Assuming the testicles are producing sperm cells, which simply can't exit because their path is blocked, your doctor will either aspirate them from the epididymis or perform direct testicular collection. The sperm he collects can then be used for assisted reproductive technolgies.

Vasectomy During vasectomy, a relatively common operation, the vas deferens is severed and the flow of sperm from the male's reproductive tract is interrupted. Given a very skilled surgeon, this situation can often be corrected microsurgically, and the connection between the testicle and the ejaculatory ducts reestablished. The operation that accomplishes this is called a *vasovasostomy*. Depending upon how successful this reconnection is, the sperm that are released and ejaculated through the urethra can accomplish a pregnancy either with normal intercourse or through direct insemination. And in the hands of a skilled urologic surgeon, reanastomosis *is* successful 75% to 80% of the time. The surgery is similar to that which is done to accomplish a tubal reanastomosis in women. But it is less invasive, since the vas deferens is reconnected in the scrotal area, and no abdominal surgery is necessary. Because of this, the operation can be done with a local anesthetic. The normal recovery time is about one week.

UNEXPLAINED—OR "IDIOPATHIC"—ABNORMALITIES

Unfortunately, most men who are subfertile, or infertile, never get any definite explanation for their lack of sperm production and function. They have no significant history of testicular trauma, infection, or surgery. They have no obvious structural or hormonal problems. Yet they still have very low sperm counts, motility, or fertilizing potential. Since the cause of the problem in these men is "idiopathic," or unexplained, it is hard for their doctors to focus on any surgical or pharmaceutical approach to treating them.

If you fall into this category, the best hope of improving your chances of impregnating your partner is by trying to enhance the function of the sperm you *do* have. In other words, since your doctor can't improve your condition as a whole, he'll concentrate on trying to improve your semen on a specimen-to-specimen basis. Happily, the eighties and nineties produced a number of advances on this front.

Many of these recently developed techniques for sperm enhancement have grown out of experimentation in the field of in vitro fertilization. Of course, for 20 to 30 years prior to the initiation of in vitro fertilization research, direct insemination procedures had been performed on individuals whose partners had borderline to low semen parameters. In these earlier attempts, gynecologists simply placed the man's sperm at the woman's cervical opening, or within her cervical canal, in hopes that by moving sperm that much closer to their goal, they would also be moving closer to successful fertilization. This technique was met with limited success—a pregnancy rate of about 5% per cycle. But the researchers who were developing in vitro technologies soon theorized that the same techniques that improved the chances of sperm fertilizing an egg in a glass dish could be equally effective in boosting the chances for fertilization following intrauterine insemination. So although techniques such as sperm separation and enhancement were originally developed for use with IVF, the improvement they are able to produce in sperm has now led to intrauterine insemination becoming a very useful alternative for men with low semen parameters, as well as for women with cervical factor abnormalities.

Sperm Separation

Sperm separation—or sperm "washing"—is the first step doctors use when they are trying to improve sperm performance. Separation selects out motile sperm from a man's ejaculate, and concentrates them into a small volume, leaving the subpar sperm behind. The reason this is important is because when a large number of unhealthy sperm are in the ejaculate, a number of them die, and the toxic waste this leaves behind may affect the performance of the healthier sperm.

Currently, "Percoll separation" is the method that is most frequently used to split sperm from ejaculate. As we discussed previously, Percoll is fluid that contains millions of microspheres. Since normally shaped, motile sperm have a heavier weight and greater cell density than abnormal, nonmotile sperm, this carries them down through the filtration fluid, leaving the lighter and less dense sperm behind. This selective migration through the Percoll solution allows doctors to separate out, and to concentrate, all of the normal, motile sperm from a man's ejaculate. Different types of Percoll solutions may be used, depending on the appearance of a patient's semen sample. A standard Percoll solution is used if the semen sample appears to be normal. If it has decreased sperm count or motility, a mini-Percoll solution will be used. If there appears to be debris in the semen, a dilute Percoll solution will probably be used. And in cases where sperm penetration needs to be enhanced, a 24-hour

Percoll solution will be used, which will give the sperm a longer incubation time during which they can undergo capacitation.

ENHANCING THE PERFORMANCE OF WASHED SPERM

Sometimes selecting out motile and normally shaped sperm is not enough. These "good" sperm may still be lacking in fertilizing ability. That's why sometimes a hamster penetration test, or sperm penetration assay, will be performed. We explained these tests previously in Chapter Five. If your hamster penetration test shows that after being washed the sperm still can't penetrate the egg, this failing can be corrected in many cases through a process in which doctors place washed sperm in various chemical solutions in hopes of enhancing their acrosome reaction, thus improving their ability to penetrate and fertilize the egg. By first testing the sperm's penetrating ability, then treating the sperm with various enhancing chemicals, and then retesting, your doctor will be able to tell whether you have a reasonable chance to succeed with intrauterine insemination.

This is one more time when the skill and experience of your doctor and his laboratory scientists is important. There is no single formula for treating sperm. The solution that will be most helpful depends on the specific problem your sperm have. To better understand how your doctor will isolate your problem and treat it, consider the case of Joe.

When Joe came to my office, his semen had already been analyzed on three different occasions. Each test showed the same results.

His sperm count ranged between 4 and 5 million sperm per milliliter of ejaculate, when the normal count is over 20 million per milliliter.

Of his sperm, around 20% had good motility; the normal percentage is 40%.

Only 15% of his sperm were properly shaped; a normal reading would be 60%.

Looking at these abnormal semen parameters, I decided to test the fertilizing ability of Joe's sperm by doing a hamster test. I isolated Joe's healthiest sperm through Percoll separation. In a normal hamster test, when the sperm and egg come together, fertilization takes place, but when Joe's sperm were tested, they scored zero—none of the hamster eggs showed evidence of penetration.

When someone like Joe fails an initial hamster test, we take a second semen specimen, separate out the healthy sperm, and then treat portions of them with different chemical solutions to try to find one that will improve their function. In Joe's case:

> One portion was treated with follicular fluid—the fluid that is collected when eggs are aspirated from the human follicle. In some men, this fluid enhances sperm membrane breakdown and improves sperm penetration.

> Another portion of Joe's ejaculate was treated with a combination of pentoxifylline and deoxyribonuclease. Pentoxifylline is a natural enzyme that should be present in the seminal fluid. It is added to increase both the sperms' movement capabilities and velocity. Deoxyribonuclease is also a natural enzyme. It occurs in seminal fluid, or possibly in the reproductive tract of the female. Because its function is to increase the acrosome membrane breakdown, it isn't added until 30 minutes before the sperm solution is placed in contact with the hamster egg.

> A final portion of Joe's sperm was separated, and then left to incubate for 18 to 24 hours before it was placed with the hamster eggs. Some men's sperm take a longer time than normal to undergo the acrosome reaction; this incubation period can improve their fertilization function.

In Joe's case, the sperm treated with the pentoxifylline and deoxyribonuclease combination had a 40% penetration rate during the second hamster test, while the sperm treated with the other methods still showed 0% penetration. Based on this result, we separated out the healthy sperm from a third semen sample, treated them with pentoxifylline and deoxyribonuclease, and used them to inseminate Joe's wife at the time of her ovulation.

Even with the help of every method of chemical sperm enhancement, some men still demonstrate 0% penetration in follow-up hamster tests. In these cases, intrauterine insemination would produce such low pregnancy rates that it isn't an acceptable alternative. For them, as well as for men whose sperm counts are extremely low, the choice that remains is between therapeutic insemination using donor sperm, or in vitro fertilization combined with micromanipulation using their own sperm.

Donor Insemination

The use of donor sperm to compensate for male factor infertility has been described in medical literature since the forties and fifties. And no doubt it was going on even before that time, it just wasn't recorded. During the period since records have been kept, they've shown that approximately 1,000,000 babies have been born as the result of donor insemination.

Even though donor insemination is being replaced with aggressive micromanipulation and in vitro fertilization approaches more and more often these days, it is still a frequently used alternative. One of the main reasons for this is cost. While the combination of micromanipulation and in vitro fertilization will commonly run between $8,000 and $12,000, a donor insemination procedure usually costs less than $500. For couples who can't afford more sophisticated procedures, simple insemination with donor sperm is an acceptable, successful, and readily available alternative.

Up until 1985, most donor inseminations were done with fresh sperm. But between 1984 and 1985, as medical researchers became increasingly aware of the possibility that sexually transmitted diseases, and life-threatening diseases such as AIDS, could be transmitted through semen, donor insemination began to be performed with frozen, thawed sperm. During the time the semen remains frozen prior to its use, the sperm donor is tested, and then retested over a six-month period, for diseases such as hepatitis and AIDS. Only when the donor is shown to be free of disease is the sperm used.

THE BIG CHILL

Using frozen sperm for intrauterine insemination produces the same pregnancy outcome as fresh sperm; overall, the same percentage of women will become pregnant with either method. But with frozen sperm it does usually take *longer* to produce a pregnancy—an average of eight to twelve cycles per pregnancy, as opposed to five to seven cycles using fresh sperm. This inconvenience is more than compensated for when you take into consideration the risk of HIV and other disease transmission through fresh donor semen. Cases of women infected by HIV after donor semen insemination occurred prior to 1985. In 1985 mandatory HIV screening of all donors and freezing and quarantining of semen became a required procedure. Since mandatory quarantining and screening has been required, there have been no recorded cases of women being infected with the HIV virus through donor insemination.

Given this possibility for infection, fresh sperm should be considered for insemination purposes only in carefully selected cases. One such situation might occur when the donor is a family member. In this instance, the couple is given the option of waiving the mandatory quarantine procedure. In another situation, when the couple uses semen donated by a very close friend, they may also waive the quarantine period and freezing process. However, even in these relatively safe scenarios, most reproductive endocrinologists still strongly recommend that sperm be frozen and quarantined for six months.

SELECTING YOUR SPERM BANK

As we write this, more than 400 sperm banks are operating in the United States alone. Since one of the most important considerations in donor insemination is the safety and quality of the sperm, it's hard to believe that until very recently, virtually anyone could set up a sperm bank. And even today, while sperm banks have come under state licensing authority and oversight in some states, both licensing and a laboratory's adherence to standards are still primarily voluntary.

Given these lax guidelines, if you're a patient who needs donor sperm, it is important to:

- Make sure that the physician performing your inseminations is comfortable with the sperm bank and their credibility.

- Thoroughly check the credentials of the sperm bank you're considering. At a minimum, make sure that they adhere to the rules of the American Association of Tissue Banks, which sets guidelines for sperm banking systems.

- Be sure that your sperm bank's donor screening includes thorough genetic screening, screening for infectious diseases, and a complete family history screening for inheritable medical conditions.

- Verify that your sperm bank freezes and quarantines all donor semen for a minimum of six months before using it for inseminations, and that they test donors at the end of this quarantine period for hepatitis, HIV, and other infectious diseases. Make sure that they continue to screen donors for as long as their frozen sperm is being released for insemination.

Beyond these very important safety considerations, there are some other areas that you will probably want to question your prospective sperm bank about. The first of these is the issue of privacy. Traditionally, sperm banks have refused to divulge any information about donors, other than brief physical and medical histories. But recently a movement has started in which progressive sperm banks offer programs that release donor identification information to children from donor insemination, upon request, once they reach the age of 18. The first U.S. sperm bank to do this was the Sperm Bank of California, in Berkeley, California. Their program releases the name, address, phone number, social security number, driver's license number, and hometown of the donor. It's possible that as time goes on, open identity will become more common; it has been mandatory in Sweden since 1989. But until it does, you can let your personal feelings and comfort level about this issue be your guide, and you can look for a sperm bank that will conform to them.

A closely related question is the amount of information various sperm banks supply about donors. In some, you will be shown only medical histories and brief summaries of physical characteristics. In others, you will be able to look through extensive questionnaires in which a donor describes not only his physical characteristics and medical history but also talks about his personality and hobbies, his IQ, education, and occupation, and his reasons for becoming a donor. Before choosing a sperm bank, you should be clear on how much information about your donor you want to have. Perhaps you're just interested in a minimal number of physical characteristics—hair and eye color, height, and country of origin. Or perhaps you're interested in knowing more—everything from his eating habits, to his history with drugs and alcohol, to whether he's right-handed or left-handed. Once you've made your decision, be sure that the sperm bank you're considering is willing to supply the type of information you want.

Another thing to discuss with your sperm bank is whether or not they set a limit on the number of children that can be sired by any one donor. While there is no legal limit in this area, the commonly used industry standard is a maximum of five children within a state, and an additional five out of state. Unfortunately, even if your clinic sets limits, there's no guarantee that a donor won't exceed them by donating at another clinic. While some countries such as Sweden and England have central registries that limit the number of children any one donor can sire, as we write this the United States does not yet monitor donations on a national basis.

Micromanipulation

As we stated earlier, the use of donor sperm is becoming less and less necessary as our ability to achieve pregnancies through a combination of in vitro fertilization and micromanipulation of sperm improves. Micromanipulation is a relatively new advance in infertility treatment, but one that holds out great promise for men whose sperm would previously have been inadequate to produce a pregnancy. Today in our IVF program, as well as in several other programs in the United States, the ability to take men who produce even a minimum number of sperm—50 to 100 cells, rather than millions—and fertilize their partner's eggs, has improved dramatically.

This is largely due to a technique known as intracytoplasmic sperm insemination (ICSI). ICSI was first introduced to the medical community in 1993, in a report from Belgium that described the injection of a single sperm into an egg. Since then, in combination with in vitro fertilization, it has revolutionized the treatment of male factor infertility. Using ICSI, doctors pick up a single sperm cell and inject it into an egg to produce an embryo, which hopefully becomes a baby nine months later. With the use of single-egg injection, the need for donor sperm has decreased dramatically. Because of this new technology, men who in the past were relegated to depending on sperm donation, or adoption, can now produce their own biological children. We will be discussing micromanipulation in greater detail in our chapter on assisted reproductive technologies (Chapter Twelve).

Alternative Medical Approaches

Since children are such an important social status symbol to the Chinese, it is not surprising that they have given a great deal of thought and attention to the problem of infertility. Practitioners of Eastern medicine have long reported that both sperm count and motility can be raised through a combination of acupuncture and herbal medicine. While these reports are largely anecdotal, there are a limited number of studies in this area that seem to bear them out. A 1986 study at the Guayang College of Traditional Chinese Medicine treated 500 subfertile men in a random fashion, with various combinations of Chinese herbs. In 442 cases (88.4%), these men's sperm parameters rose to normal. In 158 cases (31.6%), their partners got pregnant. And in 51 cases (10.2%), sperm parameters were improved, but did not become normal. The remaining seven cases showed no improvement.

A related 1987 study looking at the effects of acupuncture on male subfertility took 251 cases and succeeded in producing normal sperm parameters in 89 of them (35.5%). Another 77 men showed improvement (30.7%), while in 85 cases (33.9%), the treatment was ineffective.

Both herbal treatments and acupuncture can be potentially useful supplements to normal medical treatments, but they shouldn't replace them. If you're considering using acupuncture as an adjunct to your medical treatment, you should anticipate having at least two sessions per week, with each session lasting anywhere from 20 minutes to an hour. Acupuncture normally costs $60 to $100 per session, although some colleges do offer lower-cost treatments.

Be a Part of the Solution

Today, as you can see, there's a panoply of alternatives available for treating male factor infertility. Despite this, many men suffering from infertility report that one of the most difficult aspects of their problem is the feeling of helplessness that it brings. If you find yourself in this situation, remember that with male factor problems, as with all infertility, the more information both partners have, the lower their stress level becomes. This is especially comforting with male problems, since the information you get will assure you that, given sophisticated medical care, you can probably succeed in having a biological child.

Gathering information is a good way to reassert yourself. The more you know, the more you can participate in, and guide, the decisions that will be made concerning what's right for you and your partner. But sometimes this is still not enough. If you find that you're still troubled by certain aspects of your infertility problem, you might want to refer to Chapter Fourteen, where the emotional aspects of male infertility are discussed.

Terms We Used in This Chapter

Computer-assisted semen analysis (CASA):   the measurement of sperm number, shape, and movement by computer technology.

Cryptorchism: failure of the testicles to descend into the scrotal sac.

Donor insemination: an insemination with sperm other than the husband's. Donor insemination is used for pregnancy initiation.

Doppler stethoscope: an instrument that can detect the movement of red blood cells in a blood vessel, and then determine the velocity of that blood flow.

Electron microscopy: an instrument that can magnify structures 50,000 to 100,000 times.

Epididymis: the coiled tubules attached alongside the testicles which act as a storage system for the sperm prior to ejaculation.

Follicle-stimulating hormone (FSH):   a protein hormone produced and released by the anterior pituitary gland. FSH stimulates follicle growth in the female and sperm production in the male.

Germinal cell aplasia: a congenital condition in which the cells that are necessary for formation of gametes are not present.

Gonadotropin-releasing hormone (GnRH):   a small protein hormone produced in the hypothalamus, responsible for controlling the production and release of FSH and LH.

Gonads: the glands that produce the male and female gametes (i.e., the egg and the sperm).

Hamster penetration assay/Hamster test: see Sperm penetration assay.

Hemizona assay test: a test used to determine whether sperm binding or attachment to the zona membrane of the egg is normal.

Human chorionic gonadotropin (hCG):   a hormone produced by the placenta during pregnancy. It is used as an LH replacement during ovulation-induction therapy.

Hypospadia: a congenital defect of the penis in which the urethral opening occurs on the underside rather than at the end.

Hypospermatogenesis: low sperm production.

Hypothalamus: the midportion of the brain which produces GnRH and other hormones that control the pituitary gland.

Idiopathic: any condition that has no known cause.

Intracytoplasmic sperm insemination (ICSI):   the injection of a single sperm cell into a mature egg.

In vitro mucus penetration test: a test used to determine whether sperm mucus interaction is normal; commonly done with bovine mucus and human sperm.

Kallman's syndrome: a congenital condition in men in which the hypothalamus fails to produce GnRH, resulting in lack of FSH and LH production and lack of sperm production.

Klinefelter's syndrome: a chromosomal and developmental abnormality in the male that causes the individual to have female characteristics and male sterility.

Leydig cells: the cells in the testicles that manufacture testosterone.

Luteinizing hormone (LH): protein produced and secreted from the anterior pituitary gland which is involved in ovulation.

Micromanipulation: the use of high magnification and hydraulically controlled instrumentation to achieve fertilization in vitro.

Percoll separation: a liquid gradient that is used to filter the semen during sperm washing, prior to insemination.

Pituitary: a small gland at the base of the brain that secretes hormones that control our endocrine organs.

Prolactin: the hormone produced from the pituitary that prepares the breasts for lactation.

Receptor: the site on a cell surface where a hormone attaches to express its function.

Retrograde ejaculation: ejaculation of the sperm into the bladder instead of through the prostatic urethra.

Seminiferous tubules: the tiny tubules within the testes that are necessary for sperm production.

Sertoli cell: the cells within the testes that are involved in sperm cell production.

Sperm penetration assay (SPA): a test utilizing hamster eggs to measure the ability of the human sperm to fertilize.

Sperm washing: a technique used to separate sperm cells from seminal fluid.

Testosterone: the male hormone.

Varicocele: dilated veins around the testicle, most commonly on the left side, which can cause sperm abnormalities.

Vas deferens: the tube that connects the epididymis (sperm storage area) to the prostate gland; the pathway for sperm to leave the testicular area.

Vasectomy: a surgically created obstruction of the vas deferens that is used as a method of male sterilization.

Vasovasostomy: reversal of a vasectomy by reconnecting the vas deferens.

10

Pelvic Factor Problems

Pelvic factor infertility is one form of infertility that is exclusive to women. The good news is that in most cases of pelvic factor problems—the worst cases of massive adhesions being the exception—there is generally a high cure rate. Depending on what your condition is, and its severity, you have anywhere from a 40% to an 80% chance of conceiving after treatment.

We previously explained in Chapter Eight how we diagnose and correct problems that are found *inside* the uterus and fallopian tubes. Ultrasound can show abnormalities in the shape of the ovaries and the uterus. A hysterosalpingogram can show whether there are blockages within the tubes, but neither of these tests lets us know if problems exist on or around the *exterior* of the reproductive organs.

Stopping diagnostic procedures after an internal examination of your reproductive organs would be like asking an inspector to evaluate only the inside of a house without looking outside. He'd discover whether the interior walls are straight, and see if the ceilings are cracked, but he wouldn't know whether the exterior door locks are working, or if the yard is neat or dangerously overgrown.

In your body, the way your doctor finds out these sorts of things is by using the laparoscope to look into your pelvic cavity. By doing this, he can easily see if there are adhesions or scars connecting the surface of the ovary to the fallopian tube, which could make it impossible for the tube to pick up an egg when it's released from the ovary. Surface problems also become evident, such as irregularities in either the shape or position of the uterus and ovaries—in many cases distortions that have been caused by pelvic adhesions or endometriosis.

What's Causing Your Pelvic Problem?

Unlike some other types of infertility, pelvic problems are not caused by congenital malformations. Instead, they consist of growths that start—for any one of a number of reasons—after birth. Today, through the use of the diagnostic laparoscopic approach, we can observe, and potentially treat, the two main causes of pelvic factor infertility:

- Adhesions
- Endometriosis

PELVIC ADHESIONS

If your doctor tells you that you have adhesions within your pelvic cavity, what he's really telling you is that there are places where some of your organs are stuck together. Actually, it's not really your organs that are adhering to one another; it's the membrane that covers them—the peritoneum. Every organ within your pelvic cavity is covered with this slick, silky membrane. It completely lines the inner walls of your abdominal cavity, and it coats every millimeter of your intestines. It stretches to surround your small and large bowels, your liver and spleen, as well as your reproductive organs—your uterus, fallopian tubes, and ovaries.

The peritoneum serves a single purpose: it keeps your organs from sticking to one another. Its slippery surface separates them, even as it stretches to let them move freely. Because of the peritoneum, your 30 to 40 feet of intestine, your uterus, ovaries, and fallopian tubes, and your liver and spleen can all continue to move and function properly, despite the relatively small space they occupy within your pelvic cavity.

But when something causes a break in the peritoneum, problems can occur. During the healing phase after trauma to the peritoneum, as new peritoneal cells grow, it is very common for them to interweave themselves into any other peritoneal surfaces with which they come into contact. This is how adhesions occur. The scar tissue that is formed in this way can link together any two adjoining organs . . . an ovary to a tube, a tube to a part of the intestine, and so on.

Once adhesions are formed, their removal becomes very difficult. The very operation that takes them away may cause new peritoneal rips, which can once again knit into adhesions. Even using the best operating techniques, this vicious circle can be very hard to break.

If you have adhesions, you probably got them in one of two ways:

- Pelvic Inflammatory Disease
- Surgical Trauma

Pelvic Inflammatory Disease

One of the most common causes of adhesions is the inflammation of an organ within the pelvic cavity. As the organ becomes inflamed and swollen, it can injure the peritoneal covering that surrounds it. That area of the peritoneum can then break down, and during the healing phase, as the cells are trying to repair themselves, it is very common for it to stick to an adjoining peritoneal surface.

These infections can jeopardize your fertility, even when they don't directly involve your reproductive organs. For example, a case of acute appendicitis that doesn't rupture or become severe enough to warrant surgery, can leave the large bowel (the cecum) inflamed. Both the bowel and the appendix are located near the right ovary and right fallopian tube. Injury to them can cause adhesions that damage or block this tube. That's how something as common as a case of untreated appendicitis can interfere with your ovulation, and with the ability of an egg to move through your fallopian tube.

Another common cause of tubal and ovarian adhesions, which we discussed in Chapter Eight, is infection due to sexually transmitted diseases. Gonorrhea, for example, can create tubal inflammation during its initial stages. Depending on the severity of the infection, it may cause the fallopian tubes to stick to the ovaries, to the pelvic sidewalls or floor, or to the large and small bowel. Or the fallopian tubes may respond to their inflammation by becoming closed.

This can be further complicated by the use of an intrauterine device (IUD), a phenomenon we also discussed in that chapter. Infections that are passed upward with the assistance of an IUD can create massive adhesions that affect the tubes, the ovaries, and the entire pelvic cavity.

Surgical Trauma

The other cause of pelvic adhesions and scarring, equal to that caused by PID, is physician-produced trauma. This pelvic problem is usually the result of prior gynecologic or infertility surgeries. Trauma to the peritoneal membrane can occur during any surgery—when a general surgeon operates on a young woman for an inflamed appendix, for example, or when a gynecologic surgeon operates on a woman for an ovarian cyst. If surgery is done in such a way that it damages the peritoneal surface, standard surgical procedures can create havoc at a later date when the woman tries to conceive. Innumerable cases of pelvic factor infertility involve simple surgeries that should have been done without difficulty. Yet when these standard procedures are mishandled, they instantly create fertility problems.

With this in mind, if you are a woman in your reproductive years, and it is necessary for you to have pelvic surgery, there are some important rules to remember.

1. Find the most qualified surgeon available.

2. Whenever possible, have a laparoscopy instead of a laparotomy.

3. If you need to have a laparotomy, have microsurgery instead of standard surgery.

4. Even if you are having surgery involving your pelvic cavity performed by a nongynecologic surgeon because of no involvement of your reproductive organs, have a reproductive surgeon present in the operating room.

1. Your surgeon's qualifications

The most important thing that a woman can do if she faces any type of pelvic surgery, prior to the end of her reproductive years, is to find the most qualified reparative surgeon available. Even a simple operation, such as removing an ovarian cyst, must be done with the idea in mind that the surgeon will preserve, conserve, and promote your future fertility at the same time he is performing the surgical procedure.

You can get recommendations for surgeons through other doctors, or through several medical societies. If your operation involves your reproductive organs, you should get names of those surgeons who are qualified in reproductive surgical techniques from the Society of Reproductive Surgeons, a sub-section of the American Society for Reproductive Medicine, which is located in Birmingham, Alabama. The Society of Reproductive Surgeons reviews cases and results on all qualified reproductive surgeons. This organization, as well as Resolve, can provide you with information on surgeons throughout the country.

2. Laparoscopy versus laparotomy

Laparoscopy is an operation involving the insertion of a telescope through the abdominal wall, to allow the surgeon to view the inside of the pelvic cavity, and/or to perform surgical procedures.

Laparotomy is an operation involving an incision through the abdominal wall, to allow the surgeon to have access to the organs inside. For example, a cesarean section or a hysterectomy is done by laparotomy.

Surgical techniques through the laparoscope have improved to such a degree that it should be the method of choice for removal of adhesions and endometriosis in 99% of cases. There's an important reason why use of the laparoscope is emphasized in this way.

Any time the abdominal wall is cut open—as it is in a laparotomy—and the surgeon goes through an incision to work inside the pelvic cavity with his hands and instruments, there is a greater likelihood of trauma or damage to the sensitive peritoneal surfaces.

Because a laparotomy is done through an open incision, it requires the use of surgical instruments to hold tissues and pull them back so that the surgeon can reach the area on which he's operating. These retracting instruments can create abrasions and damage to the peritoneal surfaces, which, during the healing phase after surgery, can cause scar formation. In fact, the damage inflicted by crushing peritoneal tissue with a clamp can be as harmful as actually cutting the peritoneum. Also, when the abdominal or pelvic cavity is opened, the peritoneal surfaces can dry out, and can be sites for later adhesion formation.

3. Microsurgical techniques

The most important rule for any abdominal surgical procedure is to do everything possible to avoid postoperative scarring and adhesions. If a surgeon can avoid traumatizing tissue in the first place, it goes a long way toward accomplishing this goal. One way he can contribute to this is by operating microsurgically. What this means is that:

- The surgeon uses a magnification system, such as an operating microscope, or magnifying glasses. By doing this, he can find even tiny blood vessels and fine adhesions, and he can see every detail of the peritoneal surface. This lets him separate scar tissue and adhesions from the surrounding normal tissue more accurately.
- The surgeon uses microinstruments. These tiny surgical instruments are designed to remove adhesion bands and to separate diseased tissue with the smallest possible cuts and trauma to the normal tissue that is left behind. These microinstruments cause minimal, if any, damage—such as crushing of the peritoneal surfaces.
- The surgeon uses microsuture material, sometimes sewing with a needle as thin as a hair. This lets him close even the smallest

openings, and because the suture is so small, the body doesn't react to it as a foreign body.

- Tissue is handled gently so as not to cause trauma. The surgeon pushes carefully, and tries not to pull or tear.

- The surgeon tries to operate with minimal blood loss, since blood that is left behind in the pelvic cavity causes a chemical reaction that leads to scarring. Microinstruments close or coagulate every tiny blood vessel. And at the end of the operation, the pelvic cavity is washed free of any remaining microscopic amounts of blood.

- Tissue surfaces are constantly irrigated and moistened with a sterile solution during the surgery. If the peritoneal tissue dries, the damage to it can be as bad as a cut or being crushed.

These microsurgical techniques need to be utilized any time pelvic surgery is performed on women of reproductive age.

4. Include the reproductive surgeon

During any operation involving the pelvic cavity—whether it be for an acute problem such as an inflamed appendix, a chronic condition such as an ovarian cyst, or for something as far afield as damage due to a car accident—your doctor must remain alert to the fact that traumas created during surgery can decrease, or even completely take away, your future fertility. Because of this, women who have not yet passed their reproductive years would be well served by having a gynecologic reproductive surgeon present at the time of any pelvic surgery, even when it does not directly affect their reproductive organs. Their gynecologic reproductive surgeon will serve as a specialized advisor to their general surgeon, advising him as to what procedures may or may not cause later damage to the reproductive organs. And the gynecologic reproductive surgeon can also work directly on the reproductive organs, if this is a necessary part of the operation.

One example of a situation that benefits from this type of cooperative effort is surgery for women with inflammatory bowel disease (Crohn's disease). Crohn's disease creates massive inflammation in the small and large bowel. This inflammation can cause scarring and dense adhesions, even without surgery. When surgery *is* necessary, it becomes extremely difficult to conserve reproductive function for these young women. Women with Crohn's disease should have a gynecologic reproductive surgeon present during their bowel surgery, to try to promote and protect their reproductive potential.

The same is true when ovarian cysts require surgical removal. A condition for which this is particularly important is the removal of dermoids—pelvic tumors that are caused by embryonic cells that failed to migrate to the appropriate location when the patient was still a fetus, and that are now growing in the wrong part of the body. Dermoids are classically found in 15- to 25-year-old women, who are still in their prime reproductive years. Most gynecologists believe removing dermoids is a very simple operation. Yet if not done with gentle tissue handling, with appropriate suture material, and with appropriate protection of the peritoneal surfaces both preop and postop, massive adhesions can result. Today, nearly all dermoids can be removed laparoscopically. This significantly decreases the risk of postoperative problems, as well as decreasing the invasiveness of the surgical procedure, and the time it will take you to recover.

The problem of adhesions also holds true for uterine fibroid removal, a very common operation. Myomectomy—the removal of fibroid tissue from the uterine wall—can leave a woman with massive scars and a nonfunctional uterus, fallopian tubes, and ovaries if it is not performed by a trained and skillful surgeon who is capable of doing the operation with minimal blood loss and atraumatic tissue handling. Again, this should be someone who has expertise in preserving your future fertility.

These are just a few of the instances in which the contribution of a surgeon who specializes in fertility surgery can be an important addition, if your ob/gyn doesn't have specialized training in this area.

ENDOMETRIOSIS

Endometriosis is the most common source of problems in women with pelvic factor infertility. It's a long-known disorder, which was described in medical literature as early as the nineteenth century. The condition occurs when normal endometrial tissue relocates in an abnormal place—it migrates outside the uterus and implants itself within the pelvic cavity, where it begins to grow. In some cases this won't produce infertility, but in a large number of cases, it does.

The endometrium, as you learned in the early part of this book, is the lining of the uterine cavity. It grows during every normal ovulatory cycle in preparation for nurturing a fetus, and when one fails to implant, it breaks down, and pieces of it are shed along with menstrual blood, exiting through the cervix and the vaginal canal.

Sometimes things do not go this smoothly. A phenomenon known as retrograde menstruation occurs. Retrograde menstruation is a backing up of menstrual blood, which pushes it out through the fallopian tubes and into the pelvic cavity. We know from studies done over the last 20 to 40 years that virtually all women have retrograde menstruation during at least some part of their reproductive life.

With this retrograde release of menstrual blood, pieces of endometrial tissue are also moved out into the abdominal cavity. Sometimes this tissue implants and grows under the influence of monthly hormonal changes, just as it would if it were still inside the uterus. Unfortunately, at the end of the monthly cycle, when it begins to shed, the blood it releases into the pelvic cavity can react chemically, causing scarring and adhesions.

This is a relatively common situation. It is estimated that between 3% and 10% of all women in the reproductive age group suffer from endometriosis, although the chance of having endometriosis is less for women who have had early pregnancies. To give you some idea of its destructive potential, 24% to 35% of infertile women are found to have the disease. Four out of every thousand women between the ages of 15 and 64 are hospitalized each year with endometriosis, which is comparable to the number in the same age group that is hospitalized for breast cancer.

Most often, endometriosis involves the ovaries, the floor of the pelvis, and the fallopian tubes. But it can also migrate through the bloodstream or lymph system to virtually any part of a woman's body. It has been found in the brain, the lungs, the colon, and the bladder, where monthly bleeding can occur. It has even been detected in men who have been on high-dose estrogen therapy during treatment for prostatic carcinoma.

Mild endometriosis rarely creates problems with a woman's fertility status. But moderate to severe cases can affect a woman's fertility by causing adhesions, scarring, and fixation of the fallopian tubes and ovaries. It can even develop inside the ovary, causing what are called "chocolate cysts" or endometriomas. In its worst forms it virtually destroys ovaries and fallopian tubes because of the chronic inflammation that it causes, as well as the way it damages certain areas of the peritoneal surfaces, creating massive scarring and a type of gluing or cementing together of pelvic structures.

Diagnosis of Endometriosis

There are endless old wives'—and even old doctors'—tales that purport to describe the classic symptoms and psychological profile of a woman who is prone to endometriosis. For years, women who were goal-oriented, high-achieving, high-energy, high-stress individuals were thought to be susceptible to the disease. It was also believed to be more prevalent in white women than in black women. Classically, certain symptoms were thought to accompany endometriosis. Women who suffered from it were expected to have severe pain with their periods (dysmenorrhea). Sex, too, was expected to be painful for these women.

Today we realize that none of these symptoms necessarily holds true for every woman with endometriosis. One of the reasons it can be difficult to diagnose the disease is that women with massive amounts of endometriosis can have severe chronic pelvic pain, or can have absolutely no pain at all, including no pain with menstrual flow or with intercourse. And personality, we now know, has nothing to do with endometriosis. Instead, endometriosis is genetically passed on from mother to daughter; if you have the disease, your immune system probably developed with a genetically programmed predisposition not to attack endometrial cells when they are in the wrong place.

This genetic link provides one of the clues that help with diagnosis. Because of it, and because endometriosis is a chronic disease that persists throughout a woman's life, a thorough medical history can lead your doctor to suspect endometriosis. Physical examination can give another clue. In some cases, nodules caused by endometriosis can be felt by your doctor during your pelvic exam. But while these things might point your doctor in the direction of endometriosis, the only definite way to make a diagnosis is by actually viewing the pelvic cavity through a laparoscope. Using a laparoscope, your surgeon will actually be able to see the characteristic implants of endometriosis inside your pelvis.

Endometriosis and Infertility

The correlation between endometriosis and infertility is an area of some controversy. Certainly when massive adhesions, tubal damage, and/or ovarian damage is present, it is easy to understand how ovulation, egg pickup, and fertilization can be affected. But when endometriosis is found in minimal amounts—with one, two, or three implants scattered around the pelvic cavity—it is harder to see how this level of disease can affect tubal movement, egg pickup, fertilization, or pregnancy. Then the link to infertility is less clear.

Currently, most physicians believe that only moderate to severe endometriosis affects a woman's fertility status. However, there have been several studies over the years stating that even minimal implants of endometriosis can change the local hormonal environment, and possibly disrupt potential fertility as a result. For example, prostaglandins are produced in higher amounts in the pelvic cavity of women with endometriosis. These hormones are thought to cause the smooth muscle activity of the fallopian tube to become hyperactive, and to possibly interfere with tubal movement and egg pickup.

Also, macrophages (white blood cells that attack and destroy foreign bodies) are found in higher concentrations in the pelvic/fallopian tube environment of endometriosis patients. Some studies have demonstrated that these macrophages may also kill sperm as they move toward the egg, or embryos as they make their journey into the uterus.

These theories are still controversial, as various studies have reported differing conclusions. Since there is *no absolute proof* that mild endometriosis can actually affect fertility status, women who are diagnosed with it face some uncertainty when deciding whether or not to undergo aggressive treatment. If you have mild endometriosis, you should consider the fact that, *to date*, the majority of studies that have compared treatment versus nontreatment for mild endometriosis have found no difference in fertility outcomes. This would seem to be a good argument against women with minimal endometriosis undergoing specific treatment for the disease. If your doctor finds mild endometriosis at the time he does a diagnostic laparoscopy, he may choose to treat it by removal of the visible lesions with laser or by electrocautery. Or, alternatively, he may go directly to specific therapies designed to enhance fertility, particularly if you fall into the category of "unexplained infertility." These would include controlled ovarian stimulation followed by intrauterine insemination. If that fails to produce a pregnancy, he may opt for one of the assisted reproductive techniques.

Treating Your Pelvic Factor Infertility

Most pelvic factor infertility involves adhesions or scarring, and there is no type of medicine or hormonal treatment to date that can separate two peritoneal surfaces once they become stuck together. Therefore, pelvic factor infertility is almost always treated surgically. The exception to this rule is certain types of pelvic endometriosis. There are four different stages of endometriosis; mild stages of which do not necessarily involve adhesions or scarring. These can be treated hormonally, rather than by surgery. We'll be discussing the stages of endometriosis, and the various alternatives for their treatment, later in this chapter.

TREATING PELVIC ADHESIONS

Pelvic adhesions that interfere with fertility must be removed surgically. Over the years, the prevailing wisdom as to how this should be done has changed, as new surgical techniques have been developed and improved.

Laparotomy

Fifteen to twenty years ago, the accepted wisdom among infertility specialists was that making an abdominal incision, and then operating microsurgically, offered the best outcome in reversing pelvic adhesions. Bolstering this position was the fact that meticulous microsurgical procedures did, in some cases, reverse the adhesion process and restore a woman's fertility potential. Because of this, an increasing number of severe cases were treated using this approach.

However, when laparoscopies began to be used as a follow-up procedure after these laparotomies—as a means of checking to make sure that the surgeries had been successful—it became evident that an immediate recurrence of the adhesions that had just been removed was the norm. This was because even with the most meticulous microsurgical approach, there was still some trauma to the peritoneal tissue when the pelvic cavity was opened, and when organs were operated on through an incision. After the surgery was completed, and the incision closed, these traumatized surfaces would come into contact with each other during the two to four weeks following surgery, when those areas of the peritoneum that were cut or separated from each other grew new epithelial cells to heal the surface membrane. During this regrowth, areas traumatized during surgery simply stuck back together. So an ovary and fallopian tube that were left separate when surgery was complete, could come into contact during the tissue healing phase, and could re-adhere, producing the same problem that existed before surgery was performed.

Over the years, various coverings were experimented within an attempt to keep the traumatized areas of the membrane apart. Today, a Gore-Tex–like material is used to cover damaged peritoneal surfaces, in an attempt to block adhesion re-formation. But even with this advance, microsurgery in difficult or severe cases has been shown to be quite ineffective in correcting infertility caused by adhesions.

As a patient you should be aware of this if your doctor is recommending a conventional laparotomy and microsurgery to remove your pelvic adhesions. If this procedure is used to take apart scarring or remove adhesions, you should not expect that you will then remain free of these problems. It is important for you to understand that areas of scarring are really areas of traumatized tissue. No matter how carefully they are removed, some damaged tissue remains, which will quickly stick together again 60% to 80% of the time.

Laparoscopy

Before you become too discouraged, you should know that there is another way of operating on adhesions that produces better results. In the early eighties, as reproductive endocrinologists expanded their work with in vitro fertilization, we began using the laparoscope more and more frequently as a point of access to the pelvic cavity. As this work progressed, we dealt with increasingly difficult cases of pelvic adhesions that presented themselves during IVF, using the laparoscopic approach. Soon, with the laparoscope, we were able to remove most types of adhesions around the tubes and the ovaries, in order to reach the ovary and retrieve eggs.

In the early days of IVF, patients usually had a laparoscopy each time they had an in vitro procedure. This was before the use of ultrasound egg collection. If extensive adhesions were taken out during the first laparoscopy, we had a chance to examine the area from which they were removed during the laparoscopies that accompanied the second and third IVF attempts. We soon began to realize that the laparoscopic approach, even though it wasn't microsurgical in nature, was producing better results insofar as not having adhesions recur. It was at this point that the idea of using aggressive laparoscopic surgery for pelvic adhesions, independent of in vitro procedures, was born.

Since then, surgeons' skill in doing pelvic surgeries through the laparoscope has become so great that it is now the first choice for removing adhesions, whether they involve the uterus, tubes, ovaries, or large or small bowel. Surgical outcome isn't affected whether conventional cutting instruments, electrosurgical coagulation instruments, or various types of lasers are used. Because the pelvic abdominal cavity is never opened surgically, the chance of adhesion recurrence is much less. The laparoscope—in combination with the laser, which doesn't traumatize surrounding normal tissue as it vaporizes abnormal tissue—can also be used to remove tubal obstructions at the end of the tube. And it is now utilized in the removal of every type of ovarian cyst, including dermoids, functional ovarian cysts, and nonfunctional cysts, such as endometriomas. The chance of adhesion recurrence using a laparoscopic approach is so much less, that today (with just a few exceptions), if your surgeon can't remove your pelvic adhesions laparoscopically, you should probably not undergo pelvic surgery at all. Still, there are a few exceptions to this rule. Laparotomy may still be your procedure of choice in those extreme cases of pelvic factor adhesions where your surgeon simply cannot get access to the area through the laparoscope. Adhesions involving the colon and small bowel are one example.

And even in these cases your doctor will probably want to start your treatment with an exploratory laparoscopy, so he can evaluate your problem and confirm that you really need a laparotomy, before he operates on you.

If he determines that you do have one of those problems that requires a laparotomy, there are certain things that he can do to reduce the recurrence of adhesions. The use of certain medications following your operation—especially during the first 48 hours after surgery—promotes healing with a decrease in scar formation. The regimen you should follow combines a broad spectrum antibiotic such as Ancef to reduce bacterial contamination (which can cause both infection and inflammation), a systemic steroid such as Decadron (which also reduces inflammation), and an antihistamine such as Phenergan. Histamines are substances that are released by traumatized cells, which can cause inflammation. This trio of drugs is effective because scar formation during healing is caused by a combination of histamine release and inflammation.

Another way to avoid traumatizing peritoneal tissue during a laparotomy is by keeping it constantly moist. That's why your doctor should literally operate under water during a laparotomy. Constant irrigation with a sterile solution not only keeps all of the peritoneal surfaces moist, it also helps to wash the pelvic cavity of any microscopic amounts of blood remaining at the end of the operation. If left behind, they could produce a chemical reaction that would create scarring.

Prior to closing your peritoneal cavity, your doctor might also want to fill it with a steroid solution to keep your fallopian tubes, ovaries, and uterus floating free, so that they don't contact any of the peritoneal surfaces that have just been operated on. Your system will absorb this fluid over the first 48 hours after surgery, but while it is still in your pelvic cavity, the initial healing of tissue surfaces will have been able to take place.

Numerous studies over the years have shown the effectiveness of various combinations of antibiotics, antihistamines, and steroid solutions in retarding scar formation after pelvic laparotomy. Because of their proven value, they are often used not only for extensive laparotomy procedures, but in difficult laparoscopic procedures, as well.

TREATING PELVIC ENDOMETRIOSIS

Pelvic endometriosis is a chronic condition that persists throughout a woman's life, until she reaches menopause. If there is one thing that is consistent about endometriosis, it is that even when suppressed or re- moved surgically, it almost always recurs. It is the most difficult disorder to deal with surgically in an infertile woman. In fact, the only permanent cure for endometriosis is to remove a woman's reproductive organs—her uterus, fallopian tubes, and ovaries. And in some cases, the disease can recur even after total hysterectomy, including removal of the tubes and ovaries.

But if you're trying to get pregnant, hysterectomy obviously isn't an option. For you, the best hope is to remove or suppress your endometri- osis long enough for you to conceive and carry a pregnancy to term. Depending on how extensive your problem is, there are different ways to accomplish this.

As we explained earlier in this chapter, pelvic endometriosis can occur in various degrees of severity. Mild cases may not interfere with fertility at all, while extensive amounts of endometriosis in the pelvic cavity can create great difficulties.

Simplified Classification of Pelvic Endometriosis

Stage One:	There will be scattered spots (or "implants") of endometriosis on the surface of the pelvic peritoneum. But there will not yet be any scarring or adhesions due to the endometriosis implants.
Stage Two:	The endometriosis implants will involve the surface of the fallo- pian tubes, the ovaries, and the peritoneum. There may be areas of inflammation, or reaction, around the endometrial implants.
Stage Three:	There will be larger areas of endometriosis, including endometri- osis inside the ovaries (chocolate cysts or endometriomas), as well as adhesions around the tubes and ovaries. There can be scarring involving the pelvic floor and large intestine.
Stage Four:	There can be endometriosis lesions in both ovaries, as well as thick scarring around the pelvic organs. The endometriosis may involve the intestines, bladder, and other pelvic abdominal struc- tures. There can be obstruction of one or both fallopian tubes.

If your doctor suspects that you have endometriosis, he should start by doing an exploratory laparoscopy. This will not only confirm the pres- ence of the disease, it will let him see the severity of your case. Once he has determined this, he can decide on a treatment approach. In most cases of endometriosis, partial or complete treatment can be performed during this initial laparoscopy. Therefore, be sure the physician performing your diagnostic laparoscopy has the necessary skills to deal with the disease if he does find it. Many patients every year are told they have endometriosis, but are not treated at the time of the initial laparoscopy. These women then have to undergo the expense and discomfort of a second laparoscopy for treatment of their endometriosis.

There are two basic ways to treat endometriosis. If your disease is in Stage One or Two, your doctor may use hormonal treatment to try to shrink, or even eliminate, your endometrial lesions. However, in some Stage Two and all Stage Three situations, he will probably have to treat the disease surgically. In more advanced stages of endometriosis (Stages Three and Four), your surgeon may choose to use both hormone treatment and a surgical procedure.

Hormonal Treatment of Endometriosis

Endometriosis occurs when endometrial tissue that has migrated into the pelvic cavity is stimulated by the normal monthly cycle of estrogen to grow and bleed, just as the endometrium within the uterus does. Because of the pivotal role estrogen plays in this process, the focus of hormonal treatments to combat endometriosis is to stop the ovary from producing this hormone. When estrogen is no longer circulating in the system, endometrial tissue, whether inside the uterus or within the pelvic cavity, will no longer be stimulated to grow.

Hormonal therapy for endometriosis has undergone several changes since it was first attempted. Soon after the development of the oral contraceptive pill—in the late fifties and early sixties—Dr. Robert Kistner theorized that it could be used to suppress endometriosis. This proved to be a significant step forward in the treatment of this disease. By blocking the ovulatory cycle over a period of six to eight months, Dr. Kistner was able not only to stop the growth of endometriosis, but to actually cause the lesions to grow smaller. He did this by starting patients on one birth control pill per day, until they began menstrual bleeding. Two pills per day were then used, to suppress the bleeding and prevent them from having a complete menstrual period. This dose was continued until bleeding occurred again, at which point three pills per day were used, and so on. By constantly increasing the dose, patients could be prevented from having a full menstrual period, which in turn decreased the amount of estrogen in their systems. After six to eight months of suppression, their endometriosis would usually regress to such an extent that they could stop the pills and resume attempts to get pregnant.

Oral contraceptives continued to be the best form of medical therapy for controlling endometriosis until the late seventies, when a more effective form of hormonal suppression was discovered. It was at this point that a medication called danazol—marketed as Danocrine HCL—was developed and tested on women with endometriosis. Danazol is a hormone that is derived from the male hormone testosterone. It is chemically similar to this male hormone, but it is not as active as the male hormone. This means that when given to a female patient, danazol will cause some male hormone side effects, but these usually are controllable.

Danazol stops ovulation by blocking the hypothalamic pituitary release of luteinizing hormone. As you know, it is LH that causes a woman's follicular growth and ovulation. When LH is eliminated, and follicle growth and ovulation are suppressed, the release of estrogen from the ovaries stops as well. Once there is no estrogen circulating in a woman's bloodstream, she becomes anovulatory. As a result, all women who take danazol go through a false menopause. They may experience mood swings, hot flashes, loss of concentration, and depression.

Unfortunately, because danazol is a testosterone derivative, women who use it are also left with male-like hormones circulating in their systems. Virtually all women who take danazol for a full six-month course of treatment experience either abnormal hair growth, weight gain, oily skin, or acne, and in some cases, a deepening of the voice. All of these side effects are worrisome, as you might expect. They can be quite difficult to deal with for a significant percentage of women who take danazol—20% to 40%. While studies that compared danazol to oral contraceptives clearly demonstrated that it was a more effective endometriosis suppressant, and that it offered a better chance for pregnancy after treatment, women who were not concerned with starting a pregnancy—college-age women who suffered from endometriosis, for example—were still better served by using oral contraceptive therapy and avoiding the side effects of danazol.

Happily, by the middle to late eighties, another form of drug was developed for the treatment of endometriosis. This new form of hormonal therapy used an agonist—or longer-lived version—of gonadotropin-releasing hormone. The first GnRH agonist that was developed was leuprolide acetate, which is marketed as Lupron. Since then other forms, Synarel and Zoladex, have also become available. All of these GnRH agonists are similar to the natural hormone secreted by the hypothalamus, which stimulates the pituitary to release FSH and LH, two hormones that in turn regulate ovulation.

When a GnRH agonist is used, this hormone constantly stimulates the pituitary to pour out FSH and LH. Within two to three days, the pituitary has released so much FSH and LH that its supplies of these hormones are depleted. Within a very short period of time, a woman who is taking one of these antagonists stops ovulating and becomes menopausal, and her endometriosis begins to regress. This situation continues as long as she remains on the drug.

In contrast to danazol, the only significant side effects that women feel when their estrogen production is suppressed with Lupron, Synarel, or Zoladex are menopausal symptoms. Because these agonists aren't derivatives of a male hormone, there are none of the "male" side effects that many women find so troubling with danazol. That is why today, nearly all women who are undergoing hormonal therapy to treat their endometriosis use one of the gonadotropin-releasing hormone agonists.

All of these hormonal therapies have some things in common. Whether your doctor chooses birth control pills, danazol, or a GnRH agonist for your estrogen suppression, you will be treated for a period of six months, after which it will take another four to six weeks before you will resume regular ovulation and can begin trying to get pregnant once again. But there are differences in their success rates, convenience, and cost.

If endometriosis is the sole factor causing the infertile situation within the couple, pregnancy rates vary according to the treatment chosen. After oral contraceptive pill suppression with Stage One and Two, the success rates are 30% to 40%. However, with danazol or a GnRH agonist, 50% to 60% of Stages One and Two will conceive, and 30% to 40% of Stage Three will conceive. These success rates need to be balanced with the cost and convenience of the drugs involved. Oral contraceptive treatment averages about $30 to $60 per month, while treatment with danazol or GnRH agonist averages about $300 per month. Both oral contraceptives and danazol are administered in a pill form. GnRH agonists can be given as a once-a-month injection (Lupron and Zoladex), or as a nasal spray administered three times each day (Synarel).

When any of these hormone-suppression treatments are used for treatment of Stage One or Two endometriosis, the length of treatment should be 6 months. Following this treatment, efforts at getting pregnant should be concentrated for the next 6 to 12 months. That's because if a pregnancy has not occurred within that time, the endometriosis will usually have recurred, with a severity as extreme as it was prior to the treatment.

All of these factors, as well as each drug's side effects, should be taken into consideration as you and your doctor plan your treatment.

Surgical Treatment of Endometriosis

Almost without exception, surgery for pelvic endometriosis can be performed through the laparoscope, rather than as a more invasive laparotomy. Using the laparoscope, your doctor can usually see the extent and location of your endometrial adhesions and scars. In most cases, he will also be able to remove them via the laparoscope, using either a laser or standard surgical techniques.

As a patient, one of the questions you should ask your surgeon is whether he will be using a laser. Lasers are instruments that concentrate a beam of light energy into a small area. If you've ever used a magnifying glass to start a fire from nothing more than ordinary sunlight, you've got a general idea of how lasers work. While there are a number of different types of lasers that are used in pelvic surgery, carbon dioxide lasers and KTP lasers are the most common. Both of them have definite advantages over other surgical instruments. They can accurately vaporize even tiny implants of endometriosis, without traumatizing the surrounding normal tissue. The newer KTP laser is particularly good at doing this; it has a wavelength that is absorbed primarily by endometrial tissue, leaving normal tissue unaffected. And the KTP laser has an additional advantage. Its power is delivered through a flexible quartz fiber, which means that it can reach into almost inaccessible spots—under the ovary, for example—without difficulty. The CO_2 laser is mechanically much more difficult to use, especially for a surgeon who has minimal experience with operative laparoscopy.

Whether your doctor uses a laser or standard surgical tools, his goals should be the same. All visible lesions, scarring, and adhesions should be removed. Your ovaries should be freed of any endometrial lesions that may be adhering to their exterior. If your ovaries are enlarged with interior endometriomas—known as chocolate cysts—the ovary must be opened, the endometrial material removed, and the remaining walls of the cyst removed by laser. Once this is accomplished, your ovary will heal and function properly.

——————————— **LESS IS MORE** ———————————

Approaching chocolate cysts through laparoscopic surgery wasn't always the treatment of choice. Prior to my publishing the results of treating over 40 cases of such endometriosis through laparoscopy, the majority of gynecologic and reproductive surgeons used laparotomies to treat ovarian endometriomas. Today, with good training, most surgeons can remove chocolate cysts through the laparoscope. If your surgeon isn't comfortable doing this, you might want to seek a second

opinion. The success rate for this type of laparoscopic surgery is better than, and its invasiveness is far less than, the laparotomies that were previously done.

___

The laparoscopic techniques that have been developed over a period of years have proven to be so successful that they have completely revolutionized the treatment of pelvic endometriosis. Even most women with severe endometriosis can be treated without undergoing a laparotomy. But in rare cases—one in every 50 to 100 cases of moderate to severe endometriosis—the severity of the ovarian fixation, or the difficulty of reaching adhesions between the bowel and the ovaries, prevents treatment through the laparoscope. In these infrequent cases, a laparotomy is required.

Another thing that should be considered at the time of your surgery—irrespective of the type of surgical approach that is used—is whether steps should be taken to relieve the chronic pain your endometriosis may be causing you. If your pelvic pain is severe, your doctor may recommend that you have a procedure called a presacral neurectomy.

That means your doctor would cut the nerve fibers that go to your uterus and middle pelvic structures, so that if your endometriosis recurs, you will not feel discomfort because of it. In a high percentage of cases, a presacral neurectomy (done by laparotomy) will alleviate significant menstrual pain, menstrual cramping, and pain with intercourse. Another thing that your doctor might recommend at the time of your laparoscopic surgery is the resection, or the removal, of the uterosacral ligaments and the nerve fibers that run through them. Doing this can give relief to patients with pelvic pain, dyspareunia (pain with intercourse), and dysmenorrhea (pain with menstruation). (See Figure 10-1.)

Combination Treatment of Endometriosis

In the nineties we're able to take advantage of the experience we've gained during the last decade using GnRH agonists. We've found that in the majority of moderate to severe cases of endometriosis (Stage Three and Four), pretreating patients with either Lupron or Synarel before their surgical procedures improves their outcome. These GnRH agonists not only reduce the size of endometrial adhesions, they take down swelling in organs within the pelvic cavity that have been affected by the disease and that are inflamed as a result. This helps the surgeon in two ways. First, the endometrial adhesions that he's removing are smaller. Second, because swelling within the pelvic cavity is less, he can work

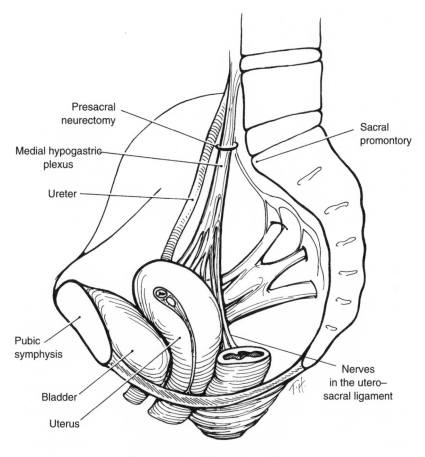

Figure 10-1: Pelvic Nerve Fibers

more aggressively as he removes adhesions, lesions, and ovarian endome-triomas. Pretreatment with GnRH agonists also improves a woman's re-covery. There is less inflammation of tissues in reaction to the surgical procedure, healing is improved, and scar formation is minimized.

COMBINED TREATMENT IS BETTER

Our group confirmed the effectiveness of combined treatment when we did a follow-up laparoscopy on severe cases of endometriosis. In each of these cases, after pretreating the patients with GnRH agonists, we performed extensive laparoscopic surgery to remove difficult en-dometrial growths in either the ovaries or other areas of the pelvic cavity. Yet despite the extensive nature of these operations, we had less than a 5% recurrence of adhesions.

Given its proven success rate, if you are going to be operated on for ovarian endometriomas, or for extensive pelvic endometriosis, you should talk to your doctor about having six to twelve weeks of agonist suppression prior to a laser laparoscopy. Using this type of combined treatment, we have been able to achieve a 50% to 60% pregnancy rate for patients with Stage Three endometriosis.

When Time's Not on Your Side

As you can see, there are a number of approaches to treating pelvic factor infertility. If your problem is pelvic adhesions caused by infection or trauma, your path is clear . . . you'll have surgery to remove them. But if you have endometriosis, you may have both hormonal and surgical options open to you. If this is your situation, and if you are in your middle thirties, you may want to factor in time as a consideration. No matter which form of hormonal therapy you're on, your ovulation will be stopped for a six- to eight-month period in order to reduce your endometriosis. After stopping your medication, it usually takes another month or two for your ovulation to resume. If you've reached the time of life when your fecundity is dropping rapidly, these are precious months for you. That's why we usually recommend that women 38 or over go directly to surgery. If this is done in a timely fashion, it is likely you will join the generally high success rate of other women who are successfully combating pelvic factor infertility.

Terms We Used in This Chapter

Adhesions: bands of scar tissue that can attach the surface of various organs to each other—for instance, a fallopian tube to the surface of an ovary.

Agonist: a drug or chemical that is designed to perform the same function as the natural, or parent, compound. For instance, Lupron is a synthetic preparation of gonadotropin-releasing hormone, but lasts longer and performs longer than the parent compound.

Anovulation: failure to ovulate.

Chlamydia: a bacteria that is considered to be sexually transmitted, which may be an underlying cause of infertility.

Chocolate cysts: ovarian cysts filled with degenerating blood that resembles melted chocolate. This occurs when endometriosis invades the ovary and bleeds cyclically, creating the cyst.

Crohn's disease: inflammatory disease of the small bowel.

Dysmenorrhea: painful menstrual periods.

Dyspareunia: painful intercourse.

Endometrioma: a cyst in the ovary caused by endometriosis; sometimes called "chocolate cysts."

Endometriosis: a disease in which normal endometrial cells get outside the uterus, stick to the surface of organs, and cause inflammation and tissue damage.

Estrogen: a category of female hormone that is necessary for female characteristics.

Fallopian tube: a narrow tubular structure connected to the uterus, which carries the egg from the ovary into the uterus after fertilization.

Gonorrhea: a sexually transmitted bacterial infection that can cause tubal damage in the male and the female.

Hysterosalpingogram (HSG): an X-ray study in which a dye visible by fluoroscopy is injected into the uterine cavity to determine the shape of the uterus and patency of the fallopian tubes.

Intrauterine device (IUD): a small, inert, usually plastic device placed in the uterine cavity to block implantation of an embryo.

Laparoscopy: a surgical procedure in which a telescope is inserted through the abdominal wall to view the inner organs.

Laparotomy: a surgical procedure in which an incision is made through the abdominal wall in order to view the inner organs.

Macrophages: cells arising from the bone marrow that kill or remove unwanted cells from the system, i.e., bacteria or tumor cells.

Microsurgery: a surgical procedure in which magnification and tiny instrumentation is used in order to improve reconstructive surgical outcome.

Myomectomy: the surgical removal of fibroids (myomas) from the uterine body.

Pelvic inflammatory disease (PID):   infection or inflammation of the female reproductive organs, usually caused by a sexually transmitted disease.

Peritoneum: the silky lining that covers the inside of the pelvic abdominal cavity.

Presacral neurectomy: the removal, or cutting, of the nerves that carry pain sensation from the uterus.

Retrograde menstruation: the back-flow of menstrual blood and tissue into the pelvic cavity.

Ultrasound: an instrument that emits pulsed sound waves which are reflected off solid tissues, to give an image of internal body structures without the use of X ray.

Uterosacral ligament: the major supporting ligament of the uterus. A common area of involvement with endometriosis.

11

Infertility and Miscarriage

"The baby's gone," he said, then quickly, "the pregnancy's gone. You knew that."

You knew that. Well, of course I knew that. I knew that from the first grab of pain. From the day the test was positive . . . because it stands to reason, doesn't it, dear, that if the truth be told, if you want a thing so badly, so nakedly, if you fasten wish and will onto it, it just stands to reason you will not actually have it.

—Jacquelyn Mitchard
Mother Less Child

It may seem strange to define a woman who is able to get pregnant as "infertile." But practically speaking, if she loses those pregnancies on a repeated basis, while she isn't infertile technically, she might as well be. Despite this, it's only relatively recently that doctors have begun to think of recurrent miscarriage as yet another aspect of the infertility picture. Women with a history of this problem now constitute a growing population of individuals seeking treatment with reproductive endocrinologists. It doesn't matter whether they lose clinically evident pregnancies, pregnancies that are too early to be detected on a clinical basis, or abort at some other time prior to fetal viability. The end result is the same. Even though conception has occurred, live birth never takes place.

━━━━━━━━━ **IT'S A QUESTION OF DEFINITION** ━━━━━━━━━

Miscarriage is the loss of a pregnancy during the first 24 weeks of gestation, or before the fetus weighs one pound. A pregnancy loss that is later than this is called a stillbirth.

In the past two decades our understanding of the causes of recurrent pregnancy loss has grown tremendously. Based on this new knowledge, doctors and researchers are beginning to explore the possibility that some of the same factors that limit a couple's ability to conceive are also involved in their inability to sustain a pregnancy. One of the more recently identified problems—immune system abnormalities—is a good example of this. In some couples, it's thought that immune system abnormalities prevent pregnancy from occurring at all. In others, they create problems with carrying the pregnancy to full term.

While immune system abnormalities are among the most recently discovered and least understood reasons for recurrent miscarriage, they are far from the only cause. Within this chapter we'll explore the diagnosis and treatment of women who are known, for any number of reasons, as "habitual aborters."

Why You?

The first thing you should realize is, if you have a miscarriage, you are not alone. Over 25% of women who are trying to conceive have a first-trimester pregnancy loss. In fact, first-trimester pregnancy loss is such a frequent complication of pregnancy that according to a 1992 study done by the World Health Organization, 150,000 spontaneous abortions occur each day. Miscarriage is so common that fully half of the eggs that are fertilized never progress to a viable pregnancy.

Since a third of these losses occur between the point of implantation and the sixth week of pregnancy, many women don't even realize they've been pregnant, much less that they've miscarried. Normally, it is only when you reach the point at which a gestational sac can be seen via ultrasound—usually around the fourth week—that you will know you are pregnant. But if you are undergoing treatment for infertility, and your doctor is testing your hCG levels, you will be aware of these very early—or "preclinical"—losses.

What's Causing Your Miscarriages?

There are a limited number of categories that account for most recurrent pregnancy loss.

1. Anatomical abnormalities in a woman's reproductive tract are responsible for 5% to 10% of miscarriages.
2. Luteal phase defects are responsible for approximately 20% of miscarriages.
3. Genetic abnormalities are responsible for 3% to 5% of miscarriages in women who have never given birth, and up to 50% of miscarriages in women who have previously given birth.
4. Immune system abnormalities are thought to account for up to 50% of miscarriages.
5. Another 15% are attributed to unknown causes.

While infections such as pelvic inflammatory disease and chlamydia are sometimes blamed for miscarriage, in fact they are only responsible about 1% of the time.

Deciding When You Have a Problem

Recurrent pregnancy losses are both frustrating and emotionally draining. Too often, this is compounded by the attitudes of the medical professionals a couple is dealing with. "Just keep trying" is the advice that is frequently given, particularly to couples who already have one child and have thus shown that they can give birth. Since this approach will prove to be successful in 95% of couples experiencing clinical pregnancy loss, and 50% experiencing preclinical loss, medical textbooks have classically stated that evaluation for recurrent pregnancy loss shouldn't be considered until after a couple loses at least three pregnancies. By that time, the odds of them carrying a pregnancy to term in the fourth attempt is somewhere around 45%.

Our new knowledge of areas such as immunological complications shows us that this may be the wrong approach. There is new evidence to show that if a first pregnancy causes an autoimmune problem, additional pregnancies will only make it worse. Added to this is the devastating emotional and physical impact of going through a second and third pregnancy loss. Taking these factors into consideration, a number of physicians now feel strongly that an evaluation looking for common factors in repeated pregnancy losses should be started after a second loss. And in a couple with a strong family history of pregnancy loss, they may even initiate the evaluation after their first miscarriage.

But since many doctors still wait until after a third miscarriage to initiate testing, it makes sense to ask your infertility expert what his policy is regarding this when you interview him.

Approaching Your Diagnosis

Similar to the logical pattern of tests for the basic workup, there is an order to this diagnostic evaluation. This priority-based testing looks for the most common reasons first, and the problems that can be corrected. Usually this testing goes as follows:

1. Structural abnormalities

2. Ovulatory or luteal phase testing

3. Immune abnormalities

4. Genetic diseases

But perhaps the most important thing to remember when approaching your diagnostic testing is that in the current medical environment, couples suffering from recurrent miscarriages can view their situation with new hope. Testing is now able to locate the cause of over 80% of these problems; and with treatment, a majority of these problems can be overcome.

Finding and Fixing the Problem

ANATOMICAL ABNORMALITIES

The types of anatomical abnormalities that can prevent a pregnancy from being carried to term are, in almost all cases, related to the uterus. The same sorts of problems that can prevent conception from occurring in the first place—Müllerian duct defects such as duplication of the uterus or abnormalities in its size and shape—can also turn the uterus into an environment that won't be able to maintain a pregnancy. With any one of these defects, even if implantation does occur, the uterus may not be able to expand and develop adequately during pregnancy to house the fetus as it grows to term.

Uterine abnormalities, and the ways in which they can sometimes be corrected, were discussed in depth in Chapter Eight. As we pointed out there, one of the more common abnormalities is the septate uterus. If your evaluation after recurrent miscarriages shows that this is your problem, it can be corrected through hysteroscopic surgery. Removing the wall of thin, fibrous tissue that divides your uterus will increase your odds for both implantation and full-term delivery.

Other structural defects, such as endometrial polyps or fibroids, that are present within the uterine cavity can be surgically removed after visualization by either hysterosalpingogram (HSG) or ultrasound. Once the polyps or fibroids are removed, implantation and a continuation of pregnancy should take place.

Unfortunately, if you have one of the other uterine abnormalities—such as DES changes, bicornuate uterus, or uterus didelphys—your condition cannot be surgically corrected. If you are an habitual aborter who has one of these problems, your doctor's only option will be to perform a cerclage, once you do get pregnant, to try to keep your cervix closed during your second and third trimesters. Hopefully, this will hold your fetus inside your uterus until a point at which it is viable and can be delivered. In addition, along with the surgery, continual bed rest after about the twenty-eighth week of pregnancy, and various medications to keep the uterus from contracting are usually recommended.

LUTEAL PHASE DEFECTS

In our chapter on ovulation (Chapter Six), we discussed the importance of the second half—or luteal phase—of your ovulatory cycle. As we have explained, the luteal phase influences not only the preparation of your uterus for the implantation of an embryo but also the maintenance of the pregnancy through its first 10 to 12 weeks. That's why most miscarriages occur when hormonal abnormalities produce deficiencies within the endometrial tissue during the first trimester of pregnancy.

Because luteal phase problems are almost always correctable, identifying them is an important step in the evaluation of women who have a history of recurrent pregnancy losses. This is done through a combination of blood tests and an endometrial biopsy. If your miscarriages are being caused by a luteal phase problem, your testing will show one of two things.

The production of progesterone and/or estradiol from your corpus luteum isn't great enough to stimulate appropriate endometrial growth and development.

The timing of your endometrium's development is out of synchrony with the days of your cycle, causing the development of your endometrium to occur too early or too late for implantation.

Fixing Luteal Phase Problems

Once a luteal phase defect is determined, your doctor will usually start clomiphene citrate therapy. Most luteal phase defects involve poor quality ovulation, a condition that clomiphene citrate can successfully remedy. This regimen is described in depth in Chapter Six.

If your ovulation mechanics are good, but your corpus luteum still isn't producing enough progesterone, your doctor will probably give you a progesterone supplement. In most cases you will receive natural progesterone, taken either in the form of vaginal suppositories, which should be used three times a day, or in the form of an oil mixture, which is injected once a day. Progesterone therapy should be continued through the tenth to twelfth week of gestation, the entire period during which the corpus luteum is responsible for producing progesterone to maintain your pregnancy. After that, your placenta will begin to produce enough progesterone to support your pregnancy on its own, and supplemental progesterone support can be ended.

In some cases, women receiving progesterone supplements still suffer miscarriages. This is often because their doctors don't fully understand that when progesterone is administered via vaginal suppositories, a great deal of it never gets into the patient's system. In fact, only about 30% of the progesterone that is concentrated in a suppository is actually absorbed. To further complicate things, the 30% of the hormone that *is* absorbed is only maintained in the tissues for a six-to-eight-hour period after the suppository is inserted. This data was clearly shown several years ago by Dr. Joyce Vargyas. She studied absorption and clearance times of vaginally administered progesterone. Dr. Vargyas found that, irrespective of the dose, the level after suppository use was maintained for only 6 to 8 hours. That's why, if you are using progesterone suppositories, they must be administered three times a day. If your doctor puts you on a once-a-day suppository regimen, or even a morning-and-evening suppository regimen, it won't be adequate to maintain the hormonal levels that are needed to protect the first 12 weeks of your pregnancy.

The blood tests that are taken to diagnose your luteal phase defect may also show that your estradiol level is too low. The ratio of estradiol to progesterone during the first 12 weeks of pregnancy should be at least a simple numerical ratio of four to one. Typically, an estradiol level of 160 pg per milliliter would relate to a progesterone level of 40 nanograms per milliliter. The small but significant number of woman who do not have an estradiol/progesterone ratio at least at this level, should be given an oral estradiol, in addition to the progesterone support they are receiving. Since estradiol production from the placenta begins earlier than progesterone production, estrogen supplements can usually be stopped by the sixth to eighth week of pregnancy. Your doctor will know that the time to stop your supplementary estrogen has arrived once he sees your estradiol levels rising, even though your dose of estrogen support remains constant.

GENETIC ABNORMALITIES

Women who miscarry are often told that it is for the best . . . that it is nature's way of ending a pregnancy that would otherwise have resulted in the birth of a child with genetic defects. Their doctors then reassure them that they should keep trying, that the same thing won't happen to them again.

In cases where a woman has had a single miscarriage, this is probably true. When fetal material that has been aborted during the first trimester is tested genetically, 70% to 80% of pregnancy losses are found to be due to genetic abnormalities. While they can be lethal to the fetus, they are not necessarily inherited from either of the parents. Genetic abnormalities such as Down syndrome (trisomy) or Turner's syndrome (45XO) occur spontaneously, on a random basis, during the developmental process of a fetus. And since these sorts of genetic abnormalities are random, rather than related to a chromosomal flaw in one of the parents, they usually don't happen again or cause recurrent miscarriages. That's why a woman who loses a pregnancy because of her fetus's abnormal genetic makeup would not usually have the same thing happen a second, third, or fourth time. The exception to this rule is women over 40 years of age, in which there is a higher likelihood that recurrent losses *are* due to chromosomal abnormalities that occur as their eggs age.

But there is another type of genetic problem that does cause a very small number of couples to have a history of recurrent pregnancy loss. Their number is so small—somewhere between 3% and 5% of recurrent pregnancy losses—that this constitutes the least common cause of multiple miscarriages. These couples usually suffer from a phenomenon called "balanced translocation": both of them have been born with the *same* defective gene. Couples whose pregnancy losses are due to balanced translocation can be identified through an examination of their chromosomes, called "karyotyping." Because balanced translocation is such a rare phenomenon, this type of testing is normally done only after all other possible causes of recurrent pregnancy loss have been eliminated. Karyotyping counts the chromosomes in cells. When done using cells from an aborted fetus, it can identify defects such as Klinefelter's, Down's, and Turner's—random problems that will probably never be repeated. When done on cells from the partners in an infertile couple, it can show defects that stem from maternal and paternal genetic abnormalities. Karyotyping costs about $300 to perform, and if balanced translocations are found, no treatment can be offered other than gamete donation.

IMMUNOLOGIC FACTORS

The medical world's understanding of immunologic function has increased dramatically during the last 20 years. We now know that immunological problems can affect all aspects of the human body—areas as diverse as the cardiovascular, respiratory, and reproductive systems. Using this new knowledge, doctors have made headway in treating a great number of diseases. Oncologists, for example, are now experimenting with immune therapy as a cancer treatment alternative. And in the field of infertility, we've begun to understand some of the difficulties the immune system can pose for human reproduction, and to find ways to help couples succeed despite them.

One of the first researchers to begin identifying immune system abnormalities, as they relate to abnormalities in pregnancy outcome, was Dr. Allen Beer, who was originally from the University of Michigan, and currently works at the University of Chicago Medical Center. It is only recently that investigators like Dr. Beer have begun to put the immunologic puzzle together. Through his work, and that of some other pioneers, we are now aware that several different aspects of the female immune system can come into play during reproduction. We are also beginning to gain an understanding of how each of these distinct components performs during conception, early pregnancy, and throughout fetal development, up until the delivery of a term pregnancy.

Because it is in its infancy, reproductive immunology is still quite controversial. While there are but a few formal scientific studies done in this area, growing data supports their validity. The knowledge that has been gained in the reproductive arena has been primarily developed by a handful of recognized reproductive immunologists. Despite their small number, they have very diverse opinions about the causes and treatment of reproductive immunological problems. Reproductive immunologists—and immunologists in general—now agree that there is a cause-and-effect relationship between immunologic disorders and pregnancy loss. But they have a harder time agreeing on exactly what that relationship is. Most accept that immunologic problems can cause miscarriage once a woman *has* conceived. But the question still exists as to whether they can create in a woman a state of infertility that will actually prevent her from conceiving in the first place.

Because of this, a very real controversy exists today as to whether couples who have unexplained infertility, and couples who have an explanation for their infertility but have gone through one or two cycles of "perfect" in vitro fertilization without having implantation or pregnancy occur, should be evaluated for immunologic disorders. Several factors contribute to this uncertainty. First, while there are only a limited number of doctors and laboratories in the United States that are qualified to do immunological testing, each one espouses radically different theories, testing techniques, and treatments, with none of them having yet been proven to be absolutely superior. Second, no matter which technique is used, all of these evaluations are expensive—running about $1,200 for the testing alone.

Given this uncertainty, if your doctor suspects that an immunologic problem may be contributing to your infertility, and he feels that testing might be beneficial, he will most likely hand you a number of scientific articles to try to make you aware of the differences in opinion that exist between various immunological experts. Even after reading them you may still be extremely confused as to what is proven and unproven in this field. Rest assured that your doctor probably is too. But despite the different theories of the experts, what should become evident to you after your reading is that a large amount of data strongly suggests that a significant relationship *does* exist between immunologic disorders, and both primary and secondary infertility. Because of this, a number of medical groups have become quite aggressive in getting a full immunologic evaluation, and treating immunologic dysfunctions, both in infertile patients and in patients who suffer from recurrent pregnancy loss. Having done this, they are beginning to find a significant percentage of individuals who have immunological dysfunction. Once these immunologic conditions are identified and treated, doctors are seeing an improvement in both implantation and birth rates when these couples undergo assisted reproductive procedures.

Hopefully, immunologic factors will become better understood in the next three to five years. Once they are, we will probably find that a significant percentage of couples with end-stage infertility have immunologic abnormalities that severely limit their ability to conceive and carry a pregnancy.

How Immune Problems Affect Reproduction

While the possible role of the immune system in infertility is still being debated, the connection between immunologic problems and miscarriages is more clear-cut. One of the first things that Dr. Beer discovered while studying habitual aborters—women who had lost at least two pregnancies prior to the end of the first trimester—was that a high percentage of these women suffer from autoimmune dysfunction. What this means is that their immune systems turn against their own bodies and begin attacking certain organs and systems, blocking them from functioning correctly. Autoimmune thyroid disease, which is both common and easily understood, is an example of this phenomenon. In a woman with this dysfunction, something triggers a response in her immune system, which causes it to manufacture antibodies that attack the cells in her own thyroid gland. Enough antibodies will eventually be built up by this autoimmune response to completely destroy the cells that produce thyroid hormone. Once that happens, she'll become severely hypothyroid and require medication to maintain a normal hormonal balance.

The reproductive system can suffer from similar types of immunologic disorders. They can manifest themselves in a number of ways.

- The mother's system can produce antibodies that attack the cells that build the placenta and its blood supply.

- The mother's system can produce antibodies that attack the nuclei of the cells of the uterus and the placenta.

- The mother's system can fail to produce the blocking antibodies that stop her immune system from attacking the fetus.

- The mother's system can have an overabundance of natural killer cells.

- The father's system can produce antibodies that attack sperm.

While each of these problems manifests itself in a different way, they all have one thing in common. If you have one or more of them, in order for you to have a greater likelihood of carrying a pregnancy to term, these problems will have to be detected and corrected prior to conception.

When Your System Attacks the Placenta and Its Blood Supply

Some cases of recurrent pregnancy loss are caused when a woman's immune system produces antibodies against the lipids and phospholipids that are in her system. Phospholipids are molecules that are found in all cell membranes. They are the "glue" that helps cells to fuse. When antibodies attack phospholipids in the uterus and placenta, they prevent the formation of cellular structures called syncytiotrophoblasts. Syncytiotrophoblasts are the building blocks of implantation: their job is to regulate nutrition for the fetus. Antiphospholipid antibodies also damage the walls of the blood vessels that provide circulation to the fetus. When this happens the vessels constrict, and the circulation of blood between the embryo and its mother is jeopardized. This can either retard the growth of the fetus or cause it to die.

Because the damage that antiphospholipid antibodies cause is so devastating, one of the first screening blood tests that should be done in women who are continually losing pregnancies is an antiphospholipid anticardiolipin screen. This test looks at whether a woman's immune system is manufacturing antibodies against important cellular materials such as phospholipids and cardiolipids.

Correcting an Antiphospholipid Problem   If your doctor finds that you are making antibodies against the glue that helps to form cells for the blood vessels and placenta, your problem is relatively easy to correct. Since the biggest threat to the fetus posed by this condition is that circulation will be inadequate, or that blood will clot, patients who are suffering from it are treated with anticoagulants. Anticoagulants help to counteract the clotting that antiphospholipid antibodies can cause.

Depending on the level of antibody activity that is found when you are tested, you will take either one baby aspirin per day throughout pregnancy, or a combination of baby aspirin and low-dose heparin. Heparin is an anticoagulant that is derived from animal tissue. It is injected subcutaneously, twice a day, in much the same way that Lupron is injected (see Chapter Six). Because its molecules are too large to pass through the placenta, heparin poses little threat to the fetus. It is normally used for at least the first 20 weeks of pregnancy.

When Your System Attacks Cell Nuclei

Some women produce antibodies against the proteins—such as DNA and histones—that are the building blocks of cells. Women with this problem very often have a history of inflammation in various organ systems, and may suffer from such conditions as rheumatoid arthritis or systemic lupus. When a woman with this problem becomes pregnant, these antibodies can attack her uterus and placenta. Once these tissues become inflamed, her fetus is jeopardized. The screening tests we utilize to find those conditions are called antinuclear antibody (ANA), anti-DNA, and antihistone antibody screens.

Treating an Antinuclear Problem   Because the threat to the fetus presented by these autoantibody conditions is inflammation, women suffering from them are treated with a corticosteroid—prednisone—in conjunction with heparin. Prednisone is an oral medication that is normally administered twice a day. It is started before conception, and the levels of antinuclear antibodies in the patient's bloodstream are monitored through follow-up tests.

When Your System Fails to Produce Blocking Antibodies

A second type of immunologic screening that is done on couples with recurrent pregnancy losses, and on couples with unexplained infertility who have failed to conceive with either GIFT or IVF procedures is an evaluation of "maternal blocking antibodies." This is an important test, because if these blocking antibodies aren't present in adequate numbers, implantation of a fertilized egg or embryo will not be able to take place.

Strange as it may sound, in order for implantation to take place, the mother's system must first perceive her embryo as a foreign material, then try to reject it and make it go away. This is a natural way for her immune system to react to an embryo whose genetic material and tissue consists of elements from the woman herself, and from her male partner also. Because these two individuals are genetically different, when their contributions combine in the embryo, it has a totally different genetic structure and tissue type from its mother.

The embryo responds to this initial rejection by its mother's immune system by sending out a signal. What exactly that signal is—whether it is hormonal or chemical—is still a mystery to researchers. But somehow, the embryo manages to tell the maternal immune system that its genetic content—its tissue makeup—although different from the mother's system, should not be rejected. This special signal encourages the mother's immune system to help the embryo remain in her uterus. To help the embryo accomplish this, the mother's immune system begins manufacturing what are called maternal blocking antibodies. These blocking antibodies coat the embryo, and protect it from attack by the maternal immune system. They continue to be produced and to provide this protection to the embryo throughout the first 16 to 20 weeks of pregnancy.

In most cases the embryo is able to send this message—"I am made up of two different things, and one part of me is from you"—because its mother and father have very different genetic and tissue makeup. But sometimes this is not true. In some couples, genetic and tissue types have enough elements in common to make the embryo's signal change. It begins telling the mother's immune system, "All of me is from you." As a result, the mother's system never sets up the initial rejection, and the signal to turn on maternal blocking antibodies never occurs.

As you can see, the way the immune system functions during reproduction is very different from the way it works at most other times. If an organ is transplanted, for example, doctors try to find the closest match they can to avoid rejection. Just the opposite is true for the embryo. The more different it is from the mother's genetic and tissue types, the harder the immune system works to help it implant.

Doctors test for a blocking antibody problem in two different ways. First, they check tissue types to try to identify couples who are too much alike. Next, using a technique called cell-flow cytometry, they test whether a woman's blood serum will manufacture blocking antibodies in response to her partner's white blood cells.

Treating a Blocking Antibody Defect   If a lack of maternal blocking antibodies is found during your immunologic screening tests, your doctor can correct the problem by taking white blood cells from your partner and immunizing you with them on a monthly basis. This should stimulate your system to produce the blocking antibodies. Using this treatment, doctors can generate production of a level of blocking antibodies that is as much as 10,000 times that normally seen in early pregnancy.

The procedure that's used for white blood cell immunization is relatively simple. Both you and your partner will be screened for infectious diseases such as hepatitis, HIV, and cytomegalovirus (CMV). This screening is a safety measure, since these diseases can be passed in blood and blood products. Once you are both shown to be disease free, a blood specimen will be taken from your partner. It will be processed through a series of steps that are designed to separate out his white blood cells, and leave his red cells, platelets, and blood serum behind. His white blood cells will then be concentrated into a very small volume of fluid, and injected under the surface layer of your skin, at about the depth that a skin test for tuberculosis would be done. Four weeks after the initial injection, the process will be repeated. And two to four weeks after this second immunization, another cell-flow cytometry test will be done to measure whether your maternal blocking antibody production has increased. If the production of antibodies still isn't adequate, a third immunization will be done using double the number of white blood cells from your male partner, and after another two to four weeks your level of blocking antibodies will be rechecked. If it's still lacking, white blood cells taken from a donor will be mixed with your partner's and used to immunize you. Eventually, enough maternal blocking antibodies will be produced in this way to protect the embryo during its initial implantation phase.

How Killer Cells Can Terminate a Pregnancy

One of the most recent areas to be investigated by reproductive immunologic researchers is that of "natural killer cells." In each of our immune systems, we have two types of white blood cells. "Helper cells" promote health, aid in the growth of normal cellular systems, and handle most protective functions—attacking a virus that invades your system, for example. Another type of cell, called a natural killer cell, is designed to attack any rapidly growing or dividing cell that it finds in your body. Killer cells are the special immune cells that work to rid us of cancer, tumors, and bacterial infections. Unfortunately, they have no ability to differentiate between a tumor that is growing in the uterus and a rapidly growing embryo. As far as they are concerned, an embryo is just one more mass of cells rapidly growing and dividing—and as such, it should be attacked.

Some women have a larger than normal number of these killer cells. On the plus side, they have very strong immune systems, and are protected against diseases such as cancer to a much greater extent than individuals with lower natural killer cell populations. The downside of having an excessively high level of natural killer cells is that they may also kill off a normal embryo as it tries to grow and develop inside your uterus.

A relatively new test, called an immunophenotype, is now able to identify women who may have this problem. An immunophenotype is a blueprint of the immune system as it relates to reproductive function. It measures five types of killer cells, each of which has to be below a certain percentage when compared to the helper cells in your system.

Treating Increased Killer Cell Activity   If you are identified as an individual with increased percentages of natural killer cells, your doctor will try to suppress them temporarily during your pregnancy, in order to protect your fetus. The most common way to do this is with monthly intravenous injections of immunoglobulins. Immunoglobulins are protein substances from the immune system. They suppress the production of the cells in your system that produce killer cells, and at the same time they enhance the production of helper cells.

As we write this, the use of intravenous immunoglobulin (IVIG) to correct immunological deficiencies is still somewhat experimental. However, more and more evidence is being gathered to strongly support its effectiveness as a means of fetal protection during pregnancy.

When Your System Attacks Sperm

As we discussed in our chapter on male factor problems (Chapter Nine), men sometimes produce antibodies against their own sperm. This happens because, unlike women—whose eggs are all present within their body at birth—men are born without sperm, and only begin to manufacture them *after* their immune systems are formed. As a result, men's immune systems perceive sperm as invaders, and treat them as such. This is not normally a problem, since a man's reproductive system is designed to keep his sperm separated from the rest of his body until they are released into his partner's vagina. It's only when something occurs that compromises this wall—an accident, infection, testicular torsion, a disease such as cystic fibrosis, or surgery such as a vasectomy—that an immune problem can arise.

While all of these things can cause immunological problems, they are most often seen in men who have had a vasectomy, and whose ejaculatory duct was blocked as a result of their operation. When sperm are released from the testicle after a vasectomy, they reach this obstruction and, unable to escape, die there in millions. As these cells die, they release protein into the circulatory system. Finding this protein in a place where it shouldn't be, the man's immune system tries to fight it by producing antibodies that attack it. Because this protein is a component of the man's sperm, his system is then filled with antibodies that will also attack his own sperm cells. These antibodies interfere with sperm movement, and possibly the ability of the sperm to fertilize the egg. This is why many men who have had their vasectomies reversed still remain infertile, even though the ejaculatory duct is successfully reconnected and sperm are being released again. Sperm antibodies may be suspected if large numbers of sperm stick together, or become "agglutinated." When a semen analysis is performed, if sperm agglutination is seen, a blood test should be done to confirm the presence of antisperm antibodies.

Treating a Sperm Antibody Problem   If high levels of antisperm antibodies are present, taking from 10 to 20 mg of prednisone a day is sometimes helpful. Having the man collect his semen specimen in a container of tissue culture fluid, and then quickly separating the sperm by sperm washing, will also provide benefit in a significant number of cases. In those men with severe antisperm antibodies, IVF with ICSI (intracytoplasmic sperm insemination) will be the only realistic alternative.

Coping Emotionally with Miscarriages

Losing any pregnancy is emotionally devastating. But the woman who is undergoing this experience for the first time will usually be able to experience the feelings of loss and separation that a premature termination brings, then comfort herself by reasoning that "these things happen" . . . that "while it just wasn't meant to be *this* time, next time things will be fine." What she's really doing is using this as a defense—she's focusing on the ways her body may possibly have failed her, and then using this focus as a way to literally "talk away" the loss. This defense isn't so easy to put up when miscarriage happens multiple times. When this happens, the idea that it's *your body* that's producing something that's incomplete, or somehow defective, begins to become internalized. Instead of blaming your body, you begin thinking that it's actually *you* who is incomplete or somehow defective. This new belief can evidence itself in physical symptoms. You might sleep too much, or not at all. You might eat too much, or not at all. This happens because on a very deep level you're no longer angry with the body that failed you, you're angry with *you*. And you're doing these things to punish yourself.

These thoughts of incompleteness and failure can begin to become entrenched in a woman's identity. The feelings they produce will commonly include:

- Depression
- Separation and loss
- Envy
- Rage

Very often the first emotion after any miscarriage is depression. It may not be accompanied by a full range of clinical symptoms. You may just feel an emotional numbness, or fatigue, or you may experience uncontrollable crying. Or you may go into a period of manic activity. Mania is the primary defense against depression. It keeps you from thinking about the things that are wrong.

"Feelings of separation and loss can quickly follow. Like many other major events in life—the death of a loved one, for example—a miscarriage can be the trigger that brings other unresolved issues to the surface . . . issues which may have built up over a lifetime. One example might be a woman's relationship with her own mother. If it's been troubled, a miscarriage can impact her even more significantly than usual by magnifying and reigniting all the unresolved feelings of failure that revolve around this topic of mother and child relationships.

"Feelings of loss and separation go hand in hand with a lack of differentiation from your mother. Especially when you anticipate a much-longed-for event—such as a pregnancy—and then feel that you didn't attain it to completion. The better your separation from your mother, the easier it is to cope with your own losses."

—Jill Model Barth, Ph.D., BCD

Another very common emotion in this situation is envy. Envy of others . . . envy of women who can make a complete baby . . . envy of *all* women who have babies . . . or envy of those who have more than one baby. Don't feel guilty if your envy makes it temporarily difficult for you to be around family members or friends who are pregnant. Your emotion is normal, and over time you'll work through it.

The final emotion you may be feeling is rage. Depression can be defined as anger turned inward. In a way it's a sign of progress when you begin to bring it out into the open. But this is not an excuse to vent it on other people. If you find yourself screaming at your husband for being ten minutes late, stop and think. Realize what the real source of your anger is, and don't transfer it to him.

While these feelings are common to almost all who've suffered miscarriages, their intensity and duration can vary significantly. Many doctors will tell their patients who have miscarried that they can begin trying for another pregnancy after three months. That's a medical model, which lets you know when your body will most likely be ready for another try. It fails to take the psychological component into account—the period of time it may take a woman to resolve her feelings of loss. Some women do better when they fill up the loss quickly. For them the three-month model may be right. Other women will take longer before they're ready to handle another try. Realize that this time frame is very individual, and understand that you need to respect it. Don't worry about whether you're moving too quickly or too slowly compared to what an expert might recommend. This can be especially difficult for older women to keep in mind—women who feel, perhaps, that time is running out. If this is your situation, don't let your anxiety rush you onward before you're ready to move on.

One reason women have very individual periods of grieving after a miscarriage is that they've reacted to their experience with different degrees of severity. Any number of things can affect the impact your miscarriage has on you. One is the stage of pregnancy at which it happened. During the first trimester of your pregnancy, you'll probably be experiencing incredible excitement as you fall in love with the idea that you're going to be a mother. But it's still a very new experience at that stage. Over a period of time, an attachment will grow. The longer the fetus continues to grow inside your body, the more you shift from thinking of it as a "fetus," to picturing it as a "baby." Also, since most women realize that the highest percentage of miscarriage is during the first 12 weeks, they know in the back of their mind that this might happen. But as the pregnancy grows more ripe, these thoughts begin to go away. They're replaced by a belief that now nothing can come and spoil the event. That's why second and third trimester miscarriages are more traumatic, and their effects can be more lasting.

Whether or not you understand the cause of your miscarriage is also something to consider. While it might seem, at first, that not definitely knowing the cause of your miscarriage would be highly frustrating and depressing, in fact this uncertainty can have just the opposite effect. Women who don't know the cause "for sure" may decide that they exercised too intensely, or worked full time when they shouldn't have. Coming up with a theory like this gives them a way to resolve the problem. They fantasize that if they just don't repeat that specific action, they'll have viable pregnancies in the future. Women who *do* know the cause of their miscarriage with certainty—be it a structural problem, a genetic problem, or an immunological problem—no longer have that imaginary way out.

Another important influence on the length and depth of your mourning period is the type of psychological support you get. Support can come from many sources . . . from your partner, from your family and friends . . . from professionals such as therapists . . . or from support groups.

Your primary source of support is your partner. Unfortunately miscarriage can affect your relationship just when it needs to be most solid. With many other issues surrounding infertility, you can try to get rid of your feelings of devastation by projecting them onto your partner. It's a relief to blame the other party. For example, your husband may be having trouble impregnating you. Certainly you're sad, but there's also a sense of relief that "it isn't me." Miscarriage doesn't allow a woman to take that out. With miscarriage, not only is there disappointment that there's no baby, there's a feeling of failure because you've deprived your husband. With this come feelings of self-doubt and incompleteness. This is a time when your capacity to function as a couple, and to be supportive, is of primary importance. Together you must realize that you're in this as a couple. While it may be the woman's body that physically lost the baby, it's the couple's issue.

Another good thing for men to keep in mind during the grieving process is that in order for a woman to work through the experience, she needs to be allowed to fully feel the loss, and to integrate its psychological meanings into her psyche. A husband who prematurely interrupts his wife's need to talk about her miscarriage, saying things like, "These things happen. It's not the end of the world, we'll do it again," works against this need. These things sound positive, but often they're a reflection of his own discomfort with the deep emotional mood swings his wife is experiencing. In an attempt to end them, he dismisses the intensity of the event. And by doing that, he keeps his wife from completing her mourning.

Your family and friends also should be made to realize that being able to work through your grieving and loss at your own pace is primary to your psychological recovery. They shouldn't feel hurt if you don't want to be around those of them who have, or are having, babies. They should realize that, as you grieve, it can be hard to be around children and babies. For your part, you should keep in mind that if this sort of situation doesn't make you feel good, it's important to be able to say no, without worrying about hurting other people's feelings. Following a miscarriage, the first priority is for you as a person (and for you and your husband as a couple) to protect yourself.

Perhaps you've felt anxious about trying again for a prolonged period. As much as you long for a baby, and as much as you realize that getting pregnant is the only way to get that baby, you're so anxious about miscarrying you're actually afraid to try. Couples with a history of losing multiple pregnancies have usually pushed their emotional strength and their denial to a level different from other infertile couples. If you're an habitual aborter and you become pregnant, your battle isn't over—it is just beginning. Your emotional stress and fear doesn't decrease, it escalates. From day to day, week to week, blood test to blood test and ultrasound to ultrasound, you wait to hear that once again the baby is dead, that its heart no longer beats. You fear going to your doctor's office for an ultrasound, yet without it, sleep and work are impossibilities. Even as you make it to the tenth week, you worry about getting to twenty weeks, and so on. If you're a patient with multiple pregnancy loss, your emotional battle is never won until you hold your baby in your arms.

When an infertility patient finally, unexpectedly, gets pregnant after years of treatment, and then loses that pregnancy early on, the emotional impact is worse than never having been pregnant at all.

If this is your situation, you may want to turn to either a therapist or a support group. We will discuss this in Chapter Fourteen. When you've miscarried, you should look for a therapist who has the capacity to deeply understand loss. Whether that person has actually been through a miscarriage doesn't matter. In just the same way that you need to find the right fit in a therapist, locating a support group that works for you may take a few tries. If the first one you go to doesn't feel right, don't give up. The next one may. Or the one after that.

When all is said and done, and you've survived the initial stages of your grieving, one of the best ways to heal is to concentrate on the positives in life. You as a couple should try to fill up on other aspects of your loving relationship. Focus on exploring your body in pleasurable ways, not just using it as a conduit for a baby. Spend alone time that's not strictly sexual. And spend sexual time that's not solely for the purpose of making a baby. Granted, that's sometimes really hard to do, especially if you have an incredible desire to get pregnant again quickly. But it will reward you by helping you to feel good about yourself and your relationship, despite the problems you've been having. Outside your relationship, associate yourself with people who are a source of comfort to you. If someone makes you feel anxious, don't spend time with them. Always remember, what you need after a miscarriage is for life to be breathed into you, not get sucked out of you.

Terms We Used in This Chapter

Antibody: a protein substance produced by the body in response to a stimulating substance (antigen).

Autoimmune dysfunction: a disease or dysfunction that occurs because the body's immune system attacks and destroys its own tissues.

Balanced translocation: the crossover of genetic material from one arm of a chromosome to the other arm. The person with a balanced translocation is clinically normal, but can pass the abnormal translocation on to offspring.

Bicornuate uterus: a malformation of the uterus resulting in two separate cavities, each with a connecting fallopian tube.

Blocking antibodies: protective antibodies that are formed by the mother's immune system in response to her embryo during implantation.

Corpus luteum: the cyst that forms after a follicle releases its egg. It produces estrogen and progesterone during the second half of the ovulatory cycle.

Deoxyribonucleic acid (DNA): the material in each cell nucleus that contains each individual's genetic code.

Diethylstilbestrol (DES): a man-made estrogen originally used to prevent miscarriages. Is known to cause abnormalities of the cervix, vagina, and uterus of the unborn fetus.

Endometrial polyps: an overgrowth of normal endometrial tissue, forming a protrusion into the uterine cavity.

Endometrium: the lining of cells inside the uterus that is sensitive to estrogen and progesterone stimulation.

Fibroids: a benign tumor made up of fibrous tissues found in the uterus.

Histones: a simple protein found in the cell nucleus that contains a high proportion of basic amino acids.

Immunophenotype: an individual's profile of natural killer cell activity, as it relates to the immune system.

Karyotyping: counting and identifying the genes in a person's cells.

Killer cells: the cells in the immune system designed to attack rapidly growing masses of cells.

Luteal phase defect: inadequate production of hormone from the corpus luteum, or poor response of the endometrial lining to hormonal stimulation, which interferes with implantation.

Miscarriage: loss of a pregnancy prior to the 20th week of gestation.

Syncytiotrophoblasts: the cells that form the placenta.

Septate uterus: a fibrous division of the uterine cavity.

Uterine didelphys: duplication of the uterus; a double uterus.

12

Assisted Reproductive Technologies

"She was born at 11:47 P.M. with a lusty yell, and it was a cry heard around the brave new world. Louise Brown, blond, blue-eyed and just under 6 pounds, was the first child in history to be conceived outside her mother's body. Her birth last week in a dowdy British mill town was in its way a first coming—variously hailed as a medical miracle, an ethical mistake and the beginning of a new age of genetic manipulation."

From Newsweek, *August 7, 1978*

Louise Brown's birth had been anticipated since November of 1977, when Dr. Robert Edwards and Dr. Patrick Steptoe of Cambridge, England, announced that they had successfully performed in vitro fertilization; they had taken an egg from a human ovary, fertilized it in a glass dish in their laboratory, and then placed the resulting embryo in the uterus of the woman who had produced the egg. Nine months later she delivered a healthy baby girl.

The news of the birth of this first "test tube baby" rocked the world. It marked the first successful human conception outside the female reproductive tract. It also ushered in the beginning of an era when medical advances would continually take place in the arena of assisted reproductive technologies. Before this incredible breakthrough, there was little doctors could do to assist couples who were hopelessly infertile. But with this medical triumph, a whole new world of possibilities opened, bringing with it an incredible inventory of moral, ethical, and legal complexities that have now—two decades later—led some to think of Steptoe and Edwards's achievement as the opening of a Pandora's box.

Much of this disenchantment with assisted reproductive technologies is the result of misinformation and misunderstanding about its success rates and techniques. While there's a constant stream of articles dealing with this subject matter in the consumer press, many of them use totally inaccurate statistics, or misinterpret valid research. That is why, before stepping into this complex and expensive arena, you should be well-versed in the realities of how these procedures work, and what you can actually expect from them.

A Thumbnail History of Assisted Reproduction

The news of a test tube baby came as an incredible shock to most of the public. But in reality, research leading toward this accomplishment had been actively under way in a number of countries for nearly fifteen years prior to Steptoe and Edwards's success. Within the year following Louise Brown's birth, a second in vitro baby was born through the efforts of Drs. Ian Johnston and Alex Lopata, in Melbourne, Australia. While other in vitro births followed, both in Australia and England during the next few years, it wasn't until March of 1982 that Howard and Georgianna Jones reported the first live birth from in vitro fertilization in the United States. Three months later our team in Los Angeles reported its own successful in vitro fertilization birth—the first in the western half of the United States. At the time of this birth, just 23 children had been born worldwide through IVF technology.

During the decade that followed, a vast array of assisted reproductive technologies (ART) were developed, tested, and perfected in rapid-fire succession. Each of these procedures allowed doctors to accomplish different reproductive cycle steps within the laboratory environment, instead of inside the patient's reproductive tract. And by doing this, each of these procedures helped infertile couples to sidestep specific physical or physiologic flaws.

Today, over 100,000 babies have been produced through the many procedures that grew out of the first IVF technology. Every new technique moved yet another reproductive step outside the human body and into a controlled laboratory setting, each technique offering hope to different groups of people who previously couldn't achieve a successful pregnancy. Since each procedure in IVF technology is best suited to work around a specific problem or problems, you should have a clear understanding of all the procedures if you're considering stepping into the arena of assisted reproductive technologies.

IN VITRO FERTILIZATION

In the early days of in vitro fertilization, eggs were collected from the woman undergoing this procedure via laparoscopy under a general anesthetic. These eggs were then mixed with the male partner's sperm in a covered glass dish called a petri dish. It's this dish that gives the procedure its name: *in vitro* is Latin for "in glass." The fertilized eggs were carefully incubated and observed within the laboratory for one to three days. By this time, the embryos they formed had begun to divide—the beginning of a stage called "cleavage development." The embryos would then be removed from the laboratory and placed in the woman's uterine cavity during a second operation, a procedure called "embryo transfer." The hope was that they would implant there and develop into a healthy baby.

With the advent of IVF, a great deal of the responsibility for the reproductive process was taken away from mother nature and placed in the hands of doctors and laboratory scientists. Sperm no longer had to make their way from the vagina, through the uterus, then up the tubes. And after fertilization, the embryo no longer had to travel through the tubes before implanting. Because of this, IVF offered great hope to women who had problems with their fallopian tubes or cervix, to men with poor or minimal sperm, and to couples with unexplained infertility. The procedure has proved to be so successful that, as we write this, approximately 27,000 IVF procedures are performed annually in the United States, with a birthrate of approximately 20% per cycle.

GAMETE INTRAFALLOPIAN TRANSFER (GIFT)

Even as IVF was being applied and improved, Drs. Ricardo Asch and Pepe Balmacedo, at the University of Texas in San Antonio, were working on what was to become the next successful ART procedure. Gamete intrafallopian transfer, which is commonly known by the acronym GIFT, was developed in 1984. Like IVF, GIFT involved retrieving eggs from an infertile patient during a laparoscopic procedure, and mixing them with her partner's sperm outside her body. But unlike IVF, this mixture of egg and sperm was not kept outside the body to fertilize in a laboratory environment. The blending was done in a catheter, and the combined eggs and sperm were immediately inserted into the patient's fallopian tubes. Because the entire procedure was accomplished in a single operation, and egg and sperm interaction took place in the nurturing environment of the fallopian tube, an improved outcome was hoped for.

Using GIFT, scientists could guarantee that the egg and sperm would indeed meet, but they weren't actually able to observe fertilization, as they could with IVF. However, they anticipated other benefits that would potentially make GIFT's success rate even greater than that of IVF. What GIFT offered was a chance for the fertilized egg to grow and develop naturally within the fallopian tube. This was an important plus. Researchers have put a great deal of effort into developing a medium to be used within the laboratory petri dish that closely mimics the nutrients, chemicals, and density of the liquid environment of the fallopian tubes. But their efforts have always fallen just a bit short. No matter the chemical blend, man-made mediums have never managed to be quite as effective as nature's.

Because GIFT requires a patient's fallopian tubes to be functional, the number of women who can use GIFT is more limited than the number who can use IVF. As we write, approximately 5,000 GIFT procedures are performed each year in the United States—considerably fewer than IVF. But in those women who are candidates, GIFT results in birth rates of approximately 30% per cycle.

ZYGOTE INTRAFALLOPIAN TRANSFER (ZIFT)

Closely following on the heels of GIFT—in the late eighties—another procedure was developed that combined some aspects of IVF with aspects of GIFT. Like GIFT, zygote intrafallopian transfer (ZIFT) can be performed only on women with functioning fallopian tubes. In this procedure, which was developed by Dr. Peter Yovich of Perth, Australia, eggs and sperm are removed from the infertile couple and combined in the laboratory. Dr. Yovich called his procedure pronuclear oocyte sperm transfer (PROST), which is synonymous with ZIFT. Fertilization is observed, just as in IVF. But there the similarities end. Instead of waiting for cleavage to begin, then putting the resulting embryos into the woman's uterus, as was done in IVF, fertilized ZIFT eggs were placed in the woman's fallopian tube within the first 24 hours after they were taken from her ovaries. All research to that point had indicated that the longer embryos remained in the artificial environment of the petri dish, the greater their failure rate became, so quickly placing them in the fallopian tube seemed like a fine idea. Other investigators allowed the fertilized eggs to divide, or cleave, before transfer. This procedure, which is called tubal embryo transfer (TET), has success rates similar to those of ZIFT or PROST (18% to 25%).

ZIFT was designed to be used with couples whose only apparent problem was with sperm quality. Since fertilization could actually be observed, physicians could confirm that the sperm had accomplished their mission. And because the woman's fallopian tubes were functional, it was thought that the embryos would be able to get the benefits of growing and developing within them as they traveled to the uterus to implant.

In actual practice, though, ZIFT proved to be a bad trade-off, when its success rates were considered in light of its additional invasiveness and cost. Like IVF, ZIFT required two separate procedures. But unlike IVF, where embryo transfer into the uterus is simple and noninvasive, ZIFT required a laparoscopic procedure to place the embryos into the fallopian tube. All this might have been justified, but for one thing. During the two or three years when ZIFT was most popular—1988 to 1990—success rates with IVF increased. Researchers continued to refine the medium in which IVF embryos grew for their first 24 to 72 hours, and succeeded to such a degree that success rates for IVF and ZIFT were, from a practical point of view, equal. Given these drawbacks, it's not surprising that ZIFT is rarely used these days. And keeping these facts in mind, you should be quick to question it if your doctor recommends this procedure for you.

EMBRYO FREEZING (CRYOPRESERVATION)

Once initial success with IVF was achieved, a number of medical groups began experimenting with ways to improve the success rate for each cycle. One of the earliest improvements was made when doctors demonstrated that they could stimulate patients to produce more than one egg per cycle. Early studies in this area were done by Dr. Carl Woods in Australia, by Dr. Georgianna Jones in Virginia, and by Dr. Joyce Vargyas, Dr. Bill Yee, and me, in Los Angeles. As it became obvious that we could consistently help patients to produce multiple eggs, and therefore multiple embryos, a new concern arose. Since not all of these embryos could be implanted during a cycle, what was to be done with all of these potential new lives?

This quandary inspired Dr. Alan Trounson of Australia to begin working on methods to safely freeze excess embryos in order to store them for future use. In 1984 he announced that a pregnancy had been achieved after producing a human embryo in vitro, then freezing, thawing, and transferring it. The first child to be born as a result of this process was delivered in Australia later that year.

My group in Los Angeles had also sought permission to begin experimental work in human embryo cryopreservation. After extensive animal trials, human use approval was given by our human research committee at the University of Southern California, and we produced the first baby from human embryo cryopreservation to be born in the United States in June 1986. Since these initial successes, embryo cryopreservation has continued to be an extremely important aspect of ART procedures.

MICROMANIPULATION OF GAMETES

In 1988, a mere decade after the first successful use of IVF, a whole new generation of infertility procedures was born. It was at this point that scientists began to work directly on gametes (another name for eggs and sperm) to assist the fertilization process. Prior to this point, only limited things could be done to help the fertilization process in a man whose sperm were sparse in number, were not motile, or were unable to penetrate an egg. Even in IVF, where sperm are physically brought into contact with an egg, a minimum of approximately 50,000 motile sperm are required. In many cases, due to poor sperm quality, men were left with no hope of producing their own biological child. *Micromanipulation techniques* changed all that.

These new procedures operated directly on the egg, a single cell just two hundredths of a millimeter in diameter, about the size of the point of a needle. Micromanipulation improved the rate of fertilization within the laboratory setting. After fertilization was accomplished, the resulting embryo—or embryos—were transferred into the uterus of the mother, using the same procedure that had been developed for IVF. By doing this, researchers vastly improved the chances for previously infertile men to father a child.

The first micromanipulation technique to be introduced was *partial zona dissection (PZD)*. In partial zona dissection an embryologist, looking through a microscope, uses a very tiny holding instrument and an equally small cutting instrument to nick a hole through the outer layer of the egg—the zona pellucida. Sperm are then added to the in vitro culture, hopefully to find their way through the man-made opening. (See Figure 12-1A.) Partial zona dissection proved to be of limited success, with 30% to 40% of eggs exposed to sperm in this manner being fertilized. However, it did have one drawback. Once the zona pellucida was broken, the natural tendency of the egg to accept one sperm, and only one, was also lost. As a result, eggs could be fertilized by multiple sperm, and embryos with abnormal numbers of chromosomes could be produced, which then had to be discarded. This defect was easily observed when the embryos were examined the day after fertilization. If more than two pronuclei are seen within the egg, it is an indication that multiple sperm penetrated and fertilized it, producing an unusable embryo.

While the fertilization rate that was obtained with PZD was encouraging, researchers continued to strive to improve it even further. They accomplished this with the next micromanipulation technique that was developed—*subzonal sperm insemination (SUSI)*. In subzonal sperm insemination, sperm are inserted into the space between the outer membrane of the egg—the zona pellucida—and the cytoplasm that forms its inner core. With this technique, sperm no longer had to find their way through a man-made hole in the zona; they were placed within this outer membrane by the physician. Fertilization rates improved marginally, but multiple sperm fertilizations increased as well. (See Figure 12-1B.)

By the early nineties micromanipulation techniques and tools had improved to such an extent that scientists attempted to extract a single sperm from a man's semen and inject it into the cytoplasm of an egg. This new technique, called *intracytoplasmic sperm insemination (ICSI)*, meant that men with an almost nonexistent sperm count could still become genetic fathers. Even those men who had no ability whatsoever to ejaculate could be treated. Sperm could be extracted directly from the testicle—either from the seminiferous tubule or from the epididymis—treated with chemicals that helped to mature them, and then injected into an egg. While ICSI has been in use since 1992, it requires such specialized equipment and skills that the number of cases that are treated with this technique annually still number in the low thousands. But in those who are treated, many of them men who would previously have had absolutely no hope of fathering a child, ICSI now yields successful fertilization in approximately 70% to 80% of the eggs injected. (See Figure 12-1C.)

OOCYTE (EGG) DONATION

ICSI has given many men suffering from difficult cases of male factor infertility the chance to contribute to fathering a child. Parallel progress has been made with women who, in the past, were unable to give birth because of poor egg quality. Because donor sperm are so easily transferred through artificial insemination, their use became common early in

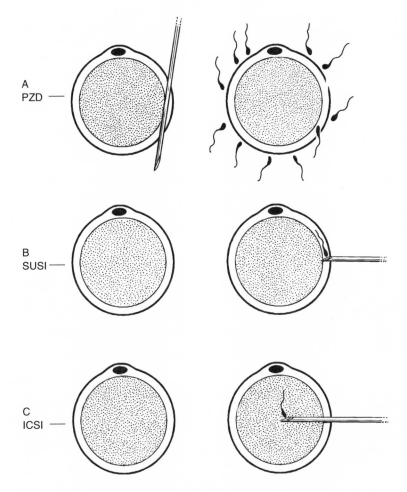

Figure 12-1:   Micromanipulation of Oocytes

the history of assisted reproduction. But the use of donor eggs, which depends on sophisticated collection procedures and precise timing, could only become feasible once ART technologies had advanced. ART procedures using donor eggs, which were first done in the late eighties, have flourished in the nineties. Because of them, women who could not become pregnant using their own eggs can now carry a baby to term. While they are not genetically linked to these children, they are their biological mothers.

Egg donation is most commonly used for women over the age of 40. Even using ART procedures, women in this age range are most often unsuccessful in their attempts to get pregnant. That's because the older a woman is, the less likely it is that her eggs will produce embryos of a high enough quality to implant and grow to term. If your age is a factor in your infertility problem, egg donation may be the right alternative for you. Because fecundity drops so precipitously after the age of forty, many doctors go directly to egg donation in women of this age, rather than spending time and money on ART attempts using the woman's own eggs. This approach has produced pregnancy in a very high percentage of cases. Programs around the world have used it to help women of all ages—some as old as 60—successfully conceive and deliver babies. However, in most ethically sound infertility centers in the United States, egg donation in women over the age of 50 to 55 is frowned upon.

GESTATIONAL SURROGACY

Egg donation helps women who have a healthy uterus, but inadequate eggs, to give birth. Gestational surrogacy does the opposite. It helps women who have healthy eggs, but who have lost their uterine function early on in their reproductive lives, to have a genetic child.

This process combines IVF with gestational surrogacy. A "surrogate gestational carrier" is a woman who carries another woman's embryo for nine months. If you are undergoing this procedure, your eggs and your husband's sperm would be retrieved, just as if you were undergoing a normal IVF procedure. But the resulting embryo would be placed in the uterus of the surrogate, rather than in your own uterus. The surrogate's purpose is to supply a uterine environment for the gestation and delivery of your embryos. If you are considering this option, you should keep in mind that since the surrogate did not produce the egg that was used to create the embryo, the future baby will have no genetic relationship to her.

Gestational surrogacy, which was first done successfully in 1985, is a good treatment alternative for women who were born without a uterus, or with an abnormal uterus that can't be corrected surgically, or who have had a hysterectomy. As long as a woman still has ovarian function and can produce eggs, this procedure is workable for her.

Is Surrogacy Legal?

One of the factors limiting the widespread use of surrogate carriers is the potential legal problems that surround it. While the medical aspects of the procedure have been mastered, ethical and legal limitations on the use of gestational surrogate carriers are still fairly significant. Adding to the confusion, rules vary from state to state. Some states have laws that make it illegal to be a surrogate carrier, or to use one. On the opposite end of the scale, there are a few states that actually identify surrogacy by state statute, and recognize it as legal. In California, for instance, surrogacy has been both legally accepted and upheld by the court system. Since there is no federal law that clarifies the role of the gestational surrogate, it is imperative that you speak with your doctor and appropriate legal counsel to ascertain your own state's rules before you step into this arena.

How Much Does Gestational Surrogacy Cost?

Another roadblock to the use of surrogate gestation is its enormous cost. Selecting an appropriate surrogate, the processing—both medical and psychological—and the pregnancy itself, normally cost around $50,000. Added to that is the cost of in vitro fertilization, approximately $10,000 to $12,000 per cycle. A total cost of $60,000 to $70,000 can be a painful shock, even when a healthy baby does result. Still, for some, determined to produce their own genetic baby, it may be the only alternative.

Making Your Personal Decisions About ART

Assisted reproductive technologies are a thriving and ever-changing area of medicine, but also a complicated one. The complexity of ART procedures has constantly increased, starting with the early procedures done by Steptoe and Edwards in the late seventies, and continuing on through the work that's currently being done in micromanipulation and other cutting-edge technologies. Today, there are a large range of treatment choices available to you. But because the human body is both delicate and complex, there are also a number of complicated decisions that you will have to make before using them. Since every couple is different, determining exactly what your best path is can be difficult. As you face these decisions, your discussion with your doctor should start by considering whether this is the right time for you to begin ART procedures.

WHEN SHOULD YOU BEGIN TRYING ART PROCEDURES?

Deciding when ART procedures should be incorporated into your treatment is a balancing act. If you wait too long, the chances for success will decline. If you start it too soon, you may be spending large amounts of money, and undergoing difficult physical procedures, that aren't really necessary.

On the surface, the timing appears simple. As soon as conventional infertility treatment fails to produce a pregnancy, you should move on to ART. That's because your age plays such a pivotal role in the ability of ART procedures to be successful. All ART procedures require healthy eggs—and as you age, your eggs age with you. So waiting too long to start ART procedures may create a situation in which the eggs can't work.

On the flip side, however, you should be wary if your doctor recommends that you move on to expensive and invasive ART procedures without first exhausting conventional treatment. A 35-year-old woman with ovulation problems should be placed on drugs for ovulation control as a first step in her treatment. She should not be directed immediately to IVF or GIFT. Yet in some infertility centers, the use of sophisticated ART technologies has run rampant. While it has obvious benefits for the doctors who are doing these expensive procedures, this "go straight to the top" treatment philosophy is not in the patient's best interest. It's bad enough that it escalates cost and invasiveness. What's worse, it doesn't produce any better pregnancy statistics than conventional therapy. While our 35-year-old woman with ovulation problems may very well get pregnant with a GIFT procedure, she should accomplish the same result with simpler, and considerably cheaper, drug therapy.

So how do you know when you're ready? In many cases, your gut will tell you. If you're feeling stuck in your treatment, it's time to discuss those feelings with your doctor. If, cycle after cycle, there's no positive outcome, it's time to reevaluate the need for ART procedures. Don't waste months—even years—with conventional therapy that's not working. It will only diminish your odds with assisted reproductive technologies. In our clinic we follow a simple rule: A maximum of six cycles of any technology should be attempted, no matter what the technology that's being used. After this point, chances of that technology producing a pregnancy diminish. So if it hasn't worked by the sixth try, cut your losses and move on to the next alternative. There has to be a concerted effort by both you and your doctor to make prudent, appropriate decisions when you're considering moving on to ART procedures. To ensure this, your discussions should include your age, the facts about your individual medical condition—giving particular consideration to the viability of your fallopian tubes and the quality of your partner's sperm—and your budget.

ASSESSING YOUR AGE AS A FACTOR IN ART PROCEDURES

ART procedures work best when a surgeon can implant multiple healthy embryos. To do that, a woman must be able to produce multiple healthy eggs. Since the status of your ovarian function is inextricably tied to your age, this is one of the first things you and your doctor should take into consideration when you start looking at ART. If you're over 40, the likelihood of your producing a large number of good-quality embryos per cycle is slim. First, you may not be able to produce a large enough number of eggs per cycle. Second, the age of your eggs, and the chromosomal changes that may have occurred in them, could mean that the quality of the embryos they create may not be good enough to give you a very high success rate in implantation and pregnancy.

Your doctor can make a fairly accurate guess about your ability to produce enough eggs. By testing your normal ovarian function, he can predict how well your ovaries will respond to hormonal stimulation. This will give him a good idea as to whether you will be able to produce the multiple eggs that are required for ART procedures. To do this, your doctor will give you a blood test on Day Two or Three of your cycle. If you have an FSH level of less than 15 mIU/ml, and an estradiol level that's less then 75 pg/ml, there's a reasonable chance that you'll respond properly to controlled ovarian hyperstimulation regimens. While this will tell you whether you can produce enough eggs to be a candidate for ART, unfortunately it can't tell you what the genetic quality of those eggs, or of the embryos they become, will be. This is something that you, as a patient, should keep in mind. Even if your ovulation function "passes the test," and you are able to move on to ART based on the results of your stimulation response, your excitement may be short-lived. The eggs you produce may still get a failing grade.

A major problem is producing eggs, but then finding out later that they won't work. By the time you make your discovery, you will already have spent a good deal of time and money, and undergone physically taxing procedures. That's why many doctors recommend proceeding directly to egg donation with women over 42 years of age. They use statistics to make their case.

- Using in vitro fertilization over the age of 40, the live birth rate per transfer of embryo averages about 10% to 12%.

• If GIFT is performed in combination with embryo transfer—
replacing a maximum of six to eight eggs and/or embryos—or if
GIFT is performed with six eggs in women over the age of 40,
live birth rates range between 12% and 20% per procedure.

As an infertile patient, all of these are alternatives that should be presented to you. One aspect of your decision-making process will be dic-
tated strictly by physical factors. Most important among those are the
condition of your fallopian tubes, and the quality of your partner's sperm.

ART PROCEDURES AND FALLOPIAN TUBE STATUS

Assuming that your ovulation is normal, the second thing to consider
when approaching ART procedures is the condition of your fallopian
tubes. Their ability to function can dictate your decision in and of itself.
Both GIFT and ZIFT involve insertion of the gametes or embryos into
the fallopian tube, through which it must then be able to travel to your
uterus. In GIFT your tubes will be receiving eggs and sperm; in ZIFT
they will be receiving embryos. Obviously, if your tubes have been surgically removed, or have been damaged beyond repair, there is no way you
can use either of these procedures. For you, in vitro fertilization is the
only alternative.

If, on the other hand, you have fallopian tubes that are open and
functional, but have some other complicating problem, GIFT may be a
better alternative than IVF. Perhaps you have ovulation problems, or
adhesions from endometriosis that prevent your fallopian tube from
picking up the ovulated egg. Having your eggs or embryos inserted
mechanically into your tubes could bypass this problem for you. Or perhaps your partner has a mild to moderate male factor problem. Having
his sperm put in direct contact with your eggs may guarantee that the
two of you will achieve fertilization.

If the condition of your tubes makes it an option, GIFT should
probably be your first choice procedure. As we discussed earlier in the
chapter, one of the great advantages of GIFT is that it allows the egg and
sperm to come together in the natural environment of the fallopian
tubes, and makes it possible for the embryo to be nourished there as it
travels to the uterus. While science is coming ever-closer to duplicating
this natural environment, it still hasn't fully succeeded. Because of this,
GIFT's success rates in women under the age of 40 who demonstrate
normal egg and sperm interaction is 30%, compared with the 20% success rate of IVF. GIFT embryos, which spend their important early days

in an optimum natural environment, are stronger and possibly more likely to implant and grow to term.

Given its higher success rate, the only argument against GIFT is its greater physical invasiveness. The average cost, in most centers, for a GIFT procedure is usually the same as that of IVF with embryo transfer. But unlike IVF, GIFT requires you to undergo a laparoscopy and general anesthetic.

SPERM REQUIREMENTS FOR ART PROCEDURES

The final thing that should be taken into account when choosing which ART procedure is right for you is your partner's sperm profile—the number of sperm he has, and their ability to function. Because your doctor will not be able to see fertilization take place with GIFT, he has to be reasonably sure before trying it that fertilization will, in fact, happen. If you have never been involved with ART procedures before, your doctor can ascertain whether your partner's sperm have the ability to fertilize your eggs through the hamster test. If you have tried in vitro previously, your doctor will look to the results of those procedures as a test of the sperm's fertilizing ability. Assuming your husband's sperm profile and function are within the normal parameters, and your tubal status is good, GIFT should be your first choice procedure.

If your sperm testing shows that abnormalities exist, and your partner's sperm function is in the range of very low or zero, GIFT is no longer an option. Once sperm defects become obvious, the age and tubal status of the female partner no longer matter. Her ability to produce good eggs means nothing if her partner's sperm can't fertilize them. Her tube's ability to transport embryos to her uterus is immaterial if no embryos are created. Under these circumstances, the logical choice is in vitro fertilization, which will allow your doctor to confirm that fertilization has taken place. In some cases, micromanipulation will also have to be used to ensure that fertilization occurs.

By utilizing this three-pronged approach—considering the condition of your eggs, tubes, and your partner's sperm—you and your doctor can take what looks to be a complex issue and simplify it. Then, once you factor in your personal, emotional, and financial considerations, you can decide what is the best and most efficient approach to your infertility treatment.

ART Procedures from the
Patient's Point of View

IF YOU'RE HAVING IN VITRO FERTILIZATION

If you are having in vitro fertilization, you will be undergoing a two-part procedure. The first step is ovarian stimulation, during which eggs will be collected from your ovaries. The second step of the procedure inserts the embryos produced from these fertilized eggs into your uterus.

Successful egg retrieval depends on accurate timing. Your eggs must be mature, and your follicle growth normal. To get this timing right, your doctor will be carefully monitoring your follicle development during the first part of your cycle. He will do this by scanning your ovaries with ultrasound. Using ultrasound, he will be able to see the development of your follicles—the fluid-filled cysts in which your eggs grow. He will also draw your blood periodically, and test it to measure your hormonal levels. If your doctor confirms proper follicle growth, he will give you an injection of hCG approximately a day and a half before ovulation would normally occur. This hCG triggers ovulation, and allows your doctor to prepare for your egg retrieval 36 hours later.

Egg retrieval is an outpatient procedure that can be done in an office setting or outpatient surgical facility. Your doctor will expect you to arrive about an hour and a half before your procedure is scheduled. In most cases you will be given an intravenous anesthetic. Many anesthesiologists use drugs called Versed and Diprivan, both of which are administered intravenously. Once you are asleep, or heavily sedated, your doctor will collect your eggs "transvaginally." What this means is that a fine needle will be inserted into your ovary through the top of your vagina. Your doctor will then use ultrasound to guide this needle to each follicle. Your doctor will insert the needle into each visible follicle, and suck out the follicular fluid and the egg that is inside. This is called *egg aspiration*, or *oocyte retrieval*. Because your ovarian function will have been stimulated with drugs prior to this procedure, your doctor will, in most cases, be retrieving more than one egg. After the retrieval is complete, your doctor will check for any bleeding. This entire procedure takes just twenty to thirty minutes. Following it, you will be moved into a recovery area, and after about an hour or two you should be ready to go home. You may notice that you feel a little washed out, or "hung over," from the anesthetic for the next day or so. But other than that minor problem, you should expect to have no negative aftereffects.

As you are recovering, your retrieved eggs are being mixed with your partner's sperm in a petri dish. The embryos that form as a result of this mixing will be carefully observed and incubated in the laboratory until "cleavage development" begins. This should take one to three days. Once the embryos reach this stage, they're removed from the laboratory and the second step of your in vitro procedure—the embryo transfer—can begin.

The exact timing of your embryo transfer will depend on your fertilization and your doctor's preferences. Most transfers are done 72 hours after egg retrieval. On the day of your transfer, you will be taken to a basic exam room in the outpatient surgery area of the hospital, or in your doctor's office. Since you won't be put under any type of anesthesia, eating and drinking prior to your transfer is permitted. But before you go ahead and do this, keep in mind that you may have to remain lying down for one to two hours after your procedure. Since going to the bathroom won't be an option, you probably won't want to have a full bladder.

During the actual procedure, your doctor places a speculum into your vagina, and cleans and prepares the cervix. He then inserts the end of a catheter, which has been preloaded with your embryos, through your cervix. Using a syringe, he gently pushes a very small amount of culture media through the catheter. This culture media carries the embryos out of the catheter and into your uterus. Embryo transfer is a painless procedure. The experience should be somewhat like undergoing a pap smear.

After the transfer, you will be placed in a Trendelenburg position—your head will be slanted down and your feet will be elevated. You may remain in this position for 30 to 60 minutes. As you lie there, the catheter that carried your embryos will be taken back to the lab, where it will be examined microscopically to confirm that all of the embryos were, in fact, transferred.

After one to three hours, you will be free to go home. But rest is recommended for the next 36 hours, and aggressive physical activity or intercourse is not suggested for about a week. Your doctor will probably be giving you luteal support, generally in the form of progesterone, until he confirms whether your procedure was successful. If it was, you may continue taking progesterone until your doctor advises you otherwise. If your procedure was not successful, your progesterone support will be stopped.

Can There Be Complications?

The only complication that could arise with an embryo transfer is the small possibility of a tubal pregnancy. It's hard to imagine how this happens, since the entire purpose of IVF and embryo transfer is to by-pass the fallopian tube completely. Nonetheless, a tubal pregnancy can, and has, resulted. Doctors think this happens because embryos migrate up out of the uterus and into the fallopian tube, where they implant, creating an ectopic or tubal pregnancy. But overall the risk of ectopic pregnancy after in vitro fertilization and embryo transfer is low. Since it happens in only 4% to 5% of pregnancies, it shouldn't be a high priority on your worry list. But it is a good reason for early pregnancy monitoring, and early identification of gestational sac location, to be included in your care after an IVF-ET procedure.

IF YOU'RE HAVING GIFT

If you are having GIFT, you will be undergoing a single laparoscopic procedure. While you will be given a general anesthetic, GIFT, like IVF, is an outpatient surgery. To perform your procedure, your surgeon will make small incisions in three places—your naval, above your pubic bone, and at some midpoint between them. The laparoscope will be passed into your pelvic cavity through the puncture in your navel. The other two incisions will be used by your doctor to place holding and transfer-ring instruments into your abdominal cavity.

Your doctor will use the laparoscope to see the interior of your pelvic cavity. To make this easier, he will use an apparatus that is attached to the scope to inflate your abdomen with gas. By doing this, he will sepa-rate your ovaries and your tubes from the other intra-abdominal struc-tures.

Once he has a clear view of your ovaries, your doctor will use a needle and suction to aspirate each mature follicle and retrieve the follic-ular fluid and egg it contains. While you are still under anesthesia, these eggs will be taken to the IVF lab and separated from their fluid. Then they are combined with prewashed sperm. These egg and sperm combi-nations are immediately placed back into a catheter, before they have had time to fertilize.

While this is going on in the laboratory, your doctor will be recon-firming that your tubes are clear and ready to receive the transferred gametes. Within one to five minutes from the time your eggs were aspi-rated from your follicles, they will be returned to the operating room, already combined with your partner's sperm. Your doctor will be handed the filled catheters from the lab. Using the laparoscope, he will transfer the sperm and eggs back into one or both fallopian tubes. Once the transfer is complete, he will suture the punctures, usually with just one stitch. Once he's finished, you'll spend one to three hours in the recovery area. You will then be able to go home. You should take it easy the next day, and resume regular physical activities in one week.

Over the next 24 hours, you may experience pain or pressure under your diaphragm or in your shoulders from the gas that was inside your abdominal cavity. You may also experience slight soreness in your abdomen, and some bruising. Be sure to check with your doctor before taking medication to alleviate the pain. He may recommend Tylenol, or prescribe a medication such as Darvocet. But he will probably tell you that Motrin, Advil, Anaprox, and other similar medications are not recommended, as there is a possibility that they can inhibit implantation.

IF YOU'RE HAVING ZIFT

ZIFT is a two-part surgical procedure. It combines elements of IVF, the removal of eggs and fertilization in the laboratory, with elements of GIFT, the return of the embryo to the fallopian tube rather than to the uterus. Unlike IVF, ZIFT involves a two-day period. On the first day, your eggs will be aspirated and put into a petri dish with washed sperm, just as they would be with IVF. Both the procedure and your recovery would be the same as with IVF. But instead of waiting two or more days before the resulting embryos are transferred back, your transfer will take place on the following day. This short waiting period will let your doctors confirm that your eggs have fertilized and that you have embryos, while the quick transfer back will let those embryos spend as many of their important early hours in the nurturing atmosphere of your tubes as is possible. The procedure and recovery from this step in the process would be identical to what you would experience with GIFT.

IF MICROMANIPULATION OF SPERM IS PART OF YOUR PLAN

Today, micromanipulation involves taking your partner's single sperm cell and injecting it into one of your eggs in the laboratory. The procedure, as we have previously described, is called ICSI (intracytoplasmic sperm insemination). After fertilization, the healthy embryo is then transferred back into your uterus. To retrieve the few needed sperm cells, your doctor can either aspirate the cells in a procedure called microscopic epididymal sperm aspiration (MESA) or perform a testicular biopsy. If your partner can ejaculate, the sperm can be produced or collected by masturbation.

Both surgical procedures are performed under either a local or general anesthetic during outpatient surgery. Your doctor would first try MESA by going into the epididymis and aspirating the sperm. If the urologist is unsuccessful, then he would enter the tissue within the testes and take out a small section that, hopefully, contains sperm. The surgery takes anywhere from one to three hours, depending on whether your surgeon has to move on to a testicular biopsy after trying to aspirate from the epididymis.

Once the sperm is retrieved, ICSI is performed, followed by an embryo transfer. Recovery from MESA and the biopsy is not difficult. You wake up from the sedation rather quickly, without a lot of side effects.

———

"It's like dental surgery, in the wrong place. You can be sore and uncomfortable for the first 24 hours. Slowly it gets better."

—*Carol J. Bennet, M.D.*

———

You are often sent home from the hospital with ice packs to reduce the inflammation. No strenuous activity, including lifting, is allowed for up to six weeks but you can resume routine activity after two weeks.

IF YOU'RE GOING TO USE DONOR EGGS

Oocyte donation is an in vitro fertilization procedure that uses eggs from a third-party (donor) to produce the embryos. While the egg retrieval, the fertilization, and the embryo transfer aspects of the process are identical to those of IVF, egg donation adds one complicating factor. As you know, a woman's uterine development must precisely match her ovarian cycle and ovulation in order for implantation to occur. Sometimes it's difficult to coordinate these two events when they're happening in one woman. It's even more difficult to coordinate them when they're happening in two different women.

If you are using egg donation, your doctor will try to accomplish this feat by holding back the ovulation time of your egg donor to appropriately develop your endometrial lining. To accomplish this, the egg donor is put on Lupron, which controls her ovulation cycle. As this is happening, you would be receiving estrogen to develop your endometrial lining. Once your endometrium is ready, the donor's ovulation is triggered with a shot of hCG. The next day you begin progesterone along with the estrogen. The donor then has her eggs collected. They are fertilized in the laboratory with sperm from your partner, and placed in your uterus, just as they would be in IVF.

Hopefully, once the transfer is complete, the embryo will implant in your uterus, where it will grow and develop for the next nine months. To help ensure this, your doctor will be supporting it hormonally with estrogen and progesterone until the eighth or tenth week.

IF YOU'VE DECIDED ON SURROGATE GESTATION

Surrogate gestation is the mirror image of egg donation. In surrogate gestation the process is reversed—the patient is the donor, while the surrogate is the recipient. In order for you to take advantage of this program, your ovaries would be stimulated, just as any donor's would, and your ovulation would be held back until the surrogate's endometrium is prepared to receive your fertilized embryos. Once this timing is correct, your surgeon will use transvaginal ultrasound to aspirate your eggs. The process and recovery would be the same as with the first step of any other ART procedure. Your eggs would then be combined with your partner's sperm in a petri dish, where fertilization would take place. The resulting embryos would then be transferred into the surrogate's uterus, in the same way that they would be in the second step of any IVF procedure.

LESS SURGERY FOR THE SURROGATE

Our group in Los Angeles was the first to utilize a ZIFT procedure with gestational surrogacy. Our hope was that the tubal environment would prove to be better for pregnancy initiation, just as it had been shown to be when GIFT was compared to in vitro fertilization. However, in a surrogate environment we found that whether you transfer embryos to the surrogate's uterus, or perform a laparoscopy on the surrogate carrier and place the embryos into the fallopian tube, pregnancy outcome was essentially the same. While there's no definite explanation for this, it's theorized that the uterine environment of the surrogate, who is by definition a woman who has been proven fertile, contributes to the high rate of success for uterine implantation. As a result of this research, today's surrogate gestational carriers receive embryo transfers into the uterus, which is a very simple, noninvasive approach.

Getting Eggs, Sperm, and Embryos
Ready for ART Procedures

Eggs, sperm, and embryos are the building blocks of ART technologies. While procedures may differ, they all require your reproductive clinic to work with gametes, and in many cases, with embryos as well. Every ART procedure involves ovarian stimulation and egg extraction. Every ART procedure involves securing sperm and making sure they're as well prepared as they possibly can be to obtain fertilization. And in many procedures, the way in which eggs and sperm are combined, and the way in which the resulting embryos are nurtured in the laboratory environment, can spell the difference between success and failure. That's why you should understand the pivotal role these tiny entities play in ART procedures.

GENERATING EGGS FOR ART PROCEDURES

Ovarian Stimulation Regimens

Even though the ovary uses up to 50 eggs each month, in the normal course of events it is programmed to develop and ovulate only one and the rest are destroyed. Steptoe and Edwards's first in vitro baby, for example, was conceived after the collection of a single egg from a natural cycle. But very early on, in the development of in vitro fertilization and other ART procedures, the logic of changing this became obvious. By producing more than one egg per cycle, doctors reasoned, a patient could create more than one embryo. And by doing this, she could increase her chances to conceive. Thus, ovarian stimulation, a process through which doctors cue a woman's body to produce multiple eggs each cycle through the use of various drugs, became an integral part of all ART procedures. With ovarian stimulation regimens, the built-in follicle selection program of the ovary is overridden.

Ironically, Steptoe and Edwards used eggs from stimulated cycles for their initial tries at in vitro fertilization. While stimulation regimens at that time were primitive, they did exist. But when their first tries at in vitro met with no success, they hypothesized that the stimulation was affecting successful implantation. They then went back to the natural cycle for their egg recovery, and the same process was used for the in vitro births that followed, in Australia.

Doctors in the United States were not so quick to lay the blame for in vitro's early failures at the door of stimulation. We began our work using stimulated cycles, and the first IVF deliveries in the United States, including those in Virginia and in our own clinic in Los Angeles, occurred with stimulated cycles. Observing this, both the British and the Australians quickly switched to stimulated cycles for in vitro fertilization, as well.

Originally, doctors were rarely able to accomplish production of four transferable embryos per patient cycle using stimulation. On average, we were happy to achieve two. Laboratory environments were far less advanced than they are today. Our knowledge of the drugs that work to encourage ovulation, and of the way in which they can be used, was minimal. In those early days, stimulation regimens were not well defined. Doctors tried different formulas, and if one proved to be successful they stuck with it, afraid to alter what seemed to be a wise approach. For instance, if Pergonal gave positive results for a few of their patients, every patient would then go on the same stimulation regimen.

Since then, stimulation regimens have been improved to the point at which doctors commonly expect to produce 10 to 20 eggs per stimulated cycle. Much of this gain is due to our improved understanding of how stimulation drugs such as clomiphene citrate and Pergonal work.

One of the primary interests of our clinic in Los Angeles was to understand stimulation alternatives. Instead of limiting ourselves to one stimulation formula, we began studying stimulation regimens scientifically. Between 1982 and 1986, Dr. Joyce Vargyas, Dr. Bill Yee, and I published a series of articles analyzing patients who had been randomly prescribed various types of stimulation regimens. Our studies showed that certain regimens performed better than others. In addition, they indicated that a certain percentage of patients responded to one regimen, but not to another. In short, we found that, as with everything else in medicine, the individual patient has individual needs. Some women respond to clomiphene, others to clomiphene plus Pergonal, and some to Pergonal alone, or combinations of GnRH agonists and gonadotrophins. Still others respond to none of the above.

This process of investigating and refining stimulation procedures is still going on today. As a patient you should keep in mind that because there is no single successful formula, ovulation stimulation can be a process of trial and error. Your doctor's experience, and his knowledge of the way in which these various stimulation drugs can affect you, alone or in various combinations, is of paramount importance in finding the right formula for you.

Your Doctor's Drug Arsenal   In the earliest days of IVF, stimulation regimens centered around two drugs. The first in vitro birth in Virginia resulted from stimulated cycles using Pergonal. The birth that quickly followed at our clinic in Los Angeles used cycles stimulated with clomiphene citrate. While both of these drugs produce a similar affect, gonadotropins such as Pergonal work the ovary harder.

As we explained in our chapter on ovulation, clomiphene citrate is an antiestrogen that stimulates the ovaries indirectly. By tricking your brain into believing that estrogen is low, it gets your body to produce more FSH to stimulate your ovaries. Gonadotropins such as Pergonal, Humegon, and Metrodin, however, are doses of the natural hormones FSH and LH. By raising these hormones to a level that's higher than what your pituitary would naturally release, your doctor can stimulate your ovaries directly. Because these drugs work in different ways, they are most effective when applied to different types of reproductive problems. For example, clomiphene citrate is often used when menstrual cycles are present but irregular. Gonadotropins, on the other hand, might be called for when women have no cycles at all. These women can sometimes be made to ovulate with gonadotropins.

While each of these drugs was effective in a number of cases, stimulation regimens remained a difficult to regulate balancing act. Doctors had to administer enough drugs to produce multiple eggs, but not so much that they overstimulated the patient's ovaries. This was very hard to do since each patient had a different amount of natural hormones in her system, and each patient reacted differently to the drugs. What was too little for one woman could be too much for another. One common side effect was premature ovulation. Using gonadotropins, 15% to 20% of stimulated cycles were lost.

This problem was largely solved in 1985, when a new form of drug— gonadotropin-releasing hormone agonist—was developed. The introduction of GnRH agonists changed stimulation regimens. By depleting the pituitary of its natural FSH and LH, it let doctors start medicating with a "clean slate," which gave them a much greater degree of control. The discovery of GnRH agonists was a major development in providing better synchronization of follicle growth. It also protected against premature ovulation, by preventing LH release. Using GnRH agonists, doctors were able to perfect the stimulation balancing act to a point at which they could help the majority of patients produce an average of eight to twelve mature eggs per cycle. Even allowing for the fact that some of these eggs didn't fertilize, in many cases more embryos were produced than could be used in a single cycle. It was this development that created the need to safely freeze and store embryos. This process, which is called cryopreservation, soon became a very significant factor in reproductive technologies.

Present-day Stimulation Regimens   Today, in virtually all reproductive centers worldwide, GnRH agonists—in the form of Lupron or Synarel—are used in combination with gonadotropins, either in the form of Pergonal, Humegon, or Metrodin, for ovarian stimulation. After years of trial and error with GnRH agonists, reproductive endocrinologists have narrowed its use to two standard regimens, which are commonly known as:

1. down regulation.
2. flare-up regimen.

In *down regulation*, Lupron is administered on Cycle Day 23 or 24, during the luteal phase of your cycle. During this phase, your pituitary gland would normally be releasing small amounts of FSH and LH in response to GnRH, which is being released by your hypothalamus. The Lupron that your doctor gives you will cause your pituitary to release all of its stored-up FSH and LH. As a result, it will become depleted of these hormones, which normally cause follicle growth in the ovaries. Doctors describe this by saying your ovaries have "down regulated," which is another way of saying they have stopped functioning. Down regulation causes an interesting phenomenon. Your follicles no longer have the hormonal fuel to prepare one follicle to be dominant. Instead, a number of follicles will begin to grow when your doctor fortifies their growth by using a gonadotropin—either Pergonal, Humegon, or Metrodin. As you can see, GnRH agonists start your follicles on a level playing field so that they grow at an equal rate, and maturity is usually reached uniformly when gonadotropins fuel that growth. Given this combination, if the stimulation regimen is done correctly, when it's time for your doctor to retrieve your eggs he should be able to find mature eggs in a majority of follicles, without having run much risk of hyperstimulation. (See Chart 12-1.)

But as we said before, different women respond to stimulation regimens in different ways. Some are so overly sensitive to down regulation that it completely—or almost completely—suppresses their follicular development. A different type of regimen, the "flare-up" regimen, was developed for these women. With the flare-up regimen, morning and evening doses of Lupron are started on the second day of the ovulatory cycle, the point at which your pituitary should just be starting to release

Chart 12-1: Down Regulation Stimulation

Date																							
Cycle Day		23	24	25	26	27	28	29	30	1	2	3	4	5	6	7	8	9	10	11			
Pergonal	A.M.									1	1	1	1	1	1	1	1	1	1	1			
(# of Ampules)	P.M.																						
Metrodin	A.M.									3	3	3	3	3	3	3	3	3	3				
(# of Ampules)	P.M.																						
Lupron (mg)	A.M.	0.5	0.5	0.5	0.5	0.5	0.5	0.5	0.5	0.1	0.1	0.1	0.1	0.1	0.1	0.1	0.1	0.1					
	P.M.																			HCG			
Blood Test (E_2)										X					X			X	X	X			
Ultrasound										X					X			X	X	X	OPU		ET

OPU = Oocyte Pick-Up (egg retrieval)
ET = Embryo Transfer

pulses of FSH to stimulate your follicles to begin a new growth cycle. They stimulate the release of additional FSH and LH from the pituitary, which encourages greater than normal follicular growth. But in a flare-up regimen, the Lupron isn't continued long enough to deplete your pituitary of its hormones. On Cycle Day 3, gonadotropin is added to support follicular growth. The flare-up regimen gives quick stimulation without suppressing follicular activity. It also protects against premature ovulation. (See Chart 12-2.)

Monitoring Stimulation Response   Today, thanks to Lupron, controlling ovarian stimulation is relatively easy. Monitoring not only protects against hyperstimulation, which can be dangerous to the patient, it helps to ensure that any eggs that are gathered are appropriately mature. Since the maturity of the egg can greatly affect the success rate of ART procedures, your doctor's careful monitoring can improve your chances for success. During your monitoring, your doctor will be looking for:

1. follicle number
2. follicle maturity
3. timing for egg collection

In the earliest days of ovarian stimulation, monitoring consisted solely of doing blood tests to measure the levels of estrogen, progesterone, and LH in a woman's system. But in 1979, our clinic began doing work with a second type of measurement—using ultrasound—in an attempt to more accurately time ovulation. Ultrasound had not been used for infertility treatment prior to that time, but once we tried it, it proved to be a very useful tool. We very quickly discovered that the information about the size and number of follicles that were developing, was somewhat limited. But when we added it to the already available biochemical monitoring methods—measurements of estrogen, progesterone, and LH in the blood—ovulation could be much more correctly timed in both natural and stimulated cycles, and collection of eggs could be timed as well. This experimentation provided the early investigators with tremendous information about follicle growth, and the physiology of follicle development.

In these early days of ovarian ultrasound work, the patient had daily blood tests and ultrasound. Because this work wasn't paid for by the patient, its cost was not a factor. But it was both invasive and time-consuming for the patient. Today, the monitoring that accompanies ovarian stimulation has been greatly simplified. Based on the early studies,

Chart 12-2: Flare-up Regimen Stimulation

	1	2	3	4	5	6	7	8	9	10	11	12	13	14	15	16	17	18	19	20	21	22	23	24	25	26	27	28
Date																												
Cycle Day	1	2	3	4	5	6	7	8	9	10	11	12	13	14	15	16	17	18	19	20	21	22	23	24	25	26	27	28
Pergonal A.M.																												
(# of Ampules) P.M.																												
Metrodin A.M.			4	4	4	4	4	4	4~4	4																		
(# of Ampules) P.M.																												
Lupron (mg) A.M.		0.5	0.5	0.5	0.5	0.5	0.5	0.5	0.5	0.5																		
P.M.		.05									HCG																	
Blood Test (E$_2$)		X			X		X		X			X																
Ultrasound		X					X		X				OPU		ET													

OPU = Oocyte Pick-Up (egg retrieval)
ET = Embryo Transfer

we know what to expect during the follicle growth and maturity phase. At different times during the first part of your IVF cycle your ovaries are scanned with ultrasound—usually on Day 2, and then again on Day 6 or 7—so that your doctor can monitor the development of your follicles, the fluid-filled cysts where your eggs grow. Your blood is also drawn, usually with each ultrasound, to measure your hormonal levels. By comparing these two factors, your doctor can confirm proper egg growth and follicle maturity. As your follicles approach maturity they will reach a size that is now known to indicate egg maturity. To make the final determination of maturity, your estrogen levels will be correlated with your follicle size. That size will differ depending on the type of stimulation used. For example, if you are stimulated with gonadotropins alone, or with agonist combinations, your follicle maturity should occur when your average follicle size reaches 18 mm in diameter. This maturity can then be confirmed by checking your hormone levels. At maturity your follicles should be producing an average of 150 to 400 pg/per milliliter of estradiol.

As you approach these levels—about a day and a half before your doctor estimates that egg recovery will take place—you'll be given a luteinizing-like hormone, in the form of hCG. This is because virtually all women preparing for an ART procedure are on Lupron. Since Lupron depletes the LH naturally found in your pituitary, a spontaneous LH release will not take place, no matter how ready or mature the follicle seems to be. This hCG is extremely important, since without it the maturation of your eggs won't take place.

Ovulation generally occurs approximately 38 to 40 hours after hCG has been administered. This ability to control the exact timing of ovulation allows your doctor to prepare for your egg retrieval, which will take place 34 to 36 hours later.

Using this regimen of stimulation plus hCG timing, over 90% of visible follicles will produce a collectible egg, and over 80% of those eggs will be mature enough to fertilize in vitro. But if monitoring is not strictly followed, the quality of your eggs can be affected even before they are collected. Poor monitoring will be reflected in a lower success rate when in vitro fertilization is performed. This is why a precise monitoring protocol is just as important to your outcome as a correct stimulation protocol.

EGG RECOVERY FOR ART PROCEDURES

Just as the ultrasound techniques that were developed during the late seventies and early eighties improved ovarian monitoring, new procedures developed during the mid to late eighties helped in recovering the eggs that were produced by stimulation regimens. Originally, doctors retrieved eggs by putting the patient under a general anesthetic, and doing a laparoscopic procedure. During this procedure the surgeon accessed the ovaries through the laparoscope. Looking at the mature follicles, he then collected the eggs simply by placing a needle into each follicle and removing the fluid and its egg. But in the mid-eighties, researchers in England and Sweden began experimenting with guiding the needle into the ovarian follicle using ultrasound directly through the abdominal wall into the ovary. As a result of their efforts, *transvaginal ultrasound aspiration* was born.

In transvaginal ultrasound aspiration, a fine needle is pushed into the pelvic cavity through the vaginal wall at the top of the vagina. It's guided to the ovary by ultrasound, where it enters each mature follicle. Once the needle is in the follicle, suction is used to empty the follicle and retrieve the fluid and mature egg inside.

This new procedure was called egg aspiration, or oocyte retrieval. Within two years of its initial use nearly all IVF centers, both overseas and in the United States, converted from a laparoscopic egg recovery procedure to a transvaginal ultrasound aspiration approach. Today, ultrasound aspiration is the standard for most assisted reproductive technologies. Using it, invasiveness, anesthesia requirements, and cost are decreased.

Identifying and Grading the Egg

When an egg is aspirated from the follicle, it is retrieved in a fluid substance. This follicular fluid is slightly thicker than water. It contains millions of sticky cells, called granulosa cells. Granulosa cells have two functions. In natural conception, they surround the egg and provide the glue that helps the fallopian tube to pick the egg up from the exterior of the ovary. These cells also produce estrogen for the female reproductive system.

With each follicle that is aspirated, two to four cc's of fluid are collected. This fluid is then inspected under a microscope in the laboratory. The scientist looks for the tiny egg, surrounded by layers of granulosa cells, as it floats within the fluid. Once the egg is located, it's given an educated—yet subjective—grading. The scientist evaluates the egg's overall maturity, and determines whether it should be placed in a petri dish with sperm almost immediately, or whether it should be held in the laboratory for another 6 to 12 hours before being placed with the sperm, a period during which it would be able to mature.

PREPARING SPERM FOR ART PROCEDURES

An equally important step in the in vitro culturing process is the preparation of sperm. As you may recall, sperm must become "activated," or "capacitated," in order to be able to break through the zona membrane of an egg and fertilize it. In order for this to happen, enzymes between the two protein layers surrounding the head of the sperm must undergo a reaction known as the acrosome reaction. In normal circumstances, activation is triggered by the fluids within the woman's reproductive tract. It occurs between the time the sperm enter the cervical mucus and the time they come into contact with the granulosa cells surrounding the egg. But when sperm are placed directly into the egg culture dish during in vitro fertilization and they bypass this important period of migration, they don't have a chance to become acrosomally reacted naturally. So doctors must try to simulate this phenomenon in the laboratory. They do this through sperm washing, a process we discussed earlier in the context of intrauterine insemination.

Sperm washing attempts to duplicate the chemicals that are found in a woman's reproductive tract. Sperm treated in this way are then activated, and are able to penetrate an egg in the in vitro environment. Chemicals that are used for sperm washing include Percoll, pentoxifylline, deoxyribonuclease, and Tes yolk buffer, to name a few. Once washing is complete, an appropriate number of motile sperm are added to the egg culture dish.

EMBRYOS AND ART

Creating In Vitro Culture Embryos

After the eggs have been graded and, if necessary, matured, they are placed in a dish with equally well prepared sperm. This dish will be filled with a fluid known as in vitro culture medium. In vitro culture medium is science's attempt to duplicate the essential elements—including amino acids and proteins—that the egg would normally be exposed to within the fallopian tube. While no one has ever been able to analyze precisely what these elements are, or precisely the combination they're found in, scientists have come quite close. Over a 15-year period preceding his first successful attempt at in vitro fertilization, Dr. Robert Edwards developed an in vitro culture environment that ultimately resulted in the birth of Louise Brown. While the basic principles that guided the formulation of his first in vitro culture are still in use today, modifications have been made since then that have created a formula even more optimal for fertilization and normal embryonic development. The formulas used by various reproductive centers may differ somewhat, but certain rules must always be observed.

1. The acid/base balance of the in vitro medium must be pH 7.4, the same as that of the fallopian tube.

2. The density of the in vitro medium must be the same as that of the fluid inside the reproductive tract—285 mosm/ml. This density is also referred to as *osmolarity*, or *osmotic pressure.*

3. The ratio between the gases that the egg, sperm, and embryo are exposed to in the in vitro medium (carbon dioxide, oxygen, and nitrogen), must be the same ratio that would be found in the fallopian tube.

There is a great deal of fine-tuning that takes place beyond these basic rules. That's one of the reasons why the talents and expertise of the scientists who work within your center's reproductive laboratories can make such a big difference in your success rate.

The culture plate where the egg is placed is a very simple dishlike container. A small depression in its center contains the culture fluid. An outer channel surrounding the depression contains a second type of fluid. This second fluid is there to provide a humidifying environment. It is important, because both the egg and any embryos that are produced require 100% humidity and a constant temperature of about 37°C—matching a human's core body temperature—in order to develop. Once the egg is placed in the petri dish, it is housed in an incubator. This incubator maintains the appropriate ratio of gases, and a consistent temperature. Several hours after the eggs are put into the culture containers, processed sperm are added, and fertilization begins.

━━━━━━━━━━━━━━━━━━━━ **THINK SMALL** ━━━━━━━━━━━━━━━━━━━━

In the early days of in vitro fertilization, anywhere from one million to two million motile sperm per egg were placed into the container. Today, just 25 to 50 thousand motile sperm are used per egg. Over time it was learned that using fewer sperm actually improves fertilization, possibly because when too many sperm are present, and a number of them die, they produce a toxin that works against the fertilization process. Using fewer sperm also decreases the risk of more than one sperm fertilizing the egg.

Once fertilization is confirmed, 18 to 24 hours later, the embryos are transferred into another dish, containing identical culture media but without sperm. This helps to reduce toxicity and prevent multiple sperm from fertilizing the same egg. Once in their new container, the embryos are allowed to grow for another one or two days before they are placed into the uterus during embryo transfer.

Embryo Transfer and Storage

Over the years, a great deal of work has been done in the area of embryo transfer, which has made this a very simple procedure. Various catheters have been designed and developed; the system in common use today is the Marrs embryo transfer catheter. Using it, the tiny embryos are loaded into the nontoxic environment of the catheter. The catheter is then threaded through the cervical opening and into the uterine cavity, where the embryos, accompanied by a very small amount of fluid, are safely placed. While this process may seem commonplace to the doctors who have done it for years, there are a number of questions that will probably occur to you as you consider it. These may include:

- At what stage of their development are the embryos transferred?
- Is there any way that the embryos can be helped to implant?
- What about your uterus? Can it be better prepared to receive the embryos?
- How many embryos should be transferred during a cycle?
- What happens if you have embryos left over?

When Are Embryos Transferred?   Embryos can be transferred as early as the pronuclear stage—within 24 hours after fertilization. This is even before the first cellular division, but it's not too early to tell whether embryo development will be normal. If your doctor sees two "moon" craters within the nucleus of the egg, it indicates that it has been fertilized. If he sees more, he will know that the fertilization is abnormal.

On the other end of the spectrum, embryos have also been transferred at the blastocyst stage, after being in culture for as long as four or five days, and have produced live births. But most often embryos are transferred at the early cleavage stage of their development, somewhere between 48 and 72 hours after fertilization. At this point, they will have attained development of between two and eight cells.

Recently, several centers have extended embryo growth time up to 72 to 80 hours. At this point, embryos have divided into 8 to 12 cells. This longer waiting period is beneficial for two reasons. It allows doctors and scientists to make a better assessment of embryo quality before transferring embryos, which is important because poor embryo quality is one of the biggest reasons success rates with IVF and embryo transfer are not as high as doctors and patients would like. It also gives doctors an opportunity to do a procedure that can help the embryos to implant. This procedure is called *assisted hatching.*

Helping Embryos Implant   Assisted hatching involves micromanipulation of the embryo. In order for an embryo to implant, it has to break out of the outer membrane—the zona pellucida—that holds the dividing cells together during its earliest stages. In assisted hatching, an opening is made in this outer membrane in the laboratory, to make it easier for the embryo to emerge. Assisted hatching has been shown to improve implantation and pregnancy rates in women over the age of 40, and in women whose embryos have an abnormally thick outer membrane.

What's the Best Way to Prepare Your Uterus?   Mechanically, embryo transfers are easy to do. Your doctor's greater challenge is knowing whether they are being done at the right time. If the ovarian stimulation that produces multiple eggs has changed the timing of endometrial development, your in vitro embryos may be entering your uterus too early or too late. This will affect implantation. This lack of synchrony caused by stimulation is the other big reason why success rates with IVF and embryo transfer are not as high as they could be.

How Many Embryos Should Be Transferred?   Over the years, as ovarian stimulation protocols have improved and the embryos available for transfer have increased, controversy has arisen around the number of embryos that should be transferred during any one cycle. While it's reassuring for a patient to think that having more embryos implanted will increase her chances of getting pregnant, there's a point at which too many transferred embryos can result in a higher risk of multiple pregnancies. In our program, a maximum of four embryos per cycle are transferred. This is a relatively uniform approach for large centers that have had long experience with ART procedures. Going beyond this number does not necessarily increase the overall chance of pregnancy, but it does increase the risk of multiple pregnancy.

What About the Remaining Embryos?   Of course, imposing this limit does present one other dilemma. To increase success rates for IVF, reproductive endocrinologists improved ovarian stimulation, in an effort to produce more mature eggs per cycle. More eggs meant that more embryos could be produced and transferred into a woman's uterus, leading to a higher chance that one of them would survive and grow into a healthy baby. But multiple embryos often meant too many embryos for surgeons to transfer into the uterus at one time. The risk of multiple pregnancies was much too high. From an ethical standpoint, to discard human embryos that were fertilized in vitro was considered to be discarding human life. What could doctors do with all of the extra embryos? That's when new technology to cryopreserve human embryos was developed.

Cryopreservation is a freeze-drying process that allows embryos to be stored for an indefinite period of time. The technology had been used for some time with animals before it was first tried with human embryos. Around the same time as the introduction of GIFT, Alan Trounson, Ph.D., at Monash University in Melbourne, Australia, was working on a technology to allow for the safe freezing and storage of the human embryo.

Initially, there were strong concerns that when embryos were cryopreserved and thawed, there would be a higher risk that abnormal babies would result. With time, it was shown that this couldn't be farther from the truth. Good embryos freeze and thaw well; abnormal embryos don't survive the process. Cryopreservation functions as a natural selection process in which only the healthiest embryos go on to produce babies.

Ironically, mastering the technical aspects of freezing human embryos took less time than sorting out all of the ethical and legal issues that accompanied this momentous step. In 1986 the National Ethics Committee of the American Society for Reproductive Medicine published their established standards regarding the use of frozen embryos in the United States. Since embryo cryopreservation is performed today in a high percentage of IVF and GIFT cycles, it's comforting to know that the issues involved in it have been identified and worked out, at least on a national level.

The Personal Dilemma

"But what happens to those embryos if you tire of the chase or if something happens to either of you? These are supposed to be joint-custody embryos, not usable by one partner alone in case of divorce; so far the courts have upheld this position. So there they sit, in liquid nitrogen, your suspended children, frozen in some twilight zone.

"The choices are daunting and I sit with the form late into the night pondering what to do. Should we give the embryos to another infertile couple? Or should we let them be used for research? Or should we simply allow them to be thawed and die? And is that the right word, anyway? Die? Isn't that too big a word? Finally, I sign, consigning my unused pre-pre-pre babies to someone else, dazzled and bedeviled both, by the thought that down the road some stranger could bring them to life, suckle them, raise them, teach them to laugh and dance and look at the moon."

—*from* Motherhood Deferred *by Anne Taylor Fleming*

The advent of embryo freezing brought momentous change to the technologies of IVF and other ART procedures. The ability to save, store, and ultimately utilize excess embryos gave infertile women a chance to conceive with fewer stimulation cycles. By doing this, it reduced the physical invasiveness of these procedures, and it also helped to cut their costs. When you've endured everything that's involved in an ART procedure, only to learn two weeks later that you're not pregnant, it's extremely disappointing. Knowing that extra embryos were cryopreserved and stored is a welcome relief. It's like getting a second chance without having to endure all the physical trauma of stimulation and egg retrieval.

Your frozen embryos can be used within months, or they can be stored for years. When the time is right for you, your embryos are thawed and transferred, just as they would be in any other embryo transfer. The only difference is your body's preparation. Most centers use the same uterine preparation with estrogen and progesterone as is commonly used for uterine preparation in egg donation cycles.

In our clinic we have stored embryos for up to five years, which when thawed and transferred produced healthy pregnancies. Because cryopreservation is relatively new, the true "shelf life" of frozen embryos has yet to be determined. The possibility exists that their viability may be open-ended.

At What Stage Is the Embryo Cryopreserved?   The survival rate of embryos does not appear to be affected by the stage at which they are frozen. It doesn't matter whether your embryos are cryopreserved 24 hours after fertilization or five days after fertilization. Seventy to eighty percent of your embryos will still be viable after thawing.

Today, the one-cell pronuclear stage is the most common time for embryos to be cryopreserved. But the four- or eight-cell stage and the blastocyst stage have also been used with equally successful results.

Micromanipulation of Embryos

In much the same way that doctors learned to micromanipulate eggs and sperm, they have now learned to micromanipulate embryos. Using these techniques, embryos can be analyzed genetically, and in some cases, structurally corrected. As you might imagine, *preimplantation genetic diagnosis* is ethically controversial. Currently, its use is confined to genetic diseases such as Tay-Sachs and cystic fibrosis. This type of diagnosis is done by removing one of the cells (blastomeres) during embryonic development. This cell is then analyzed to determine the embryo's genetics. It can be determined whether the embryo has a normal number of chromosomes, and whether it's a carrier of a certain genetic disorders. Preimplantation genetic diagnosis will be discussed more fully in our chapter on controversies in reproductive technologies (Chapter Fifteen).

Success Rates . . . Whom Can You Trust?

Newsweek, September 6, 1995 . . . assisted reproduction is front-page news. INFERTILITY . . . HAS THE HYPE OUTWEIGHED THE HOPE? reads the cover. Inside, a table lists declining success rates with successive in vitro attempts, from a high of 13% to a low of 4.3%. A good thing to know if you're a prospective patient. And, unfortunately, dead wrong. On another page, there's a list of success rates and costs for various ART procedures. A useful guide, to be sure. But again, totally inaccurate on both counts. Apparently, a well-respected publication has gotten it all wrong. An isolated incident? Hardly. The unfortunate fact is that ART is such a quickly changing field, and in such a stage of infancy, that snippets of information are often taken out of context, misinterpreted, and then incorrectly communicated to the public.

So if you can't trust the media, whom *can* you trust? How about your doctor? Well . . . not necessarily. For a number of reasons, there's no definite consensus, either on the true effectiveness of many ART procedures or on who will most benefit from them.

IT'S A YOUNG SCIENCE

Because so much has already been accomplished in the arena of assisted reproductive technologies, it is often difficult to remember that it is still—from a scientific perspective—almost a newborn itself. The first successes with in vitro fertilization are less than two decades in the past, and the procedures that followed them are even younger. As in any developing scientific field, the researchers, and in this case the physicians, who pioneered ART had strong emotional feelings, biases, and superstitions as to why they had achieved successful outcomes. And each of them strongly defended his own work and his personal philosophy.

It was very difficult for the validity of these various theories to be demonstrated in the human system. The procedures were labor-intensive. Because they were difficult to do, both the skill level of the individual physician and the sophistication of his equipment had a great influence on their success or failure. And the patients who underwent them had multiple variables, any one of which might have had a bearing on the result. Given these factors, it's not surprising that reproductive science has seen conflicting and confusing interpretations of its research data since its very beginnings.

Because of this lack of consensus, during ART's early days researchers often fell back on anecdotal information to support their scientific contentions. For instance, a paper published by Steptoe and Edwards in the early eighties reported that transferring embryos at midnight, instead of during the morning hours, improved implantation and pregnancy rates. Not surprisingly, many other doctors and scientists were quite skeptical, but Steptoe and Edwards strongly stood by their theory. In doing so, they ignored an important scientific principle—they based their conclusion on the results from a mere handful of patients. It wasn't until some time had passed, and they had completed more implantation cycles, that they realized their theory wasn't accurate. But by that time, a number of other physicians were religiously following their advice.

Variations of this mistake were common during the early days. Since only a minuscule number of patients had undergone *any* of these procedures, theories were, of necessity, always based on a small sampling of results. While this way of reaching conclusions wasn't scientifically correct, it was the only possible approach at the time.

This kind of trial and error often takes place when new ground is being broken. What does this mean to a patient? Unlike some medical technologies, which are painstakingly tested over a period of years before being used in the patient population, ART procedures were frequently used on patients as quickly as they were developed. And women who wanted to get pregnant were willing to try anything, even if it meant being part of an experiment.

Fortunately for those of you reading this book today, a great deal more work has now been done to test the early theories, and to perfect the procedures that go along with them. While more still needs to done, you will, at the very least, be able to look at statistics based on results from an appropriately large patient population.

IT HAS TOO MANY CLINICS, AND TOO FEW RESEARCH LABS

In 1982 a grand total of two clinics in the United States had ever performed an assisted reproductive procedure. Each of them—the Jones Clinic in Virginia, and our own clinic in Los Angeles—had been successful with the first of the new technologies, IVF. It took two years for the number of infertility clinics in the U.S. to grow to twenty. By that time, public excitement over this new science was so enthusiastic that its careful and measured growth rate flew out the window. Over the next ten years, clinics specializing in the commercial application of in vitro technologies began to spring up rapidly throughout the country. Some would say too rapidly. By 1994, the Society for Assisted Reproductive Technology registry stated that there were over 300 clinics performing IVF and ART procedures within the United States. But of this large population of infertility clinics, only a small number of them—fewer than 50—were actively doing research or investigative work to validate and improve their patient procedures.

With so many clinics commercially applying technology without making any effort to improve it, success rates have leveled, even as the number of procedures being performed has gone up. Ironically, the rapid growth in the number of clinics participating in ART has slowed the growth of knowledge in this new field. And as a result, the clinical outcomes of today are suffering.

COMPETITION MEANS SURVIVAL OF THE FITTEST

Another problem that rapid growth in the number of infertility clinics has caused is a fierce competition for patients. Sad to say, this has produced a number of instances in which centers have manipulated and exaggerated the data on their procedures and success rates.

So, How Do *You Get a Straight Answer?*

One source you can go to for statistical information on infertility procedures is the Society for Assisted Reproductive Technology. This subgroup of the American Society for Reproductive Medicine had published an annual compilation of statistical outcomes for all ART procedures performed in the United States. To prevent clinics from reporting inaccurate success rates, SART has attempted to build random auditing into their reporting process. However, this auditing process has never come about. Moreover, because validation of the data has never occurred, questions of accuracy have arisen. Its purpose is to provide you, the patient, with reliable, factual, honest data so that you can make decisions as to where and how you want to be treated. Unfortunately, after ten years of working to provide you, the patient, with honest, factual, accurate outcome data. I feel that once again, we have failed to accomplish that goal. To give you an idea of what this report can tell you, we've summarized one in the tables.

Assisted Reproductive Technologies—Clinical Outcome

	IVF	GIFT	ZIFT	FET
#CYCLES	31,900	4,992	1,792	6,672
#RETRIEVALS	27,443	4,202	1,557	—
#PREGNANCIES	6,321	1,472	466	984
%SAB	19.0	20.6	18.5	19.6
%DELIVERIES	18.6	28.1	24.4	12.8

Modified from *Fertility Sterility* 1995: 64:13-21

As you can see, the SART registry tells you what the average outcome per cycle is for any infertility procedure on a national basis. By doing this, it can give you a sense of what is considered to be a reasonable or standard outcome. But since the results obtained by each of the 300 centers working in this field differ individually, you will still need to gather specific information from the clinics you're considering. The center that you're interviewing should be able to give you accurate data as to:

1. The number of cycles they perform on an annual basis.

2. What their clinical pregnancy rate is.

3. What their live birthrate is for various procedures . . . IVF, GIFT, surrogate gestational carriers, and egg or sperm donation cycles, for example.

Don't hesitate to ask for these numbers. The time you spend attempting pregnancy through infertility procedures is irreplaceable. Failure can mean more than the loss of significant amounts of money—it may mean that you're out of the game.

As you look at the statistics your clinic presents to you, pay special attention to their success rate for the procedure you're actually considering. It's important that you be treated in the place that's best for your particular problem. Some clinics do exceptionally well with GIFT but poorly with IVF. Some programs don't even do GIFT, but have good success rates with IVF. Some programs have wonderful results with ICSI procedures, while others aren't equipped to do any type of micromanipulation for male factor problems. If the center you're looking at doesn't perform the procedure that best suits your needs—either because they're not equipped to do it, or they're biased against it—you're at the wrong place. Check to see if there is another center nearby that does have a proven success record.

There are several other things you should be alert to as you review your clinic's statistical outcomes. While success rates are important, live birthrates are what really count. That's why SART's registry reports live births, not just positive pregnancy results. Yet some centers persist in showing you positive pregnancy rates, rather then baby rates. The reason for this is obvious—pregnancy rates are higher than birthrates. Clinics show them to you in an effort to make themselves look better. To get an accurate idea of what's really happening, make sure that your clinic is giving you their actual live births per procedure.

As you review the statistics that your clinic presents to you, you should keep your own situation in mind and try to have realistic expectations. You should remember that each infertile couple is unique. Each one is made up of two different people, with individual problems and individual treatment responses. Even though you're looking at "average" results, there is no such thing as an "average" couple. While a GIFT procedure performed on a 22-year-old woman may produce an average success rate of 40%, it will have a far smaller success rate when performed on a 42-year-old woman. That's why even when success rates with ART procedures are reported accurately, they can still be very difficult to interpret. Applying the best case success rate to yourself, when you're not a best case patient, will only lead to unrealistic expectations and possible disappointment.

And Don't Forget About the Laboratory Scientist

Another question you might want to ask your prospective clinic, particularly if their success rate is good, is whether they are still working with the same lab scientists who were with them when those results were produced. These scientists are usually trained in animal sciences, in embryology in particular, and have at least a Ph.D. degree. National pregnancy rates from assisted reproductive technologies reflect not only the ability of physicians performing the procedures, but equally important, the ability of the scientists who work alongside them in their laboratories. Many patients don't realize that no matter how accomplished the surgeon, the skills of a center's laboratory scientists are pivotal to the success of its program. But infertility specialists know that their success rates depend equally on the talents of their lab scientists. Your doctor can retrieve wonderfully healthy and mature eggs, but if the petri dish is prepared incorrectly, or the sperm isn't washed properly, or the incubation process isn't handled appropriately and in synchrony with your body, your procedure will most likely fail.

A Personal Note from Dr. Marrs

No other chapter in this book has affected me personally as much as this one. I've been involved in the development of assisted reproductive technologies since their very beginning. In January of 1981 I walked into the office of the chairman of the Department of Obstetrics and Gynecology at the University of Southern California, where I was teaching, and asked for permission to set up an in vitro fertilization program at Los Angeles County Women's Hospital. While he was supportive, he was discouraging. ART was a totally experimental area; only one other clinic in the United States was working in it at that time. While he told me that whatever I could do on my own I was welcome to do, he could give me no funding. Given this sliver of an opening, I went directly to the operating room supervisor.

I surveyed the operating room facilities, and found an old storage closet filled with operating room equipment dating back at least 50 years.

I went back to my department head, and told him that if I was allowed to use that storage closet for a laboratory, we could start our in vitro program. Not surprisingly, he was quite skeptical. But he told me that if I could find a place to get rid of all the old equipment, I could do what I wanted with the room. I did find one—the roof of the hospital.

I spent my first weekend in my new "laboratory" with Jody Greene, my laboratory associate, scouring it with disinfectant and wire brushes. We then "borrowed" from other laboratories equipment that wasn't in use at the time . . . a microscope, an incubator that, while old and decrepit, could maintain a controlled temperature reasonably well, and a centrifuge for sperm washing and processing. After announcing to my department chairman that I was now ready to begin patient studies, I went through the Institutional Review Board and Ethics Committee at USC and obtained approval to do experimental trials with egg collection and in vitro fertilization.

Prior to treating the first patient, I went back to my department chairman and asked permission to attend a private conference in Melbourne, Australia, where they had already been successful in producing a pregnancy using in vitro fertilization. I offered to pay my own expenses to go there and learn about what they were doing. I was allowed time away from my teaching responsibilities, and left for Australia with my research fellow, Dr. Joyce Vargyas, who had just become my wife. We worked there for six weeks, with Drs. Alex Lopata and Ian Johnston.

Upon returning to Los Angeles, in August of 1981, I modified my laboratory approach and began stimulating a group of volunteer patients with clomiphene citrate. Joyce, I, and my friend and associate, Dr. Bill Gibbons, did our first egg recovery procedure in September of 1981. With the fifth procedure that we performed, the patient conceived after embryo transfer, and we delivered our first in vitro baby in June of 1982. After the birth of that first baby, I moved out of my broom closet into a more refined laboratory, and we began working with an increasing number of patients. During that first year we performed 24 procedures, four of which resulted in pregnancy, and two of which resulted in the birth of a baby.

In these early years, success rates with ART procedures did not improve significantly. But assisted reproductive technologies have now been around for almost 20 years, and procedures have changed dramatically. During that time, advances have been made and knowledge has increased. Viewing the physiologic process of human reproduction through the in vitro window has improved not only our ability to increase pregnancy outcomes using ART, but to treat routine infertility disorders.

Still, as a patient, you should remember that assisted reproductive technologies should only be utilized as a last step. They cannot, and should not, replace conventional therapy.

If you and your doctor do come to the conclusion that you would be helped by an ART procedure, make sure you understand which one is best for you. Be clear about its cost, as the financial impact can be overwhelming. And make sure you understand its success rate, not only nationally but at the center you've chosen. All ART procedures fail more often than they succeed. If you've done this homework, your expectations will be hopeful but realistic.

Terms We Used in This Chapter

Abdominal ultrasound aspiration: a procedure used to remove the egg from the ovary, with visualization by external ultrasound viewing. This was the original procedure developed to replace laparoscopic collection of eggs for IVF. During this procedure the aspirating needle is passed through the abdominal wall into the ovarian follicle to collect the egg.

Assisted hatching: a windowlike opening made in the zona pellucida of the embryo to improve implantation or attachment of the embryo to the uterine lining.

Assisted reproductive technologies (ART): a term used to identify procedures such as IVF, GIFT, and ZIFT.

Cleavage: the process of embryo cell division.

Cryopreservation: storing of tissue or cells by freezing.

Culture medium: the fluid solution used for growth of cells or tissue in vitro.

Down regulation: the use of GnRH agonist to stop the pituitary gland from producing and releasing FSH and LH, causing the ovaries to stop developing follicles and estrogen. Thus the ovaries are "down regulated."

Egg aspiration: the removal of the egg from the follicle during the in vitro fertilization procedure.

Extracorporeal fertilization: another term for in vitro fertilization; fertilization outside of the female's reproductive tract.

Flare-up regimen: one of the types of drug protocols used to stimulate multiple follicle production.

Follicle aspiration: see Egg aspiration.

Gamete intrafallopian transfer (GIFT): a surgical procedure whereby the egg and the sperm are laparoscopically placed into the fallopian tube.

Gestational surrogacy: the use of a woman to carry a genetically unrelated embryo for an infertile couple.

Incubation: maintaining a controlled environment to allow cell growth and development.

Intracytoplasmic sperm insemination (ICSI): the injection of a single sperm cell into a mature egg.

In vitro fertilization and embryo transfer (IVF-ET): the procedure in which the egg is removed from the ovary, fertilized in the laboratory environment, and the resulting embryo placed into the egg donor's uterine cavity.

Microfertilization: see Intracytoplasmic sperm insemination.

Micromanipulation: the use of high magnification and hydraulically controlled instrumentation to achieve fertilization in vitro.

Microscopic epididymal sperm aspiration (MESA): aspiration of the epididymis to procure sperm for use in microfertilization.

Oocyte donation: see Egg donation.

Osmolarity: the pressure created by a liquid due to the concentration of various particles within it.

Ovarian stimulation: the use of fertility drugs to either regulate single egg ovulation or multiple egg production.

Partial zona dissection (PZD): a form of micromanipulation in which the zona pellucida is opened to allow sperm to swim through.

Perivitelline space: the space between the zona pellucida and the surface of the egg cytoplasm.

Petri dish: the plastic or glass container in which embryos grow and develop during in vitro fertilization procedures.

Preimplantation genetic diagnosis: a removal of an embryonic cell prior to implantation to determine whether the genetic makeup of the embryo is normal.

Pronuclear oocyte sperm transfer (PROST): another term for ZIFT.

Pronuclear stage: the stage in embryonic development that occurs after sperm penetration of the egg.

Subzonal sperm insemination (SUSI): a micromanipulation technique whereby the sperm is injected into the perivitelline space of the egg.

Transvaginal ultrasound aspiration: a technique used to aspirate eggs from the ovary for in vitro fertilization.

Tubal embryo transfer (TET): the placement of the embryo into the fallopian tube after in vitro fertilization.

Zona pellucida: the outer protein covering of the egg that the sperm first comes in contact with during fertilization.

Zygote intrafallopian transfer (ZIFT): placement of a fertilized egg into the fallopian tube; see PROST or TET.

13

Is Infertility Treatment Only for the Wealthy?

In a recent worldwide survey, it was estimated that one in every six couples of reproductive age has some kind of problem with fertility. A 1991 survey by the Centers for Disease Control, in Atlanta, reported that in the United States alone, over five million couples have some form of infertility. It went on to say that only around 40% of those infertile couples will ever attempt to find out what their problem is, or to seek treatment for it. Why do the remaining 60% choose to remain in the dark about their condition? Some don't seek out care probably because they have misperceptions about the way infertility treatment is done or about its effectiveness. But a great many others remain untreated because they're fearful of the financial aspects of their care. . . . While they don't understand what costs are really involved, they *have* heard that infertility treatments are prohibitively expensive.

As an infertile couple, you need to realize that while some types of treatment are very expensive, others are more reasonable. To avoid misconceptions, and to prepare yourself for future financial demands as you're about to embark on treatment, you should educate yourself about the actual costs of the wide range of services you might be using. This chapter will help you do that by reviewing the costs involved in the basic workup, in a number of treatment options, and in assisted reproductive technologies.

As you look at these figures, you should keep in mind that what is actually charged will vary from center to center. This is largely due to the fact that the cost of doing business is different in various parts of the country. The price of equipment, office space, and medications can be higher or lower, depending upon your doctor's geographic location. And since the cost of living varies throughout the country, the charge for his professional services, and those of his staff, will vary too. In this review we'll identify a range of costs which should reflect a high and low for the United States. And in some cases, we'll also give you a comparison to overseas costs.

Initial Consultations

As you may remember from our chapter on the basic workup (Chapter Five), the first step that you will be undertaking in your infertility treatment is interviewing subspecialists in reproductive endocrinology. The cost for these initial consultations can range anywhere from a low of $150 to a high of $400, depending on where in the country you're located. While the cost of initial consultations is minimal compared to the expense of the treatment that will follow, this is one place in the process where you can still reduce your expenses by doing your homework. Try to do as much background work, and make as many decisions as possible, before you actually make appointments to speak to physicians. If you can eliminate some obviously unsuitable doctors from consideration by doing this, you will have saved yourself the cost of their initial consultation fee. To accomplish this, discuss the physicians you're considering with national and local organizations. Find out as much about their practices as you can from Resolve, the American Society for Reproductive Medicine (ASRM), the Society for Assisted Reproductive Technology (SART), and the Society for Reproductive Surgeons (SRS). These groups can often help you to narrow the field by giving you the names of physicians who specialize in your particular type of problem. If you have close friends who have been involved in an infertility situation for a long time, discussing physicians with them may also be helpful. But while these discussions can help you to limit the number of physicians you'll be talking to, ultimately it is up to you to make the final decision as to whom you'll be working with, and the only way you can do that is by actually meeting with your finalists. If you don't feel satisfied during your initial consultation with the first doctor you meet, set up an appointment for a consultation with another. Try not to waste money on an overly large number of initial consultations, but do spend enough to be sure you've made a decision with which you're comfortable.

The Basic Workup

Once your initial consultations are finished and you've chosen a physician, his first step will be to come up with a game plan for your treatment. A variety of tests are routinely done on new infertility patients, to help a doctor devise this plan. The ones you should anticipate having include:

- Infectious disease screening
- Hormonal screening
- Routine semen analysis
- Ovulation testing
- Ultrasound
- Endometrial biopsy
- Postcoital test
- Hysterosalpingogram
- Laparoscopy

With the exception of laparoscopy, infertility screening tests are not covered by your insurance carrier unless specifically stated to be so. Companies' policies on this can be far-ranging. While some companies deny *all* coverage for infertility—both its diagnosis and treatment—others will pay for diagnostic testing but not for the treatment the diagnosis calls for. So take a good look at your insurance policy before stepping into the diagnostic testing environment. Become acquainted with your policy restrictions, and find out exactly what you can count on financially as you begin this costly process.

The cost of a blood test to screen for infectious diseases (most states now require hepatitis, HIV, and cytomegalovirus [CMV] screening for both male and female patients) will be $200 to $300 per person. The cost of an initial screening to establish your baseline levels of hormones such as estradiol, FSH, TSH, and prolactin averages $180 to $300.

Usually, the first test to be performed beyond the baseline hormonal and infectious disease screens is a routine semen analysis. This should cost anywhere from $45 to $120, depending on the laboratory that does it and the method they use. A computerized semen analysis is more expensive, but the less expensive manual test is also less accurate.

As a semen analysis is being done on your male partner, your physician will concurrently be checking to see if you are ovulating normally.

Testing your ovulation function will cost roughly $350 to $500 depending upon how your physician observes your cycle. This can be done with a simple basal body temperature chart, which costs nothing. But, usually, ovulation-induction kits are used to more accurately time the LH surge. The cost of ovulation-induction kits will be around $40 to $60 for a six-day test kit, and $60 to $90 for a nine-day test kit. When you are buying your kits, keep in mind that even though you may only use two or three of a kit's test days during the first month that you are timing your ovulation, you can continue to use the same kit from month to month until it is completely used up. Some kits have a single control stick, or tube, which continues to be used every test day. If this is the way your kits are designed, you will need to save it from month to month. Other kits have individual control dots on each day's test.

Mid–luteal phase estrogen and progesterone testing, ultrasound, and endometrial biopsy are three other possible steps your doctor might want to do while analyzing your ovulation. Additional blood tests to measure hormone levels at the time of ovulation, or during your luteal phase, will range anywhere from $45 to $100 per test. The cost of an ultrasound will range anywhere from $75 to $200. And an endometrial biopsy, which is done to confirm endometrial development, can range anywhere from $75 to $150. If you're having an endometrial biopsy, you will also incur charges from a pathology laboratory, which will range anywhere from $50 to $150.

If your semen and ovulation tests seem normal, and your physician then decides to perform a postcoital test, it will be done during an office visit. The charge will vary, depending upon your physician and his geographic location, but it should be somewhere between $45 and $120.

If these tests have been performed, and your problem still hasn't been found, a hysterosalpingogram is usually the next step in the evaluation. This is done by a radiologist, either in a hospital or in a private office. The cost for a hysterosalpingogram ranges anywhere from $200 to $400. In cases where proximal tubal obstruction is found during the hysterosalpingogram, and the radiologist then attempts to open the fallopian tube, selective catheterization will probably add another $300 to $400 to the cost of the HSG.

The final step in a routine evaluation is a diagnostic laparoscopy. A laparoscopy is performed in a hospital, on an outpatient basis. The hospital charges for outpatient laparoscopy can range anywhere from $1,400 to $3,500. Anesthesiologists' fees usually average an additional $450 to $600. And your surgeon's fee for a laparoscopy can range anywhere from $1,000 to $4,000, depending on whether corrective procedures are done during the laparoscopy or whether it is used merely for diagnostic purposes. If hysteroscopy is performed in conjunction with your laparoscopy, the cost usually increases by another $1,000 to $2,000, depending on your surgeon's fees and additional operating room charges.

If you were to add up all of these charges, from the cost of the initial visit through a complete workup, you might expect to pay a minimum of $4,410, and a maximum of approximately $11,000.

Costs of the Basic Workup

	Low	High
Initial consultation	150.00	400.00
Infectious disease screening	200.00	300.00
Hormonal screening	180.00	300.00
Semen analysis	45.00	120.00
Ovulation test kit	40.00	90.00
Ultrasound	75.00	200.00
Endometrial biopsy procedure	75.00	150.00
Endometrial biopsy tissue analysis	50.00	150.00
Postcoital test (PCT)	45.00	120.00
Hysterosalpingogram (HSG)	200.00	400.00
HSG with cannulization	500.00	800.00
Laparoscopy		
Anesthesia	450.00	600.00
Hospital	1,400.00	3,500.00
Surgeon's fees	1,000.00	4,000.00
Subtotal	2,850.00	8,100.00
Estimated total:	$4,410.00	11,130.00

Advanced Testing

If no abnormalities have been found by the time you finish your laparoscopy, other, more advanced testing—such as sperm function testing and immune testing—may be performed. The sperm penetration assay, or hamster test, is fairly expensive. It will cost anywhere from $250 to $400, depending on how many sperm preparations are tested. A hemizona assay is another sperm penetration test that can be performed. This test will range anywhere from $200 to $400.

Antibody testing, to detect antibodies directed at sperm protein, may be done on both the male and female partner. This testing can be done using a man's semen or blood, or using the blood of the woman. It usually costs from $75 to $150 per test, regardless of whether it is semen or blood that is tested.

If the immunologic system is suspect, further immune testing will be performed. A complete screening of the immune system—which looks at ANA, antiphospholipids, anti-DNA, histones, leukocyte antibody detection, and reproductive immunophenotype—can run upward of $1,000 to $1,800.

Tests for Couples with Unexplained Infertility

	Low	High
Sperm penetration tests		
Hamster test	250.00	400.00
Hemizona test	200.00	400.00
Antisperm antibody	75.00	150.00
Immune series	1,000.00	1,800.00
Total	$1,525.00	$2,750.00

The costs of the first phase of treatment, the basic workup that identifies the cause of your infertility problem, are fairly straightforward. Still, you should keep in mind that some procedures need to be repeated more than once, and remember to multiply accordingly.

Treatment Costs

Once your basic diagnostic testing is done and a game plan is put into motion, you should estimate what the costs for your recommended treatment will be. Because costs can mount up so quickly, it is extremely important at this stage of your decision-making process to get a complete picture.

COSTS FOR OVULATION INDUCTION

Ovulation induction, or ovulatory control, is by far the most commonly used treatment for infertile couples. If your doctor recommends it to you, you should take two factors into account in estimating its cost—the cost of ovulation-enhancing drugs, and the cost of monitoring their effects on your body. The treatment first prescribed for these disorders is usually the drug clomiphene citrate (marketed under the brand names Clomid or Serophene), which helps a woman to ovulate.

A simple ovulation control cycle using clomiphene citrate is relatively inexpensive when you consider just the cost of the necessary drugs. Clomiphene citrate can cost anywhere from $4 to $8 per 50 mg tablet. Most patients take a 50 mg tablet of clomiphene per day for five days, for a total drug cost of $20 to $40 per cycle. But if you require monitoring for intrauterine insemination, or merely to correctly time your intercourse, it adds on additional dollars.

The minimum monitoring you will need to time ovulation is an ovulation predictor kit. These can run anywhere from $40 to $90. And in some cases, where ultrasound and intrauterine insemination is necessary, these costs also have to be added to the per cycle cost. Usually more than one ultrasound will be performed in these cycles, and your costs increase in proportion to the number that are actually done.

Clomiphene Citrate Cycle Costs

	Low	High
Medication (Clomid, Serophene)	20.00	40.00
LH Kit(s)	40.00	90.00
Ultrasound (per scan)	75.00	200.00
Total	$135.00	$330.00

If clomiphene isn't appropriate for you, or if it has to be used in combination with menopausal gonadotropin (Pergonal or Humegon), or with urinary FSH (Metrodin), costs rise considerably. In the United States, a single ampule of human menopausal gonadotropin costs $52 on average. The same is true for Metrodin. The cost of these drugs can be much less when they are purchased outside the borders of the United States, and many patients who travel take advantage of this fact. In England, for instance, the cost of an ampule of hMG or FSH averages $18 to $20. In Mexico, the cost per ampule may be as low as $17. In South America, the cost may be an even lower, $8 to $11. But purchasing drugs outside the United States is something your doctor cannot legally recommend to you. Physicians who are licensed and practicing in the United States are required to use drugs that have been approved by the FDA, and that have been purchased within the U.S. borders. So in calculating your per cycle cost, you should assume that you will be paying the

United States price of approximately $52 per ampule for drugs, and that you will be using 15 to 40 ampules per cycle, for a total cost of $780 to $2,120.

Monitoring also has to be taken into account. The monitoring that is done for hMG and FSH cycles is much more extensive than the monitoring that is done when clomiphene citrate is used for ovulatory timing. One variable in your monitoring costs is the experience of the physician you're working with. Physicians who are well versed in monitoring patients on gonadotropins need do only a minimum of testing. Ultrasound and blood testing two to three times apiece during the ovulation-induction cycle should be enough to let them determine when ovulation is approaching, and to tell them exactly how soon after hCG is administered that it will occur. Under this regimen, monitoring the average cycle of Pergonal ovulation induction would cost an additional $300 to $800 for four ultrasounds, depending on the cost per scan. Blood tests done on four occasions would add another $180 to $400 to the cost of the ovulation-induction cycle. But an inexperienced physician might need to monitor by ultrasound and blood tests as many as seven times per cycle. If this is the case, your cost for ultrasounds would be between $525 and $1,400. And your blood tests could run anywhere from $315 to $700. In order to calculate what your cycle will cost, ask your doctor how many ultrasounds and blood tests he anticipates doing. The cost of monitoring will be directly related to how many of these tests are done.

Cost of Gonadotropin Cycle

	Low	High
HMG or FSH ($52/Ampule)	780.00	2,248.00
Ultrasound		
Experienced M.D. (Approx. 4 scans)	300.00	800.00
Inexperienced M.D. (Approx. 7 scans)	525.00	1,400.00
Lab monitoring		
Experienced M.D.	180.00	400.00
Inexperienced M.D.	315.00	700.00
Total - Experienced M.D.	1,260.00	3,448.00
Total - Inexperienced M.D.	$1,620.00	$4,348.00

Always keep in mind that there are twelve cycles per year . . . twelve chances to get pregnant, twelve chances for your doctor to evaluate and observe your system, and twelve testing and treatment cycles that will potentially have to be paid for. That's why you should be clear on the nature of your treatment, and establish with your doctor ahead of time the number of cycles that fit within your financial limitations. As you step up to more advanced stages of treatment, you should be aware that *all* procedures will include one of these drug therapies, to help increase ovulation function and increase your chances for a healthy pregnancy.

COSTS FOR INTRAUTERINE INSEMINATION

In a high percentage of ovulation-induction cycles, intrauterine insemination (IUI) is also performed. This adds a number of other costs to your cycle. Your ovulation will have to be triggered by an injection of hCG, which will cost from $20 to $40. The cost of sperm preparation will vary from as low as $75 in some laboratories to as high as $250 in others—again, laboratories that do a greater volume of these procedures charge less than ones that do only a few. The insemination itself is usually the cost of an office visit, which will be anywhere from $45 to $100. And the cost of luteal phase support—given either in the form of progesterone suppositories (which cost approximately fifty cents to $1 per suppository), or daily injections of progesterone (a vial of progesterone costs around $20, and contains enough hormone for ten injections at a normal dosage) will average about $40 for the cycle. If boosters of hCG are needed once or twice during the luteal phase, these will run approximately $40 per cycle. Adding these items to the cost of drugs and monitoring, the total bill for an ovulation-induction cycle including insemination will be somewhere between $1,440 and $4,858. A great deal of this variation will depend on the experience of the physician, and amount of drugs utilized per cycle.

The Cost of Intrauterine Insemination as Part of an Induced Cycle

	Low	High
hCG shot	20.00	40.00
Sperm preparation	75.00	250.00
IUI	45.00	100.00
Luteal support	40.00	120.00
Total	$180.00	$510.00

Perhaps your tests have shown that your ovulation is normal and ovulation induction isn't necessary, but that intrauterine insemination is called for because of a cervical mucus–sperm interaction problem, or because of sperm abnormalities that were discovered during semen analysis. In your case, the cost of ovulation timing can be minimized by using a home ovulation predictor kit, which should be accurate enough to help a pregnancy take place. The morning after the kit indicates that the LH surge has occurred, you would go to your doctor's office for an insemination with prepared sperm. Costs for sperm preparation, and for the insemination procedure itself, will be the same as with an induced cycle— anywhere from $75 to $250. If an ultrasound is performed to determine the status of ovulation, an additional $75 to $200 will be added to the cost of the insemination.

The Cost of Intrauterine Insemination Without an Induced Cycle

	Low	High
Ovulation testing	40.00	90.00
Sperm preparation	75.00	250.00
IUI	45.00	100.00
Ultrasound	75.00	200.00
Total	$235.00	$640.00

SURGICAL COSTS

Perhaps, following your basic workup, you were told that your infertility problem is one that requires surgery. If this is the case, you will have to take hospital charges, surgeons' fees, and anesthesiologists' fees into account, as you try to estimate the costs you will be incurring. All of these costs should be available to you through your physician's office, or through your hospital when you preregister for your procedure. Make a point of getting exact fees—or the maximum and minimum range of fees—so you will know what you are facing. And also clarify what the insurance reimbursement process will be for your procedures.

The cost of surgical procedures varies widely. In any given geographic area, both hospital fees and surgeons' fees are somewhat consistent within a given range, but that range can be a large one. For instance, if you are having a hysteroscopic myomectomy, hospital charges can range anywhere from a low of $1,200 to a high of $3,500 or more. Surgeons' fees will vary to the same degree. Your surgeon's charge may be as low as $1,500 or as high as $4,000 for a simple hysteroscopic myomectomy. And your anesthesiologist's fee can range between $400 and $600.

Costs for Hysteroscopy/Myomectomy

	Low	High
Hospital fees	1,200	3,500
Anesthesia	400	600
Surgeon's fee	1,500	4,000
Total	$3,100	$8,100

The same is true when operative laparoscopy is performed. Hospital costs for laparoscopy may vary from a low of $1,800 to $2,000, to a high of $4,000 or $5,000. If a laser is used, there is normally an additional charge added to your hospital fee of anywhere from $500 to $1,500, depending upon the type of laser that is used and the amount of time it's used. Anesthesia charges will average $400 to $600, but they could be more if the case is complicated and the surgery goes beyond an hour and a half or two hours. In longer cases, anesthesia charges can go as high as $1,000. Surgeons' fees for an operative laparoscopy vary between $1,200 and $4,000, depending on the surgeon, and geographic area in which you live.

Costs for Operative Laparoscopy

	Low	High
Hospital fees	1,800	5,000
Laser	500	1,500
Anesthesia	400	1,000
Surgeon's fee	1,200	4,000
Total	$3,900	$11,500

If an abdominal surgery, such as exploratory laparotomy, is necessary—either for myomectomy, for tubal reanastomosis, or for treatment of extensive pelvic endometriosis—additional charges and fees will be encountered. Hospital fees for exploratory laparotomy will include anywhere from $2,500 to $4,000 for operating room charges alone. And you will have to remain in the hospital for two or three days after the procedure, at a cost of $1,000 to $3,000 per day; your daily charge will depend on your hospital, and whether they have a contract agreement with your insurance carrier. It's important to discuss this with the hospital's accounting department ahead of time, so that you understand what their charges are, how your insurance carrier interacts with them, and what percentage of the costs your carrier will cover. Anesthesia fees average $800 to $1,000, while surgeons' fees will range from $1,800 to $4,000 for these sorts of cases.

Costs for Exploratory Laparotomy

	Low	High
Hospital fees/OR	2,500	4,000
Hospital fees/Recovery	2,000	9,000
Anesthesia	800	1,000
Surgeon's fee	1,800	4,000
Total	$7,100	$18,000

As you can see, abdominal surgery is significantly more expensive than laparoscopic or endoscopic surgery. Not to mention that a surgery that requires you to be in the hospital for two or three days, and then recovering at home for four to six weeks, is far more draining physically than one in which you leave the hospital the same day as your procedure.

One factor that can never be predicted when you are estimating costs is surgical complications. If there are any, they may require you to stay in the hospital for a much more prolonged period than you originally anticipated. Maybe you'd like to look at a worst case scenario, and try to figure out what those costs might be. This isn't easy to do. Hospitals will have a hard time giving you an exact cost, since they charge separately for every article and every medication you use. For instance, a box of Kleenex in your room after surgery will show up on your itemized bill. So will every sanitary napkin and IV antibiotic you use. That's why you should examine your bill carefully. You may be horrified when you do—with markup for overhead, a box of Kleenex can cost as much as $10. But you need to verify that the things that are itemized there were actually used by you. Many times mistakes are made. Your hospital charges can sometimes be reduced significantly if you review what was billed for. Remember, even if your insurance is covering much of your expense, you will be paying at least a portion of your bill.

THE COST OF ASSISTED REPRODUCTIVE TECHNOLOGIES

Another option you might be faced with is one of the assisted reproductive technologies (ARTs). While a number of insurance companies cover surgery for infertility, only a few lucky individuals have insurance coverage for assisted reproductive technologies such as IVF, GIFT, and ZIFT. Often your carrier will exclude all these costs, and they will be a totally out-of-pocket expense.

That's why when you are contemplating any ART procedure— whether it's in vitro fertilization with embryo transfer, gamete intrafallopian transfer, IVF combined with a surrogate carrier, or IVF with egg donor—it is extremely important to fully understand the process. You should examine not only how the medical steps will affect you physically and emotionally, but their financial impact, as well. Patients who question the price of infertility treatment often focus on the cost of assisted reproductive technology, which is admittedly high since each attempt involves a number of labor-intensive steps. But as you have seen, when you look at the cost of conventional therapy, it can be quite costly as well. Even cycles of the simplest therapies, like routine ovulation induction with intrauterine insemination, can add up very quickly when they're repeated month after month. In fact, the expense of a few months of ovulation-induction cycles can meet, or even exceed, the expense of a cycle of IVF or GIFT. You should remember this when you're making your decisions as to which type of treatment you will choose.

The average cost of an IVF cycle in the United States, not including the cost of ovulation stimulating drugs, is about $6,500 to $6,800. Add to that another $2,000 for the cost of ovulation-inducing drugs, and you get an average total cost of about $8,500 to $9,000. Again, the geographic location where you live will determine, to a large extent, what you pay. Within a given community the cost of IVF is usually fairly constant from center to center. But if you compare the cost of a routine IVF procedure in regions throughout the United States, it can range anywhere from a low of about $3,500 (not including medication costs), to a high of $10,000 to $11,000 (not including medication costs).

All of the steps and costs in a GIFT cycle are similar to an IVF cycle, with the exception of egg recovery. The laparoscopy that is required for GIFT is usually slightly more expensive than the ultrasound aspiration of eggs that is done for an IVF cycle.

Frozen Embryo Procedures

The cost of freezing embryos will range anywhere from $100 to $500. Some laboratories start charging an annual storage fee immediately, while others give you a grace period during which you can use your frozen embryos before annual storage charges begin to be incurred. Embryo storage costs can be charged either monthly or annually. Monthly costs range from $10 to $50, and annual fees can be anywhere from $75 to $300. In our laboratory, patients are given a one-year grace period from the time of their initial transfer, during which they can use their frozen embryos for a second pregnancy. If they choose to delay longer than that, an annual fee of $120 is charged.

In most cases, the cost of doing frozen embryo transfers following a GIFT or IVF procedure is significantly less than that of doing an entire IVF cycle from scratch. Since most centers today use an estrogen-and-progesterone preparative cycle, the blood testing and ultrasound monitoring that is performed is very minimal. Because of this, and because you don't have to pay for ovulation induction, the average cost of doing a frozen embryo transfer cycle with estrogen-progesterone preparation of the uterine lining ranges anywhere from $600 to $2,000. That includes preparation of the uterus, monitoring and timing, the thawing of the embryos, and the embryo transfer itself, as well as blood monitoring and luteal phase support. The lower cost of cycles using frozen embryos helps to increase the cost-efficiency ratio of ART cycles in general.

Third-Party Procedures

The burden of cost in an ART procedure is even greater when it involves a third party, such as an egg donor or surrogate. In the case of egg donation, the cost of doing a cycle is increased in several ways. First, the screening, selection and preparation of the donor will cost anywhere from $500 to $1,000. This pays for the advertising that locates prospective donors, for their psychological and medical screening, and for the process which matches them with an infertile couple. Once the donor is selected, she is paid a fee for donating her eggs. Currently, in Los Angeles, the standard fee is about $2,500 per cycle. She will also have to undergo stimulation, at a cost of about $2,000 per cycle. The rest of the costs match those of a normal IVF cycle, with the exception of double monitoring, since blood and ultrasound checks will have to be performed both on the recipient and on the donor. Given these extra costs, using an egg donor adds $3,000 to $4,000 to the cost of an IVF cycle.

If you need to use a surrogate gestational carrier, costs become even more markedly increased. Much of this added expense is due to the legal complications of surrogacy, resulting from the fact that an unrelated woman is going to carry a pregnancy to term. A standard surrogate carrier cycle is detailed below.

Costs for a Surrogate Gestational Carrier

	Low	High
Administrative	4,500	8,000
Legal fees		
Couple	2,500	5,000
Surrogate	500	1,500
Birth documents	1,000	2,500
Surrogate screening		
Medical	2,200	3,000
Psychological	1,200	1,600
Ongoing support	2,000	3,000
Surrogate payments		
Delivery	12,000	15,000
Insurance	1,200	4,000
Medical expense	1,000	1,500
Obstetrical fees (assumes insurance coverage)	1,250	2,500
Total	$29,350	$50,600

As you can see, the cost of going through an IVF cycle with a surrogate gestational carrier can range anywhere from $30,000 to $60,000 not including the cost of the IVF cycle. If the cycle is successful, and a pregnancy results, obstetrical costs to deliver the baby can sometimes be borne by the surrogate's health insurance carrier. This possibility should be discussed at the time you interview prospective donors.

THE ART OF GETTING ALL THE COSTS

ART procedures are complicated techniques, necessitating a number of individual steps. So when you are presented with a cost analysis by your doctor or clinic, you should make sure that it includes *all* of the expenses that will be involved. Some programs only give the hospital costs, egg recovery costs, operating room costs, anesthesia charges, laboratory culturing fees, and medication costs. When you look at this analysis, you assume that it includes all your fees. Imagine your surprise when you then receive a bill with additional charges for professional services—your doctors' charges—which weren't reflected in the cost analysis you were given.

To avoid this, insist that your clinic detail every step of the process they're recommending to you. The estimated charges that they show you should include:

- any administrative fees that they charge to start an IVF cycle.

- all professional service fees for the physician(s) overseeing your cycle. These fees should be broken down and listed individually.

- charges for the evaluation and testing that will have to be done before your cycle starts. These should include HIV and hepatitis tests, CMV testing, semen analysis, and bacterial culture.

- ovulation-induction costs. These should include both drug and monitoring costs. Per test charges for blood testing and ultrasound should be detailed out, with an estimate of the number of times they foresee doing those tests per cycle.

- charges for stimulation with hCG.

- cost of egg recovery. And if it is to be done in a hospital setting, any hospital charges that will be involved.

- laboratory charges for IVF culturing. Micromanipulation fees, if sperm injection is to be performed. The cost of assisted hatching, if that is to be performed.

- fees for embryo freezing and storage.

- embryo transfer fees. Again, if this is to be done in a hospital setting, a list of anticipated hospital charges.

- charges for any additional blood testing and monitoring of the luteal phase that they anticipate doing.

Using these guidelines, a typical cost breakdown would look a great deal like the following list of charges:

Costs of ART Cycles

	Low	High
Screening labs	200.00	300.00
Ovulation drugs	1,500.00	3,000.00
Monitoring (lab, ultrasound)	1,200.00	2,400.00
Egg recovery	800.00	1,500.00
IVF lab		
Routine	800.00	2,000.00
ICSI	500.00	2,000.00
Assisted hatching	500.00	1,000.00
Freezing	100.00	500.00
Embryo transfer	600.00	1,000.00

Lately, some centers have begun to use marketing approaches that offer a package price for two or three cycles of IVF, with a guarantee that you will either have a baby as a result of your cycles or will be able to adopt a baby through them. Typically, this is offered for a fixed price of $30,000 or $40,000, all of which must be paid in advance. If you're considering one of these packages, it's extremely important that you read all of the details in the center's contract. In some cases it may include steps you won't want to participate in. If you enter into the contract without understanding that, and then don't fulfill each of its required steps, you can be left with no baby, and with no way of getting back any of the money you paid. This is not to say that offers of prepackaged services are bad. Some can be very helpful. But it behooves you to look at each plan on an individual basis, and to carefully review all of the paperwork that's involved in it so that you fully understand the contractual commitment you're making.

Helping People Pay

It's impossible to leave our discussion about the costs of care without taking into account the pivotal role insurance plays in infertility treatment. Obviously, infertility treatment is expensive. So expensive, in fact, that unless a large portion of the cost is borne by a couple's insurance carrier, many can't afford to even try it. Given that fact, it's unfortunate that coverage for infertility treatment is so spotty. Some carriers don't cover it at all. Others will cover the costs of your basic evaluation, but won't cover therapy. And some cover certain types of therapies but not others. One of the reasons for this disparity is that there are no national guidelines within the insurance industry for infertility treatment.

Nor are there any for the state and federal agencies that control third-party payment for infertility treatment. As a result, there are only ten states in the U.S. with legislation that either requires insurance carriers to offer coverage for infertility treatment or actually mandates them to cover infertility services, including assisted technologies. The state that has taken the most aggressive stance in this regard is Massachusetts, where insurance carriers must provide benefits for all forms of infertility treatment, including 100% coverage for multiple ART cycles. Nine other states have policies requiring various degrees of coverage. But in many, even though state legislation has been passed and signed into law, enactment of the law has never taken place. A case in point is California, which has a state mandate requiring carriers to offer coverage, but which has yet to act to enforce this mandate. As a result, the majority of insurance companies in California don't include infertility coverage as part of their health care packages. And in those plans that do offer coverage, employers can elect to delete it and reduce their premium rates. So in most cases, despite a state law requiring it, employees in California still don't have coverage for infertility services. The state of Oregon is another example. Oregon has an exemplary health care plan, under which the state controls the provision of health care services. But of a total of 720 health needs listed for coverage, Oregon has given infertility a priority of 609. Oregon doesn't reimburse for infertility diagnosis or treatment in their present health care plan, and doesn't propose to do so in the future.

This tendency to consider infertility treatment as a luxury, rather than a necessity, puts the United States somewhat behind many other countries. In Canada, for instance, IVF is mandated, and is covered by national health insurance, although the government will only pay if the treatment is done at a particular institute in Ontario. Assuming it is, the government will cover 100% of costs for up to three IVF cycles. Alternatively, patients can choose to do IVF in private centers in Canada, and to pay for these costs out-of-pocket. The average cost for a cycle there is about $3,000. Similar government involvement can be found in Europe. France mandates coverage, and does 30,000 cycles per year on average, all of which are paid for by national health insurance. England requires approval before covering IVF, but with approval, their public hospitals perform IVF procedures under their national health plan. There are also a number of private hospitals that do IVF in England, for patients who are willing to pay personally, at a cost of $6,000 to $8,000 a cycle. Australia does a large number of IVF cycles each year, the costs of which are paid by national health insurance. Private IVF procedures are also done in Australia, at the expense of the couple. The average cost per cycle is around $4,000 in private centers in Australia.

As you can see, a number of other countries are doing more than we are to help infertile couples fund their infertility treatment. But even in the most enlightened countries, where government mandate provides help, a great deal of the cost is still borne by the couples themselves. This situation won't change until both the insurance industry and state and federal agencies become more aware of the problems infertility can cause for couples. This is something we can all work on together.

In 1992 and 1993 I was active in heading a group of physicians that lobbied Washington during President Clinton's attempt at national health care reform. We encouraged inclusion of both diagnostic procedures and treatment, including coverage for assisted reproductive technology procedures, in the health care provisions that were being drafted. We were successful in educating legislators, and in changing their stance on providing coverage for infertility services, including the recognition of IVF and GIFT. Unfortunately, President Clinton's health care reform package never came to fruition.

Until we get reform, there is a very good chance that you will be largely on your own when the bill for infertility services arrives. The more you understand about the cost of your treatment, the better prepared you will be to go into it. Many couples don't realize, as they begin their infertility work, that its financial impact can be just as stressful as infertility itself. Couples that borrow money to undergo infertility treatment—even taking second and third mortgages out on their homes—should ask for realistic counseling on their chances and risks before embarking on this extreme course.

Early in your evaluation, it is important either to have your physician's office call and verify what your insurance will or won't cover, or for you to personally call your insurance carrier, or contact the insurance advisor in your company, to determine what percentage of cost or reimbursement will be available for you.

When treatment options lead to surgical treatment of uterine, tubal, or pelvic factor infertility, it is important to fully understand what level of coverage, if any, your insurance carrier will provide, and exactly what costs you are facing personally—from hospital facility costs, to professional service costs from your operating physician, anesthesiologist, and any other physicians that may be involved in your care.

If you're approaching surgery, you should have a very thorough discussion with your doctor. With some problems, more than one surgical choice is available. Making the right decision could save you thousands of dollars.

For example, if you require tubal microsurgery or laser surgery to reconstruct the end of your fallopian tube, you may be told that your procedure can be done either with a laparotomy (an abdominal incision like a cesarean section), or with a laparoscope (using a telescopic type of instrument that is inserted through the navel and does not require a large external incision). The average charges for an exploratory laparotomy and tubal microsurgery run between $1,500 and $3,000 for surgeon's fees, and from $5,000 to $15,000 for hospital and surgical care costs. While the surgeon's fees would remain the same if the procedure is done laparoscopically, the hospital fees would be reduced to $5,000 to $10,000—a $5,000 savings to you. Obviously, understanding the financial ramifications of the procedure you choose can save you money. In this expensive environment, every penny counts. That's why you should talk to your doctor about options that might decrease the overall costs of certain types of treatments.

In all infertility cases, but especially where surgery is involved, it is imperative that you inform your insurance company of the chosen procedures in advance, and get their approval or clearance. Most insurance companies require preauthorization for treatment, especially for surgery. Having an approval in place ahead of time will help to ensure your reimbursement. If your doctor's office has a professional medical insurance biller, he or she will be able to give you diagnosis codes, charges, and procedure codes to forward to your insurance company.

It's easy to understand how some doctors, in their enthusiasm, can work toward the possibility of getting you pregnant, without focusing on the costs that are involved. That's why it's important for you to question the price of becoming pregnant, and then go further and find out what it will cost to stay pregnant and safely deliver a healthy child.

Be sure that your insurance covers obstetrical care and any complications that can occur during pregnancy. If it doesn't, get good health insurance with obstetrical coverage before undertaking a treatment cycle of IVF or any other infertility treatment.

The majority of couples facing infertility procedures aren't wealthy. They can't afford to ignore the cost of treatment. Since insurance coverage is almost universally nonexistent, having a detailed understanding of your projected costs before you start treatment is one of the most important things you can do.

PART FOUR

THINKING ABOUT
INFERTILITY

14

Infertility and Your Emotions

Let's go back in time to Sidney's party. Remember the intense pain that came with the discovery that your period had begun? . . . proof you were once again not pregnant. This has probably happened to you more times than you care to acknowledge. But your career, your marriage, and your lifestyle are so comfortable. You really don't want to face the fact that you are having difficulty conceiving. Or maybe *you* recognize that a problem exists, but your mate chooses to lessen its importance. Whatever the case, it can be terrifying to entertain the thought that your body, your husband's body, or your coupling, isn't working. It's as if you've failed, and how can you fail at a birthright? Fertility, or the lack thereof, becomes a burden. It's even taxing to talk about your "failure," let alone to find out what's not working. So you continue on as is. After all, there's always next month.

Eventually, too many "next months" pass, and you decide to see a doctor. He'll be able to help you get "better." After all, isn't that what you've been raised to expect? And with all of the innovations that infertility treatment offers today, of course you'll be "cured," right? Well . . . not always. In fact, not often enough. Depending on your age, it may not happen even half the time. And if there isn't a "cure," then time and understanding is needed as you decide what alternative is best for you. Regardless of which way your personal road leads, the trip can take a long time.

It also can involve a great many emotional responses. To help you negotiate your way through them, we'll start by explaining what you might feel as you're going through treatment. How you'll have to accept that infertility is a crisis, and then be prepared to work your way through the stages of grief it brings with it. We'll give you some insights into the different reactions men and women have to their infertility diagnosis, and then help you to anticipate some of the feelings you'll be experiencing as you go through your treatment. We'll explore your relationship as a couple, and with the world around you—with your parents, your siblings, your friends, your religion, and your medical caregivers. We'll give you some tips for coping with your emotions, and tell you how to go about finding professional psychological help, if you think you need it. Finally, we'll explain some ways in which you can try to reach resolution if you're not successful in having your own biological child.

What You're Going to Feel

The emotional aspects of infertility are as complex, in their own way, as its medical aspects. The best way to weather them as you go through your treatment is to be aware, ahead of time, of what you will be facing.

TRUST US . . . IT'S A CRISIS

The first bump in your road can come up when you and your partner must actually face the fact that you're having an infertility problem. Some couples try to shrug it off, unwilling to admit that it's of much importance. But infertility doesn't just affect your medical well-being. It can affect your psychological health as well, and it usually does. So much so, that most mental health professionals consider it to be a real crisis.

What is a Crisis?

"A stressful event that poses a problem that is insoluble in the immediate future. The problem overtaxes the existing resources of the persons involved because it is beyond traditional problem solving methods. The problem is perceived as a threat to important life goals of the persons involved. The crisis situation reawakens unsolved key problems from both the near and distant past."

—B. E. Menning
Infertility: A Guide for the Childless Couple, *1977*

This definition was found in one of the first books ever published dealing with infertility's relationship to emotional health. But does it really relate to *your* infertility situation? Some of you may argue that although getting pregnant is a challenge, it's not a crisis. You may say that you're dealing with it well, managing within the normal confines of your daily life. However, the majority of you *are* having difficulty with it, whether you consciously recognize the struggle or not.

You'll cope with your crisis better if you're willing to acknowledge that it exists. Once you understand yourself emotionally, you can find tools which will assist you on what may become a very difficult journey. You should start this process of acknowledgment by breaking down Menning's definition of crisis, and relating it to your own infertility situation.

It's Insoluble in the Immediate Future.

When you discover that you and/or your spouse is infertile, you also quickly discover that the problem can't be instantly cured. In fact, you can't even be given an approximate date—some vague idea of when things might work out. And not only is the solution to your problem in question from the standpoint of time, worse yet, you can't even be sure that your treatment will have a positive outcome.

It's a Stressful Event.

Admit it. The inability to immediately solve your problem, or to even have some control in solving the problem, is causing you a great deal of stress.

It's a Threat to Important Life Goals.

And the depth of this stress is further magnified by the fact that having children, an important life goal for you, is being threatened.

———

"Fertility is revered in almost all cultures, and pregnancy is a mile-stone in adult development. It is the bridge between generations, rich in symbolism and central in human experience."

—M. T. Notman, Reproduction and Pregnancy:
A Psychodynamic Developmental Perspective, *1990*

———

Of course you expected to become pregnant. It's probably been a goal since you were a child. You've waited a long time. You've most likely planned for it to happen at the right moment in your life—after school is finished, your career is under way, and you've found the right partner to share all of the happiness it will bring. But what promised to be a happy, joyous event in your life, has turned into a frustrating and depressing experience.

It's Beyond Traditional Problem-Solving Methods.

Naturally, you will employ all the resources you are aware of to help you deal with the pain you're experiencing. But not only are you unprepared for the news of your infertility, the traditional methods that you've used to deal with problems in the past can't help you through this process. Your family and friends, if you feel comfortable sharing your pain, may not be able to soothe your hurt. In fact, without realizing it, they may even say the wrong thing and further aggravate the pain. Nothing in your schooling, or in your socialization, has taught you how to cope when you're faced with not having a baby. The only thing that education stresses when it tells you about fertility is the need to protect yourself with birth control, since a baby could appear in an untimely manner. So you struggle to conduct your life in your usual fashion, while trying to cope with the pain. But you just may find that it slips beyond normal boundaries, and pierces the very core of your being.

It Just Came Over Me

I remember going to a first birthday party for my best friend's son. My husband and I had been trying to conceive, but had met with no success. I knew it was going to be uncomfortable at times, but I thought I could handle it. After all I had been in worse situations. Or so I thought. As other one-year-old children filled her backyard, I found myself creeping toward the corner. When the cake was brought out, I looked into my friend's eyes. They were filled with joy. It was one of the happiest moments of her life, and unfairly, one of my saddest. After quickly sneaking out, I sat in my car and cried my eyes out, I'd never realized the intensity of my pain. I hadn't allowed myself to feel it, until it exploded out of me.

—Eileen, age 30

Eileen was in the midst of a crisis she didn't realize existed. In trying to cope with her pain she had denied, even to herself, the extent of it.

But when she entered a situation that she thought wouldn't cause her pain, she suddenly discovered that she couldn't control herself. Had she honestly examined her feelings about her infertility, and thought about how she might react during the party, she may have been better prepared to handle her emotions. By thinking through the situation ahead of time, Eileen might have realized that a first birthday party was an inappropriate place for her to be. And had she discussed that possibility with her best friend, the delicacy of her emotional condition would probably have been acknowledged and understood.

It's a Situation That Reawakens Unsolved Key Problems from Both the Near and Distant Past.

Your awareness of pain can be intensified even further if there are unresolved issues from your near and distant past, especially issues that involve disappointment and loss. In other words, the pain that you experience with infertility may open up old wounds, intensifying your feelings. In these instances, both hurts come from the same place in the heart. For example, if you were adopted as a baby, and never had the ability to get close to a biological parent or sibling, you may have always longed for a biological connection . . . one that you hoped to find with your own genetic child. Learning that you're infertile would only serve to deepen your already aching wound. Another example is the couple that learns they're infertile due to a male factor condition. Their problem could be amplified if the husband's father had passed away a short time before they got this news. Learning of his infertility could make the husband feel that his dream—or unconscious wish—to have his father reborn in his own new baby is lost forever. In both of these cases the pain of infertility trips the previous pain, escalating the entire trauma into something beyond what you had ever imagined or had ever been prepared for.

Perhaps, after reading this, you now accept that you're in the midst of a crisis situation. Even if you don't, you can be certain about one thing. The moment you realize you're infertile, an enormous emotional expedition begins, an expedition that affects every person differently. So let's describe in more detail some of the feelings you may experience, and then learn how you can better cope with them. Your goal is to reach some sort of emotional resolution, even as you are striving to resolve your infertility crisis.

NEGOTIATING THE STAGES OF GRIEF

"Infertility is an emotional crisis that precipitates the cycle of grief."

—Linda Callahan
*"The Crisis of Infertility and Its Effect
on the Couple Relationship"*

In her book *On Death and Dying,* Elisabeth Kubler Ross, M.D., describes the various stages of dying. It's very common for people who are faced with a diagnosis of infertility to experience the same deep sense of loss that they would feel with the death of a loved one, and it's not unusual for them to travel through stages of grief that are comparable to those a death or other loss would bring on, as well as through some others that are unique to infertility. The stages you might experience include:

- Shock

- Denial

- Isolation

- Guilt and Blame

- Loss of Control, Anger, and Rage

- Depression and Hopelessness

- Acceptance

You may experience some of these feelings, but not all. You may experience them simultaneously, or you may go through one, and then shift to another, and even shift back again. You should be aware that any of these emotions can hit you at any stage of the process—from your infertility diagnosis, through your medical treatment, or even as you're reaching resolution. And most important, you should always keep in mind that these reactions to infertility are normal!

It's a Shock!

Shock is usually the first reaction to an infertility diagnosis. Learning that a life goal and a birthright may have been snatched away from you is definitely a jolt to the system.

It's a Mistake . . . It's Got to Be!

I couldn't believe my ears when our doctor told us that my hystero-salpingogram showed severe tubal blockage. I wanted to run out of his office and start all over again, in another infertility specialist's office. It's a mistake, it's got to be. How could my tubes have gotten this bad without my knowing? This kind of thing happens to other people, but not to me, right? After I calmed down, my doctor showed me my actual tests results. Why me? Why not some of the other girls I went through school with who slept around, definitely much more than I did?

—Carly, age 36

Carly was exposed to a silent infection when she used an IUD. Since she hadn't experienced any real symptoms, it was natural that she'd be shocked by this upsetting news. Like the great majority of infertile women, Carly had been relatively healthy throughout most of her life. So it was a nasty surprise when she suddenly learned that something was terribly wrong with her body. Maybe you've had a similar experience. And maybe you've had, or are continuing to have, feelings of shock and disbelief. The good news is that they generally last only a short time, and they don't cause any long-term emotional harm, especially if you learn to understand why you are feeling the shock, and to accept it.

If, on the other hand, you've been aware of a previous condition that could affect your infertility, or you've simply delayed having a family until too late in life, your doctor's diagnosis won't be as shocking. Or maybe you're someone who put off seeking treatment, as you continued to deny that you had a problem. In that case you've probably already sensed that you're going to learn of a problem. In fact, you've already been coping with the pain of it by using a mechanism of denial. This will help to pad the shock. But while your diagnosis won't be such a surprise, it is still traumatic, nonetheless.

And It Can't Be True!

Denial comes in many forms. You may totally deny you have a problem, or you may only deny certain aspects of your infertility. Don't worry. Denial is a common coping mechanism. It comes into play when you find yourself in a situation that's too overwhelming for you to deal with.

Later, Later

Even though we had been trying to conceive for over a year and a half, my husband and I used every excuse in the book to rationalize why we were unsuccessful. Finally, when the alarm on our biological clock started to sound loudly, it became time to find out why we were infertile. By denying our problem, we couldn't begin to solve it. We just postponed the inevitable.

—Karen, age 38

Denial can occur through all stages of infertility treatment: from taking the first step into medical treatment, through accepting the need to have invasive treatment such as ART procedures, to understanding that the time to examine donation practices has arrived . . . even through deciding to stop treatment altogether. Hopefully, your personal journey won't be an arduous one. But if it is, it's good to recognize that denial can fill a need in helping you get through it. How? Denial gives you time to adjust to your emotional crisis at your own pace, as you work at resolving your infertility.

Karen and her husband couldn't accept the pain of not being fertile, so they denied the possibility. Eventually, as time passed and they weren't getting pregnant, the reality of their situation, combined with Karen's biological time clock, helped them to accept their situation and to seek treatment. Their months of denial helped them to ease into their problem.

While this is a healthy way of using denial, there is also an unhealthy one. Instead of using denial as a way to cushion their transitions, some couples use it as a tool to push down the truth and keep it from rearing its ugly head. Couples who unrealistically continue to believe that they will find success by continuing to repeat ART procedures, when they've had no luck with them in the past, are typical examples. The telltale signs of trouble are the passage of time, and an insistence on ignoring the experienced doctor who's trying to tell them of the declining success rates that they're facing.

It'll Happen Next Time, I Just Know It

After my fifth GIFT procedure, I begged my doctor to let me try it one more time. I didn't care that I was 42 and never pregnant. I didn't care that the odds for me to get pregnant with GIFT in my situation were practically

*zero. I knew in my heart that the next time was going to be it. Yeah, right
. . . If I had only listened to my doctor and to my husband. If I had only
seen what was really happening in my life. I wish I was young and could
start the whole process over again. I would have spent my money, and my
time, much differently.*

—Suzanne, age 42

Listen to Suzanne. Don't let denial blind you to the reality of your
infertility situation for too long. At some point, refusing to accept things
can close off your other options.

Isolation . . . It's My Problem, Just Leave Me Alone!

As you accept your situation—and for some of you, that in itself can
be a long process—you may discover that you're separating yourself from
most of your world. Why? Because being infertile is still considered
something to be hidden. While it is true that times are changing, and you
can occasionally find yourself at a dinner party openly discussing infertility treatment, for most of you being infertile is still a topic that makes
you uneasy at best. Many of you are embarrassed and ashamed that you
are "stricken" with this condition. Especially if you're in a circle of
friends who openly discuss how easy it is to get pregnant.

The Big-Mouth Bitch

*It's happened to me more than once. I'm sitting with a group of ladies.
One is talking about another woman who is having trouble getting pregnant. Sure enough, she says it: "I just don't get it. My husband just looks at
me and I get pregnant." Not only is it an insensitive comment, but a painful
one too. It makes me shy away. I'm ashamed of being an inadequate
woman, and I'm forced to realize how different and separated I am from
the norm.*

—Colleen, age 35

You may find yourself withdrawing from every aspect of the fertile
world where children's activities rule. This may be true even if you
aren't actively trying to get pregnant. And if you are—if being infertile is
an acute problem that you're painfully trying to work through—the need
to separate from your extended family and friends who *are* fertile, and

who neither understand nor empathize with your situation, is that much greater.

While these protective mechanisms can be helpful, you should always keep in mind that isolating yourself to an extreme can be very damaging. If you find yourself avoiding life whenever children are present, you may be risking the loss of special friendships and familial relationships. The best thing to do is carefully choose the people in your life with whom you can communicate. Tell them what you are going through. Help them to understand why you are stepping back. Together, figure out how to pick and choose your outings with their children. This may seem difficult at first, but eventually you will find that given your circumstances it's the best thing to do.

Regardless of these adjustments, you may find as you endure treatment, and despite your best efforts not to, you're fixating on why you're not making a baby. Why are you the one who isn't able to reproduce naturally? Is it your fault?

Guilt and Blame

Was it the things you did in college? Was it that stupid one-night stand? Was it the infection you didn't take care of in time? Was it that IUD you decided to use, just so sex would be more convenient? Was it that abortion that you had to have? . . . If only you'd used birth control! Or is it simply that you kept waiting and waiting for the "right time" to start a family? Waiting too long.

Guilt is an uncomfortable feeling. It makes you scrutinize your past and agonize over what you should have, could have, would have done differently, had you only known what your future might bring. Is your infertility a punishment for the bad choices you made in the past? Most likely not. But the guilt and self-blame that you feel is still painfully present. Unfortunately, it's an all-too-common accompaniment to infertility. In some cases—if the cause of the infertility problem is you, and not your partner—you may feel that you're depriving your mate of children. You know how much he longs for them. No wonder you have that horrible feeling of guilt.

On the other hand, if it's your partner who's infertile, it's not uncommon for you to blame him. This blame can grow out of something your partner did in the past, or just out of pure frustration. Try not to fall into this. It's extremely destructive to your relationship. If you have these thoughts, just imagine how you would feel if your partner laid the blame on you. And remember, no one is to blame because being infertile is not the result of a deliberate action. It just happens.

Even if you don't blame your partner for being the cause of your joint infertility, you may blame him for not reacting to the problem as you would expect . . . for not fully understanding the many shades of your pain and suffering. Resentment can grow out of this, sometimes reaching such mammoth proportions that the desire to have a child becomes overshadowed by larger problems within your relationship as a couple. When you hold it in, you enter a danger zone. Try to talk out your feelings with your partner, so you understand each other and can grow together in the process. And don't underestimate the extent to which *both* of you feel a loss of control over your life choices as a result of infertility and its treatment.

Loss of Control, Anger, and Rage . . . I've Got to Take It Out on Someone!

Most of you made a definite decision about when you were going to have a baby. You put it into action by doing away with your birth control pills, condoms, diaphragms, and IUDs. It was an exciting time in your life. Until disappointment set in, as a positive pregnancy continually failed to appear. That's when you learned the process of getting pregnant is very much out of your control.

This realization hurts! After all, you've exercised control over every part of your life up until now. You chose your mate, picked your career, decided where to live, and picked your friends. Now everything seems to be on hold, as you endure endless treatment. You feel that you can't control your body. This is especially true when you do everything your doctor tells you to do, and the results still aren't what you were hoping for. Add to that the fact that you can't make decisions about other parts of your daily life. You're feeling and acting in ways that aren't recognizable to you. And you're paralyzed by the thought that you don't know what your future will hold.

How do you react? Most likely, you continue putting your life on hold, and avoid making any kind of decisions. Instead, you focus your energies on gaining control over your infertility. Only to learn that, unfortunately, aside from listening to your doctors, there isn't much you can do to assure yourself of whether, or when, you're going to have a baby. So you try to refocus your energies. You try to stop neglecting other parts of your life. At least in those areas, you have more of a chance of controlling the situation.

And yet, with all of this refocusing, and despite all of your efforts to stay somewhat in control during this emotional crisis, you can't help but notice all the other couples around you who are getting pregnant and planning wonderful lives with their new babies. Life's so unfair! No wonder you're angry at everyone and everything around you.

I Wanted to Punch Her

A woman that I work with who became pregnant while I was desperately trying to conceive would rattle on and on about the difficulties of her pregnancy. I decided to just tune her out. Then one day she cornered me in the bathroom, and proceeded to complain that her baby was breech, and that she was most likely going to have a cesarean. She dreaded the operation. She worked herself into a frenzy over what I thought was nothing. Big deal, she has an incision. It's not that painful. But she went on and on about how unfair life is. Finally I screamed, "Shut up, you idiot! You're getting a baby out of it, aren't you?" She stared back at me as if I had hit her with a 200-pound weight. Days later she apologized, as did I for my outburst. But to be perfectly honest, I wasn't sorry for how I felt.

—Missy, age 34

Why wasn't Missy sorry for what she felt? Because deep down she believed that she was dealt an unfair hand in the game of life. It's easy to fall into that attitude when you expect things to happen, want them to happen, truly desire to have them happen, and they don't. Anger can grow out of this lack of control, this sense that infertility is unfair. Many times, just looking at another pregnant woman, seeing a woman breast-feeding a baby, watching a baby pushed in a stroller, or running into a person buying disposable diapers in the market can create resentment.

Car Trouble

I remember not really concentrating on the fact that I wasn't getting pregnant. My work kept my thoughts occupied. But every day, as I left my office and drove away to lunch, I inevitably found myself stuck at a traffic light. And day after day, I found myself looking at the car next to me, where a brightly colored car seat always perched in the backseat. Usually I didn't look to see what was inside. But sometimes I couldn't help myself. There would always be a newborn or a toddler, happily drinking juice or playing with small toys. Ouch, it hurt. As I drove away in lonely silence, I would sit there wondering, "Why couldn't I have a baby? How come that mother could? Why was she luckier than me?" And then, what really got to me was "Why did she have to come along and remind me?" Remind me of what I didn't have, but wanted more than anything in the world. Was I really asking for so much? Once I found myself cutting off a car when the next light changed, so I didn't have to see the car seats in the back.

—Susie, age 33

It's natural to feel anger and resentment toward those around you who've already been handed their birthright, when you're still coming up empty month after month. You may also feel resentment toward people around you who, you're sure, couldn't possibly understand what you're going through. You may find yourself overreacting to a seemingly incompetent nurse, an ill-advised friend, or an overbearing mother. Try not to redirect your anger toward people who are genuinely trying to help you. Realize that the real source of your anger is your lack of control over your infertility. Remember that the "nice you," who's still there underneath all the anger, would act differently, given a chance.

Sometimes your feelings of anger can become so extreme that they erupt in a type of a rage.

Dumpster Baby

I remember driving home from work on the freeway a couple of days after I learned that my wife's IVF procedure was not successful. A news broadcast came on the radio. Another baby was found in a Dumpster in New York. I lost it. I started screaming at the radio like a lunatic. "Are you fucking kidding, you threw it away!" It was incredible to me. Here I was doing everything I could in life to get my wife pregnant, and some sick person threw away their baby. Their own flesh and blood. How could it be that they could have it and discard it like a piece of trash, something we wanted more than anything in the whole world? Preoccupied with the broadcast, I got too close to the car in front of me. Fortunately, I still had a split second to slam on my brakes. Otherwise, that little broadcast could have put me over the top.

—Matthew, age 40

My Monthly Fling

A couple of days before my period was due, I felt that I wasn't pregnant. So I went to a flea market and bought many incomplete sets of broken dishes. When the nurse called me to say I wasn't pregnant for the fifteenth time, I went to the box of dishes, picked it up, and carried it outside. Then I proceeded to throw each dish against my garage door like a madwoman. At the time it was the only thing I could do.

—Linda, age 41

These feelings of loss of control, anger, and rage are normal reactions to infertility. But don't underestimate the power of your emotions during this crisis. You may need to consider seeking professional help to guide you through. If you don't, and if you internalize your anger, it can become a form of depression.

Depression and Hopelessness . . . I Give Up

It's bad enough that infertility causes you great emotional pain. What's even more unfair is that it makes you relive it every month, each time that you bump into a failure. As you undergo treatment, you find your menstrual cycle has two parts—the two weeks after ovulation, and the two weeks prior to it. The part that comes after you ovulate is marked by a nervous excitement, a hopefulness that this month you'll find out that you're pregnant. All you can do is wait. The second part begins when your period appears, as do powerful feelings of letdown and pain. After a while they begin to subside, at least a little. All you can do at that point is try to pick yourself up again, and prepare for your next ovulation. As Jan Crosby, wife of singing star David Crosby, describes it:

Riding the Roller Coaster

Each month, each cycle, I would be aware of a two-week period of very high hopes. I would go up this hill of hope, and get to the top and peak out the day before finding out whether I was pregnant or not. Then the next day, I would find out that I wasn't, and I would come sliding down the other side of the hill, and kind of crash into this pool of disappointment. It was like I was in a little roller coaster. Two weeks of the month I'd be going up, and two weeks I'd be coming down the other side.

As month after month passes, the great mountain of hope you started with slowly erodes. And as twelve months pass, and you have to begin thinking in terms of years, instead of months, it may become impossible to remain positive. This is when you can fall into depression.

Depression can't be taken lightly. If you're depressed, everything seems to take extra effort. And unlike the past, nothing seems to bring you any pleasure. You can put on a show for your colleagues at work, or even in social situations, but your close friends and family will notice something is off balance in your behavior. You may have feelings of sadness, malaise, fatigue, and pessimism. And privately, you may be doing a lot of crying. You can become apathetic toward your everyday routine, pushing aside personal hygiene, your house, and your work responsibilities. This can create a vicious circle. Because you've let yourself and your surroundings go, you feel inadequate, incompetent, and undesirable. This lowers your self-esteem even more, which then makes your depression even deeper. If your depression develops into a severe condition, hopelessness will begin to dominate your entire world. This can be extremely dangerous. Since there's no answer as to when your infertility condition will be resolved, your depression could also continue indefinitely.

Many people, in an effort to cope with their depression, avoid their problems by indulging themselves. If you're falling into this trap, you may begin to spend excessive amounts of money, or to look for temporary relief through drugs or alcohol. But these temporary solutions will only increase your depression in the long run . . . they underestimate the power of the feelings of pain that surround your infertility. And, of course, drugs and excessive alcohol will only make the physiological problems worse.

The best way to snap out of your depression, or to deal with any of your other emotional reactions to infertility, is by confronting your pain head-on. In order to accomplish this you should:

1. Acknowledge and accept your feelings. Don't judge them. They are the way you feel.

2. Allow yourself to really feel what is hurting you. Don't block it out.

3. Talk about your feelings with someone—your spouse, a close family member or friend, a therapist, or a support group.

4. Discuss the use of antidepressant medications with your doctor. Short-term use may be of help to you.

These steps will assist you, as you try to understand your reactions to your crisis. If you don't take positive steps such as these, your feelings will continue to circle through your head like travelers stuck in a revolving door. This will never help you to maneuver toward some type of resolution.

Physical Reactions

You're not feeling like yourself. Maybe you're more tired than usual, or have a sense that you lack energy. Perhaps you're experiencing breathlessness, a tightness in your chest, or a hollowness in your stomach. You may become irritable. You may feel a weakness in your muscles, or experience a sense of being off balance at times. And in some instances, you may feel dry-mouthed, have a tightness in your throat, or an oversensitivity to noise. Any of these physical sensations can occur, and can be attributed to your infertility, so don't be alarmed.

In addition, you may find yourself acting somewhat differently. For example, you may become a bit forgetful, preoccupied with your infertility. You may find that your sleep patterns shift, and that you're becoming lethargic. Your interest in sex, eating, socializing, may change. You may find yourself more anxious than usual, especially when waking up. Your obsessions may intensify. And most of all, you may find that you are doing a lot of crying.

These behaviors may sound foreign to you. But chances are, many of them are all too familiar. Don't panic. Just keep in mind they're all within the normal realm of reactions to infertility.

THE DIFFERENCE BETWEEN MEN AND WOMEN

Not only are you experiencing strong emotions when faced with infertility, so is your partner. This may not always be obvious, since men and women have very different ways of reacting to some situations. Keep in mind that no two people are alike. Each one carries distinct past experiences with them . . . not to mention a different personality, different coping mechanisms, and different expectations. And our sexuality gives us very dissimilar viewpoints. The sexes are unalike, both physically and mentally. Each of them has had specific mores and values passed down to them by society through the generations.

Even the medical treatment you face is different, depending on your sex. This starts right from the beginning—the diagnostic workup. For a man, once a semen analysis has been performed, no additional procedures are required, unless he falls into the small category where further analysis or surgery needs to be performed. Still, the one test that he does have to continually perform, masturbating in a doctor's office until orgasm is reached, is not a comfortable experience for most men. For women the procedures are very much different. Diagnostic evaluations are almost always comprised of a number of physically invasive procedures. These can include surgeries to view, confirm, and repair a problem. But while the burden to "deliver" a baby rests with the woman, the fact that he isn't enduring the same degree of physical invasion as his partner doesn't necessarily negate the stress that a man experiences. Particularly if he is the cause of the infertility.

Given all this, it's a wonder that any couple can survive infertility and its treatment. The difficulty lies in understanding the ways in which gender influences the experience.

Men's Reactions

Men have a tendency to hide their feelings and keep them to themselves, even when asked to speak frankly by medical personnel. Women, on the other hand, are more inclined to talk about their feelings. So when their partner doesn't, misunderstandings and conflicts can present themselves.

It's a Secret

". . . Men require more secrecy, believing infertility to be a private marital matter that should not be discussed outside the relationship. These secrecy demands leave their partners feeling angry and resentful, as well as increasing their isolation from possible support networks."

—Linda Callahan, M.A., 1992
"The Crisis of Infertility and Its Effect
on the Couple Relationship"

If a man is diagnosed as infertile, he may withdraw from his partner, brood, blame himself for his sterility, lose interest in sex, or even become impotent. He often interprets his infertility as a failure, even though he failed at something he had no control over. This lack of control only magnifies the problem. Since a man's self-esteem is inextricably linked to an ability to be "in charge," it may decrease, and he may inwardly obsess about his adequacy as a man.

If your husband reacts like this, and doesn't communicate his pain, you may incorrectly interpret his reactions as a lack of concern, as an inability to accept the diagnosis, or as an unwillingness to cooperate in the treatment process. Understand that he is not only concerned about the situation, he is painfully disappointed and saddened by his inability to easily reproduce, or to reproduce at all. He probably expects to find assistance through his usual methods of coping, but this is a crisis, and as we explained earlier, those methods won't necessarily work in this type of situation. Most likely he won't feel comfortable discussing his problem with family or friends. And his upbringing never prepared him for the possibility that one of his life goals could be threatened. With his usual way of doing things stripped away, how does he react? Usually he withdraws and doesn't communicate his feelings. That's why studies have shown that marriages are more at risk with male infertility than with female causes.

One of the forces that drives a man's negative reaction to his own infertility is society's ideals. Nowhere in the history books or in literature is it made clearly acceptable for a man to be infertile. In some cultures it simply isn't accepted, even today.

ROYAL MISCONCEPTION

I once had the honor of treating a patient from another part of the world. He had an infertility problem that was, unfortunately, not correctable. And yet every time he came into town, he would bring another woman with him, in the hope that she would be the one who was able to deliver him a child. I remember discussing with him, more than once, the fact that changing women wasn't going to help the situation, because the infertility problem was his. But tradition had placed a heavy burden on him. He never could accept it.

Male sterility has traditionally been associated with male impotence, even though, as we discussed in Chapter Nine, a man's ability to have an erection and intercourse rarely have anything to do with his fertility. Unfortunately, one of the ways society judges men's masculinity is whether they can reproduce. So it's only natural for a man who receives a diagnosis of infertility to believe his masculinity is being threatened. And don't kid yourself, the women around him can have the same reaction.

The Virile Stud

My husband was diagnosed with a severely low sperm count. I remember going to a cocktail party and overhearing another man being congratulated on his wife's recent pregnancy. The news of the pregnancy wasn't as painful as witnessing both men and women commenting to him, "What a stud." And when it became known that their baby was conceived the first month they tried, a woman cozied up to the future father and said, "You're

awesome, you virile guy, you." I gave my husband a pained look, which he
returned. No wonder he was feeling so isolated and depressed.

—*Carol, age 31*

Notice how Carol was just as pained by the remark as was her husband? This is a healthy reaction to the diagnosis of male infertility. By
internalizing his problem and being sensitive to it, Carol had accepted
his problem as their problem. This union of forces is a positive approach
to male infertility.

Paul and Cathy's story isn't.

The day that I met Paul and Cathy was stressful for all of us. The
tension that had taken over their relationship was obvious from
the moment they sat down in my office. Discussing their history and
the evaluation that had been made prior to their meeting with me, it
seemed obvious that a low sperm count was the cause of their infertility. But it's one thing to recognize poor sperm count as the cause of a
couple's problem, and quite another to decide on the best way to deal
with it.

In the case of Paul and Cathy, the approach their previous doctor
had taken had not only failed to solve the problem, it had created an
unhealthy strain in their relationship. Cathy had been undergoing
some fairly invasive treatments in an attempt to produce a pregnancy
using Paul's inadequate sperm. She'd been on hormone treatments.
She'd been evaluated by laboratories. She'd been probed and injected
daily. And since she herself had previously been proven to be fertile,
all of this was an attempt to remedy a problem she perceived as his.
Her frustration had led to a negative view of her marriage, and even
of Paul. In her mind all he had been doing was masturbating, while
she was undergoing painful and physically demanding procedures.

Although she didn't say so, Cathy was angry at Paul. His subfertile condition had put her into this position. To Paul, this seemed
unreasonable. If he could have taken the shots . . . undergone the
ultrasound . . . given the blood samples . . . he would have,
gladly. But since no doctor had ever offered any alternatives, he was
limited to entering the semen collection room, masturbating, and collecting specimens. He was angry too. At himself.

What neither of them wanted to look at was the fact that their
confrontational situation, filled with fighting and innuendo, was creating such severe stress between them that not only might their infertility situation not be correctable, their marriage might disintegrate to
an irretrievable point as well.

This is a very common situation, and one which needs to be dealt
with directly and aggressively. So even though Cathy and Paul had

**come in to talk about the science and technology of what could be
done for them medically, we spent most of their first visit dealing with
the interpersonal aspects of their infertility problem.**

One thing we should learn from Paul and Cathy is that male factor
infertility can magnify problems that already exist within a relationship.
If you weren't totally happy with your mate to begin with, you now have
a tangible focus for your dissatisfaction. If the two of you didn't communicate well before you found out you're subfertile, things will probably
get worse once you do.

One reason for this is the "shame factor." The shame factor can
affect how men see themselves—even men who previously felt confident and healthy.

As John Gray, Ph.D., pointed out in *Men Are from Mars, Women Are
from Venus*, "Martians value power, competency, efficiency, and achievement. They are always doing things to prove themselves and develop
their power and skills. Their sense of self is defined through their ability
to achieve results. They experience fulfillment primarily through success
and accomplishments."

Of course, in Gray's terms, Martians are men. And as we in the field
of infertility know, in a "Martian's" eyes, one of a man's most important
accomplishments is fathering a family. Women can suffer from the shame
factor too. But it's more common, and more devastating, among men.
And that's just *one* of the ways that men and women react differently to
infertility.

- *Men have a tendency to feel uncomfortable when answering the personal
  questions that are posed by medical personnel. Many men think that
  infertility is a private matter, which shouldn't be exposed outside the
  marital relationship.*

- *Men have a tendency to internalize stress and to become withdrawn
  when dealing with it. Women are more prone to vocalize and to
  respond emotionally.*

- *Men often think they should be able to solve their problems themselves.
  As Gray points out, to men ". . . autonomy is a symbol of efficiency,
  power, and competence." Because of this, some men may feel that asking
  others to aid them reveals their own inadequacy.*

Given men's nature, the physical process of an infertility evaluation
and diagnosis can only make things worse. Men are marched into a room
in a crowded doctor's office, and told to masturbate and ejaculate into a

specimen cup. This is the ultimate invasion of privacy—everyone not only knows what they're doing, but how they're doing it. The experience is both difficult and embarrassing. Not surprisingly, it makes many men want to withdraw even further.

———

"Run that by me once more," Marissa called to him. "I don't think I heard you correctly."

"It's simple," he said. "I'm not going to the clinic this morning. I'm not up to it today. I'm not some kind of sperm dispenser."

—Robin Cook
Vital Signs

———

Worst of all, in many cases infertile men feel that they've let down their partner, who's yearning for a child. Considering all of these things in combination, it's no wonder that the great majority of subfertile men suffer from feelings of inadequacy, inferiority, guilt, and lowered self-esteem. Unfortunately, the same masculine traits that have contributed to these emotional difficulties—things like a difficulty in communicating personal feelings, and a do-it-yourself attitude—can also keep men from seeking help.

Given the speed with which medical technology is advancing, at some point in the future men whose reproductive systems don't even manufacture sperm cells should be able to fertilize an egg. Once that is a reality, the term *male factor infertility* may cease to be part of our jargon, and the emotional baggage it carries with it may also disappear. But that has yet to happen, and for most subfertile men, difficult issues of ego, self-esteem, and virility still complicate the purely technical aspects of their problem.

If you're diagnosed with male infertility, this presumption of a lack of masculinity is one more emotional issue you'll have to contend with. The more you prepare for it, the stronger you'll be. Keep in mind, as we have said before, that if you're infertile, you aren't alone. Remember the statistics? . . . Forty percent of all infertility is male; it's just something no one talks about.

Even armed with this knowledge, there may come a time when a man will need to seek psychological help in order to cope with infertility. If you think your partner may have reached that point, ask him to look at this list, and to see if he recognizes himself in it.

- You now see yourself as less healthy than you use to.
- You're less confident in business and social situations.
- You've suffered from bouts of unexplained anxiety.
- You've had nightmares, or other problems with your sleep.
- You're trying to compensate for your infertility by fulfilling your partner's every material demand.
- You want to be left alone more often than you used to.
- You're having problems talking to your partner, or to your close friends.
- You're short-tempered and impatient.
- You're finding it difficult to make plans for the future.
- You're less interested in sex.
- You're sometimes impotent.
- You're becoming more sexually aggressive to try to prove that you're still potent.

If he feels that a number of the items on this checklist describe him, it may be time to turn to a psychologist, a psychiatrist, or a group, and he shouldn't put it off. Remind him that repressing his feelings about a loss of fertility can affect both his mental and physical health.

The Special Emotional Problems of Donor Insemination

———

"Now I know what it feels like to play second string. At the moment of creation, I'll be sitting on the bench."

—*Bob, age 37*

———

With doctors' new ability to aggressively use even minimal numbers of sperm to produce successful fertilization, most subfertile men no longer have to face the specter of donor sperm as their only alternative for producing a family. This can make those cases where donor sperm is still necessary even more difficult from an emotional and psychological point of view. Some of these problems—for example, a man's concern over his partner's safety, or his confusion over how a donor match is made—can be alleviated by sitting down and discussing in detail how the process works. Men considering using donor sperm should understand the new openness of information about donors which some sperm banks offer. They should be made aware of how the quarantining of specimens ensures safety for their partners. In the majority of cases, making things like this clear can help men more easily accept the process.

"It doesn't matter who my father was; it matters who I remembered he was."

—Anne Sexton
"All God's Children Need Radios"

But even well-informed men may still resist having a child that is not genetically their own. If you find you can't accept donor sperm as an alternative, rather than forcing the issue, adoption may be a better alternative. It's at this point that you as a couple need to try to pull together. In cases where a man's partner is totally prepared to accept donor sperm, but he can't, strife and division in the relationship can easily occur. Most of the time, with good psychological counseling and support, these issues can be dealt with, and a compromise can be made so that the relationship will survive.

Women's Reactions

Society is less prone to connect female infertility to a woman's sexuality than it does to a man. Women who can't reproduce are still considered to be feminine. But while infertility may be less threatening to women sexually, they do feel it more deeply as a life crisis.

It's All Her Problem

"The general public, the infertile couple as well as the physician, often tend to see infertility as the woman's problem, even if both partners carry the diagnosis."

—Linda Callahan, M.A.
"The Crisis of Infertility and Its Effects
on the Couple Relationship," 1992

In studying twenty-two cases, Greil, Leitko, and Porter discovered that it was the woman who initially raised the subject of infertility when the couple was finding no success after months of trying to conceive. In twenty-one of those cases, she made the first contact with a doctor, and took the leadership role throughout the treatment process. She was also more likely to view infertility as a devastating experience. Even in situations where the male partners were diagnosed as infertile, very often the women viewed the problem as being something having to do with the functioning of their own bodies. And finally, when the women evaluated their mate's role in terms of support, a supportive partner was defined as one who didn't interfere with treatment. Why is it that the majority of the women interviewed took the aggressive step forward? One reason is society's view of infertility as a "female problem." After all, it is the woman who delivers the baby. So isn't it her responsibility? Given this, it's incumbent for the female to act on it. And that action offers a bonus to women: it gives them some sense of control over an uncontrollable phenomenon in their lives.

Another problem women face during the infertility process is their wish for everyone around them to be happy. This can cause some interesting behavior, especially in respect to male infertility.

Lie to Cover

"Some women with infertile partners report they lie to friends and family, saying they themselves have the problem, to protect the man and his sense of potency."

—*S. H. McDaniel, Ph.D., J. Hepworth, Ph.D., and W. Doherty, Ph.D., "Medical Family Therapy with Couples Facing Infertility," 1992*

These women are feeling guilty for the pain that their spouses are experiencing. By taking the blame for the problem, at least in society's eyes, these women hope to strip the worry from their mates' minds, while they're attempting to answer the unresolved question of Why? They're hoping that once there's an understandable reason for their mate's infertility, he'll feel less frustrated, less angry, and less depressed.

These have been just a few examples of the stages a typical couple may experience, as they journey through their infertility treatment. Whether it's society's influence, or simply the nature of our sexual makeup, there are definite differences in the way the sexes react to each of them.

Battle of the Sexes

"Infertile wives are reported to suffer more significant damage to self-esteem, and to marital, sexual, and life satisfaction. Infertile men are reported to have more intense feelings of guilt, anger, frustration and isolation than do infertile women, but both feel increased guilt and blame."

—A. G. Sadler, R.N., M.S., and
C. H. Syrop, M.D. "The Stress of Infertility:
Recommendations for Assessment and
Intervention," 1987

Do you recognize yourself and your partner in these discussions on gender differences? Most likely you do. Now let's move on to what happens when you have to work together, in union, to solve your problem.

HOW TREATMENT WILL MAKE YOU FEEL WITHIN YOUR RELATIONSHIP

As infertility treatment begins, your life changes dramatically. You're forced to mold your days around your medical treatment. You lose your independence . . . as well as the enormous amounts of money that have to be expended in the hopes of getting pregnant. Your personal space is repeatedly trespassed during examination and treatment. The intimate details of your sexual activities become part of an impersonal medical record. Inwardly, you start quietly focusing your attention on your failure. Not only do you experience the emotional stages of grief, but your self-esteem, your confidence, your health, your relationship, your security, and your ambitions are probably impacted as well. By the very nature of your condition, your sex life will most likely be affected too. This can put additional stress on your marriage.

Sounds pretty gloomy, doesn't it? Our goal is to help you to understand the scope of what you are going through, to recognize danger areas, and to realize that everything you're experiencing is within the norm for infertile couples.

As you realize by now, you and your mate are two distinct people. Infertility is going to affect you differently. Your emotional upheavals most likely won't hit at the same times. And because of the nature of your past experiences, once they do hit, each of you will cope with them in your own way. This can give you a sense of disconnection, out of which problems can arise. For example, each of you may have your own periods of calmness, and then explode from the underlying stress that's been building up below the surface. These eruptions may seem unexpected, but they're actually the fallout from your extended treatment, your monthly reminders of failure, and your inability to make clear plans for the rest of your life. Each explosion has to be recognized for what it is. Instead of taking your partner's outbursts personally, you have to help them calm down and work through the episode. If you panic at the first signs of an explosion or disagreement, you'll never understand its true cause, and the result may serve to further complicate matters.

Gender differences cause another type of couples pattern. If your husband retreats, you may want to talk about the problem. But your husband, feeling powerless in the situation, will sometimes avoid listening to your complaints and retreat further. As he does this, you feel abandoned. In response, you complain more. Then he feels overwhelmed because he's not meeting your needs. Friction arises out of the resentment each one of you has toward the other. As a result, you both feel depressed, not only because of your inability to make a baby, but because of the distance that's been created between the two of you.

If you feel this happening, nip it in the bud by talking out your feelings. Understand that the two of you have come to this point in your life with different past experiences, and be sensitive to the fact that both of you are in great pain. If the two of you find talking out your feelings to be a frustrating experience, search for a third party to mediate while you reconnect.

Your Sex Life

Your sex life is one of the aspects of your relationship that can suffer as a result of infertility, and in some cases severely. Just at the time when you most need to be intimate with your partner, you may experience a separation and loss of interest. Many times your sexual desire lessens or becomes nonexistent. This is typical. Hopefully it will be a temporary phenomenon. Talk about it, and understand each other's needs. Deal with the issue of intimacy openly. Unresolved anger and poor communication between you and your partner are likely culprits that can affect or destroy your sex life.

Another way your sex life can suffer is if your image of your body suffers. Your body image was formed in early childhood. It reflects your feelings about your physical well-being, your physical abilities, and your fantasies about what may someday be possible.

"People with a positive body image feel attractive, normal, and acceptable to others, both inwardly and outwardly. The discovery of a physical defect such as infertility threatens the stability of that image."

—*Patricia P. Mahlstedt, Ed.D.*
"The Psychological Issues of Infertility
and Assisted Reproductive Technologies," August 1994

Then along comes an infertility diagnosis. You're not only told that you're defective, you're defective in an area that will impact one of your most cherished life goals. For men, infertility is a deficiency that makes you question your masculinity. For women, it's a condition that leaves you feeling unable to rise to the traditional maternal role. Either way, your body image is stripped, leaving you feeling negative about your physical self. Then as you go through treatment, you are asked to tolerate all types of medications, procedures, and surgeries . . . things that further contribute to poor body image. This can make you feel depressed and angry, and cause you to lose self-esteem. And even when you aren't medicated or recovering from a surgery, someone else is controlling your sex life. You're told when to have sex, and when not to. When you *are* permitted to have it, it becomes a mechanical experience, devoid of passion or caring. In response to this strict regimen you, and/or your partner, will most likely feel self-conscious and apprehensive toward sex.

Sex? No, Thank You

In a study reported in 1988 of approximately 35 infertile couples, almost sixty percent of the women and men experienced decreased frequency of sexual intercourse and almost fifty percent experienced decreased sexual satisfaction after diagnosis.

—*Based upon R. Sabatelli, R. Meth, and S. Gavazzi*
"Factors Mediating the Adjustment to Involun-
tary Childlessness," 1988

Suddenly sex is a job with one purpose, and it becomes a difficult task to perform. The very act that's supposed to be an enjoyable tension-reliever now reminds you of what you don't have but want more than anything in the world. Not surprisingly, you find yourself losing interest in it altogether. Avoiding sex sometimes becomes the easiest way to protect yourself from the monthly pain and disappointment of not conceiving.

When a man is diagnosed as infertile, or when he becomes frustrated with the strict bedroom regimen that's been prescribed, he may react, just not vocally. How can all of this sexual invasion not affect him? Generally speaking, if men aren't comfortable vocalizing their other fears and anxieties, sex rarely comes up for discussion. And if a man doesn't speak out, frustration generally rears its ugly head in the area of performance. He may experience performance problems that leave him feeling even more inadequate sexually.

I Couldn't Even Get It Up

After several cancellations because of early morning meetings, we were finally able to schedule a postcoital test. Next we needed to have intercourse. We got started late, and as we did, my boss called on the machine, which I could hear, saying he needed me in the office. Next I had a tough time with an erection, which bummed me out. Then I wasn't able to ejaculate, despite all of our efforts. My wife even tried to slip in a dirty movie, but nothing worked. I remember being drenched in sweat, not out of pleasure, but frustration. Finally I got dressed for work as my wife called the doctor's office to say we were unsuccessful. It was so demeaning, so humiliating. I did everything I could not to put my fist through the wall. The only reason I considered doing it again was because I really wanted a kid. The next month we were lucky. My wife ovulated over a weekend. We were better prepared and a little more relaxed. Thank God it worked.

—David, age 38

Had it not worked, this couple might have found themselves in a bad place in their relationship. David was feeling embarrassed, frustrated, and enraged. Both he and his wife would have resented the other for the failure . . . after all, you have to place blame for not getting to the next step somewhere. And you may already have been secretely blaming each other for not getting pregnant.

Sexual degeneration isn't just limited to men. Women, too, become disenchanted, but for different reasons. To begin with, infertility can affect a woman's emotional responses, making her feel preoccupied, disinterested, and asexual. And the side effects of medical intervention don't contribute to a great sex life either.

———

Not Tonight, I've Got a Headache

In a study involving a group of 118 women undergoing infertility evaluation and treatment done in 1992, the women indicated that their sexual pleasure, interest in sex, and the ease in reaching orgasm had decreased. They reported increased feelings of sadness, changes in how close they felt to their partners, and changes in how worthwhile they felt as people.

—*Based upon J. Downey and M. McKinney*
"The Psychiatric Status of Women Presenting for Infertility Evaluation," 1992

———

Often, either because of the aftereffects of medical intervention or the issues surrounding programmed sex, couples may react in a way that is counter to their normal natures. It is not unheard of for a spouse to seek healthy, undisturbed sex with an outside partner. If they do, they are probably seeking to bring back their feelings of pride about their bodies, to regain a positive body image. They are also seeking to regain control over their lives. This is not unlike the person who develops substance abuse or eating problems as a result of infertility treatment. In each one of these instances, they are dealing with an uncontrollable situation by acting out in areas that *are* within their control. Keep in mind, reactions such as these can and will cause you great harm in the end, so please don't attempt them.

Even if your partner doesn't entertain these thoughts, you may experience guilt, and slowly begin to doubt the affection of your partner. This is especially true if you are the one who has been diagnosed as infertile. You may dwell on the idea that if your partner had another mate, he could then have a baby. And if you believe that, you may find yourself subconsciously encouraging your partner to look for someone else.

———

"It is common for the infertile spouse to either overtly or subtly encourage the fertile spouse to seek a partner with whom he or she may bear children."

—*Linda Callahan*
"The Crisis of Infertility and Its Effects on the Couple Relationship," 1992

Revisiting Old Turf

I remember traveling on business to the city where I grew up. My wife, who had extreme endometriosis, asked if I planned to see my old girlfriend. She then encouraged me to have coffee with her . . . you know, discuss old times, show off what's going on in my career. At the time I thought it was a good idea. As a matter of fact I enjoyed it. But today, with two boys, I have no desire to see her. Looking back, I can now see that my wife and I were both in a bad spot.

—Jake, age 42

Why did Jake enjoy revisiting his old girlfriend while he was going through infertility treatment? And why does he have no interest today? Back then, feeling somewhat inadequate, he probably flirted with the fantasy that maybe he could impregnate his old flame. So he explored it a little. Why not? After all, it *was* his wife's idea. And why not try something a little different to spark some energy in his life, since the infertility seemed to drain him? Had his life taken another turn . . . had he married his old flame . . . maybe he wouldn't be going through the stress of trying to have children. But today his life is complete. He and his wife have two boys. Jake's experience is a common one. Many patients tell themselves that if they'd ended up with a different partner, they wouldn't be having an infertility problem.

There are many permutations to this thinking.

The Department Store Stud

I remember walking through a department store one day, a couple of months after my husband was diagnosed with poor sperm motility. I saw this really cute guy buying a sweater and I thought, "Motile? Could he get me pregnant?"

—Randi, age 30

Suffice it to say, if you and your mate aren't finding success in getting pregnant, it's a normal reaction to fantasize about someone else stepping into your spouse's shoes and delivering the goods. Just keep in mind, fantasy is one thing, actually crossing the line is another.

Can Infertility Break Up a Marriage?

Whether an affair does occur or not, can infertility break up a marriage? It's very possible. Infertility is a crisis, a trauma in a couple's life, and to some even a tragedy. If a couple breaks up during infertility treatment, it's because the bonds within their marriage weren't strong enough to endure this, or possibly any other crisis.

The riskiest type of pairing to bring into an infertility situation is one where the most basic component of the marriage is parenting. When that is threatened, so is the very concept of the marriage. If you're in this category, renegotiating your marriage goals can be very difficult. What happens when your need to become a parent stems from your family of origin . . . when the very environment that you developed in molded your need to parent? Then you learn that you, as a couple, have an infertility problem—one that may not be reversible. You have to choose between what you've always believed in, and the possibly childless future that you and your spouse are now contending with. This shift may be extremely difficult for you, and marital strife may result. At this point you may react emotionally to the crisis. If you don't understand your responses, and communicate your thoughts, you can compound the problem by creating even greater distance between yourself and your partner.

Fortunately, some couples have complementary styles, and a confiding relationship that allows them to increase their bond during this crisis. But for those of you who are having serious difficulty in coping as a couple, there are many alternatives offered today, that can help you to compromise between your emotional need to parent, and what's now possible within your marriage. You may have to move from expecting to become pregnant, to recognizing you won't be able to have biological children. If you can't make this shift, it demonstrates that the need to have your own genetic and biological baby outweighs all other needs in your life, even your marriage. Serious marital problems and divorce usually follow this realization.

There can be a tendency to blame everything in the marriage on not having children. This is a dangerous form of escape. It lets you avoid looking at other, very real problems in your marriage. Children rarely resolve marital issues. Raising them often doesn't relieve stress, it increases it. So if infertility has unmasked other problems in your marriage, take the time to figure out what's really wrong, and fix it if you can, before children arrive and complicate matters even further.

To keep your pairing intact during infertility, you must first of all understand, and be sensitive to, the gender differences in your marriage. You have to remain balanced, trying not to neglect your other goals and needs. In other words stay in control as the two of you are faced with infertility decisions—both about your daily treatment, and your long-term goals. And throughout it all, focus on the reasons why both you and your partner want a child.

INTERACTING WITH THE WORLD OUTSIDE YOUR RELATIONSHIP

Obviously it's so difficult to cope with the problems within a couple, it's almost inhumane to add on yet another layer of potential emotional upheaval. But in the real world, you don't have the luxury of experiencing your condition privately. You have to integrate it into all the public aspects of your life, as well. This means that you're going to have to decide what you'll tell, or not tell, your family and friends. And you'll also have to be prepared for the varying ways in which they will react to your problem.

Interacting with Your Parents

It isn't easy to cast aside your most traditional views. Since the dawn of civilization, a premium has been placed on being fertile. The Book of Genesis tells us, "Be fruitful and multiply," and most would-be grand-parents agree. Having children is such an ordinary part of adult life, it's only natural for most parents to look forward to the joy of becoming grandparents. It's this desire that makes infertility an intergenerational crisis. To your parents, especially, infertility can mean the loss of your family line's future.

The Music Stopped with Me

I remember an intense feeling that surfaced while my wife and I were being treated for our infertility, but hadn't yet found success. I was constantly thinking about my family line . . . my father, his father, and his father before him. I was caught up in how each generation had reproduced to form our family of today. How could it be that every couple in my family's history, in my entire bloodline, had had no problem getting pregnant? But when it came to me, it stopped. Reproduction was a natural event, that no one before me had bungled. And yet I was unable to carry on that tradition. It felt like I was driving one night and came to a dead end. Or as if I was playing musical chairs, and the music stopped with me. Someone had

swiped my chair from underneath me, for reasons unknown. I was devas-
tated.

—*Matthew, age 40*

———

Becoming a parent is a developmental need for most people. Children enable you to become an adult in the eyes of the previous generation, and to project yourself in your progeny. Infertility can disrupt your life's plan. No wonder Matthew had such a difficult time integrating his traditional views into the crisis he was living.

Some parents of infertile couples wonder if they themselves might have caused the problem. In a small percentage of cases—with DES babies, for example—this may be true. But no parent consciously sets out to cause their children to be infertile. In addition to this guilt and self blame, parents experience many of the same emotional responses as the infertile couple—responses such as shock, denial, loss of control, anger, and depression. It's not uncommon for a parent, once their circle of friends has begun to become grandparents, to be constantly questioned as to why their children aren't getting pregnant, too. They may be one step removed from infertility, but society's mores and traditions combine to make their experience just as painful as yours. And compounding the pain is the fact that since they have had the experience, they understand the joy of having children, unlike you who can only fantasize about it.

Grandchildren offer everyone an opportunity to rebalance the family ledger. Maybe part of your reason for wanting a family is your wish to repay your parents for your own good childhood, by giving them loving grandchildren. Maybe your parents were very busy with work during your childhood, and they yearn to give grandchildren the love and attention they were unfortunately unable to give you. These needs to rebalance the family can't be met when infertility strikes.

Try to understand your parents' response to your infertility. When their reactions aren't what you might want, expect, or hope for, understand that they are hurting too. You might even pinch yourself when your mother or mother-in-law asks you, "Are you sure you're doing everything?" . . . implying that you aren't. This is their only way of combating their helplessness. Remember, you and your husband are actively working through your grieving process every step of the way . . . whether you're considering exploratory surgery, ART procedures, alternative means of biological parenting, adoption, or child-free living. Your parents and in-laws have even less control than you do.

On the other hand, keep things in perspective. Recognizing parents' role in this unfortunate crisis, doesn't give them the license to hurt you.

It doesn't allow them to pressure you, or nag you to do what they want. Your infertility problem is primarily yours, and you need to satisfy your own needs first.

Interacting with Your Siblings

Infertility can also strain your sibling relationships. For example, if your sister has had a child recently, it may be hard for her to understand when you tell her you can't attend the baby christening. If your brother just had a baby boy, and you decide at the last moment not to show up for the bris, he may be extremely disappointed. Another uncomfortable situation can arise when your sister, your *only* sister, wants to share stories about her daughter's birth or breast-feeding issues. But it's too painful for you to listen, so you tell her to stop, and this causes a rift in your relationship.

Unfortunately, the infertile couple stands out at family gatherings. Why? Because these are the times when it's natural that children take the spotlight. Very often they are the topic of conversation. Attention and respect is given to those with children, making you extrasensitive to being without, especially since you want children so much. And there's always the well-meaning family member or dear friend, who catches you in a corner at a family gathering or social event. The purpose? . . . to whisper advice about getting pregnant, or to find out why no announcements have been made. If this situation has happened to you, and most likely it has in one way or another, know that it is a natural reaction, and that no harm is meant. But always be prepared, and have ready a response you are comfortable with. For example, "Yes, we've thought about children. And when we have an announcement, you'll be one of the first to hear."

You can help to head these things off at the pass by making sure your family members know and understand the pain you are experiencing. You don't want to have to contend with more grief, frustration, and sadness as a result of your family not understanding you. It's important to remember that when you are going through infertility, you need your family's emotional support more than ever.

Interacting with Your Friends

Depending on your relationship and on their personalities, friends can either be extremely helpful or very hurtful. Don't always expect their reactions to be what you need. Especially if you don't help them understand the scope of what you are going through. If you choose not to share, for reasons which you feel are sound, then understand the consequences may be painful. Friends may say and do the wrong things, simply because they don't understand what it is you need.

Shut Up with Your "Just Relax"

Too many people told me as I was going through infertility that all I had to do was relax. "You're too stressed about having a baby. Have your husband take you away." One time I almost smashed my fist into someone's mouth. Damn it! Doesn't anyone get that it's a medical problem?

—Nicole, age 39

Unfortunately, at some point you get to an age where all your friends seem to be getting pregnant. Maybe that's one of the reasons you decided to try yourself. Eventually, as it becomes clear, particularly to close friends, that you are having difficulty conceiving, this can distance you. Especially as your friends are about to move on to their second child. This drawing apart isn't intentional on their parts. It's just that more often than not, their daily goings on, weekend social engagements, and everyday conversations revolve around children. So you are left out. Soon you stop being invited to social occasions. Or you're invited with the caveat that you probably won't have a good time, since all of the planned activities will revolve around the children. Understandably, this hurts. You experience feelings of inadequacy, injured pride, and isolation.

What About Us?

I remember going through a phase where I was invited to different parties on the weekend, either children's birthday parties or Sunday night barbecues. Children were everywhere, and the topics of conversations were all about child rearing. My husband and I felt so left out. Then we stopped getting invitations. It was a lonely and sad experience. Either way we felt like losers.

—Patricia, age 41

And then there is the very close friend with whom you've chosen to share your infertility predicament. The friend who tries to say the right thing even if, at times, she doesn't. The friend who listens to your daily pain, and doesn't complain. The friend who asks you in what ways she can help you to be comfortable. These friends are hard to find, but they do exist. If you have one, be careful not to step over your boundaries and overwhelm her with your pain. After all, it is *your* problem.

There is also the friend you may not talk to every day, but who is still there for you whenever you need the help.

An Understanding Friend

We'd been trying for over two years when Geri, an old friend, gave birth. Although we didn't discuss it often, we knew we both were suffering from an infertility diagnosis. Lucky for her, she found success. All of our friends were invited to the hospital to see the new baby. I didn't want to miss this moment in her life, nor miss the gathering of our old friends. But mostly I wanted to give her a hug, and show her how truly happy I was for her. She was thrilled when I appeared, and I watched her glow with happiness. After we talked a bit amidst all of our friends, she pulled me to the side of her bed and said, "You really must love me to be here. You are a true friend." She was right. It took enormous strength to be there. But I couldn't respond to her recognizing my efforts, because my eyes quickly welled up and I ran from the room. It's a moment neither of us will ever forget.

—Mary, age 30

These two women understood the extreme pain they had each suffered, and the true happiness that Geri was now experiencing. The reason Mary was emotionally overcome was that Geri, in her moment of glory, took a moment away from her new baby—the very thing she had been desperate to have—to be compassionate and sensitive to Mary's feelings.

But not everyone is like Geri. Not everyone can empathize with what you're going through. Often, as a reaction to the feeling of losing control over your life, you obsess over every little hurt you feel that your friends are dealing you. That's when you know you're too caught up in the emotional and physical aspects of your infertility. The loss of important relationships . . . the loss of self-esteem . . . the loss of your positive body image . . . the loss of your self-confidence . . . these all contribute to a feeling of insecurity and instability in your life. Soon you start to wonder if anything is predictable and secure. When this happens, you may turn to a close friend, or to a family member who acts as a friend. Be careful not to overload this person with too much. If you do, you may add to your list of woes by losing their support.

Too Blind to See It

My friend Jane works around the corner from my office building. Almost every day we would meet for lunch. When I was diagnosed as infertile, she listened to me cry. When I started treatment, she listened to me complain and carry on. When my ART procedure was set, she listened to my fears. And when it failed, she stood by me, even though I was a basket case. But slowly she began to make doctors' appointments during lunch, and to accept other lunch invitations she said she couldn't turn down. Eventually, we stopped having lunch altogether. I was extremely hurt. I felt abandoned, and swore never to talk to her again. Today I can see I deserved what I got. I was so out of control, no one in their right mind would have hung in as my friend.

—Terri, age 35

Unfortunately, Terri lost her friend when she needed her the most. Her emotions had ballooned to a point at which she didn't even realize the extent of her painful obsession. She should have sought counseling, either one-on-one or within a support group. Professionals are trained to help you negotiate your feelings; a friend can only listen, and try to soothe your pain. Friends can't guide you through your crisis. They're not armed with the tools that are needed to help you. Don't give such an impossible task to anyone you really care about.

Interacting with Your Religion

Throughout history, people have turned to religion to help them understand why certain things in their lives are beyond their control. It follows, then, that religion would hold out some hope to you, as you desperately try to become fertile. And yet, religion can often saddle you with even more frustration and conflict. If you believe that God created the universe, life on earth and human beings—and that he gave them the responsibility to reproduce—then it would figure that God would give you the power to become pregnant. If he hasn't, you may wonder if you've done something wrong to deserve this punishment.

Many people struggle with the question, "Why me?" You may have been raised believing that if you were a good and moral person, you would be rewarded, and bad things wouldn't come your way. So you try to atone for whatever sin you committed . . . whatever transgression has led to your deprivation. Soon you find yourself trying to strike bargains with God. These deals can involve prayers, penance, and "good behavior." When desperation really sets in, you may even find yourself wishing for a miracle, or doing silly things that you would never do at other times in your life.

Wish Upon a Star

Every time I went outside and the stars were shining, I would focus on the first star that I laid my eyes on and I would make a wish. Once, after a business dinner, we were outside waiting for our cars when I started reciting out loud, "Star light, star bright . . ." My boss thought I'd lost my mind, and tried to interrupt me. But I stood there and finished my little prayer, then closed my eyes and finished my wish. It was unprofessional, but I didn't care. My will to get pregnant took over every aspect of my being. When I opened my eyes, I turned to him and the others and said, "You've got to do what you've got to do." And to his surprise and my comfort, another V.P. said "Hear, hear!"

—*Fae, age 26*

You begin to wonder, as you pray, wish, and hope month after month, why you're still meeting with failure. How can God create all of the wonderful miracles around you, then keep you from having the one thing you want . . . the baby he seems to be giving to everyone else? At this point, it's common to become disillusioned and doubt your religion. Some even begin to question the very existence of God.

Hopefully, at some point along the road, you'll take a look at all the tragedies that are happening in the lives around you, and begin to realize that you're not alone. Life just isn't fair, no matter how good you are. For some of you, your infertility may be your first real awakening to life's realities. Once you face this, you can begin to search for the strength to endure the treatment you must go through in order to overcome your infertility. This begins to lead some people back to the notion of reconciling their infertility with their belief in God.

For many of you, religion offers a place to find strength, though sometimes you may have to redefine your interpretation of God in order to discover it. Strength is essential to a successful infertility experience. You need to be strong to confront, overcome, and accept your infertility situation.

Maybe a part of your new interpretation of God has grown from the necessity to negotiate where, and how, infertility treatments (in particular, ART procedures) fit within your religion and its traditions. To many religions, these new technologies aren't acceptable ways to conceive, because they manipulate human life. The rule seems to be that the more traditional and strict the religion, the greater its opposition to infertility treatments will be. It can create a difficult dilemma when your medical treatment conflicts with your religious beliefs. To move ahead toward resolution you must sometimes choose between them, and for some it is a painful choice. Most often, people compromise by maintaining the general tenets of their religious beliefs, while accepting the fact that they can't possibly follow every rule that religion lays down. Ultimately, they follow their own consciences. From a practical standpoint, you should make sure your doctor knows and understands your religious constraints, if there are any, early on in your relationship.

Infertility is not only a medical problem, there are those who consider it to be a medical crisis. You respond to infertility in much the same way as a chronic illness. Although it's not life threatening, you're in constant contact with doctors, hospitals, nurses, ovulatory technicians, medications, injections, ultrasound examinations, and surgery. Your intimate relationship is also affected, as the treatment invades almost every aspect of your sex life. And let's not forget how lengthy and expensive your treatment can become, which can severely strain your financial resources and your quality of life. To ensure the best possible experience under difficult circumstances, the relationship that you develop with your medical team should be handled with care. This is critical.

If you and your husband see your medical team to be competent as professionals and supportive of you as individuals, then this is one area of your infertility treatment that shouldn't create conflict. If you don't, take steps to change doctors and ensure the most harmonious experience possible. You're stepping into a world that's engulfed by conflicts. At the very least, you need to be in sync with your own team. In order to work against a common "enemy" you need to share common goals. To be sure you're always doing this you need to have an understanding as to the rules you'll follow in resolving conflicts.

If communication has diminished—or was nonexistent to begin with—the relationship can turn into a standoff of "us" versus "them" when problems arise. Once this occurs, it is the patients who end up the losers. Don't let this happen to you. Communicate what you're feeling to your medical caregivers. Ask questions, after doing your homework. And try not to take your frustrations out on your team. They are not your enemy.

Remember that your day-to-day care may become very confusing to you if you don't have good communication with your doctor's office. In most practices, much of this communication is handled by nurses or support staff. Your road will be a little less bumpy if you pay attention to their advice.

THE NURSES' LIST OF DO'S AND DON'TS

- *DO*   become familiar with the routine of the office you're working with. Most offices have specific hours when the phones are answered by the staff, and others when their service takes messages. If there's a specific time of day that's devoted to communicating with patients, find out what it is. If there are times when it is best to speak to your doctor, find that out too. And find out when test results are normally received. Why spend all morning calling for a result that won't arrive in your doctor's office until the afternoon?

- *DON'T*   keep pushing your nurse for an answer once she tells you your question should really be answered by your doctor. Understand that she's doing it because she wants you to get the most accurate information, not because she doesn't want to take the time to answer you.

- *DO*   educate yourself to some extent about your condition. It will help you to ask the right questions, and it will make it easier for you to understand the things your nurse is trying to explain. If you are well-informed, the questions you ask of the staff will be appropriate, logical, and well received.

- *DO*   plan ahead. Take the time before you place your call to write down all the questions you want answered. Calling your nurse over and over again during a busy day because you "forgot to ask her one more thing that's really important," will only make her want to stop taking your calls.

- *DON'T*   think you're the only patient your nurse is working with. If she's not available for you exactly when you want her, it's probably because she's trying to help someone else who's just as much in need of information and comfort as you are.

- *DO*   be polite. Most infertility nurses have chosen their job because they really care about the couples who come to them. It's not their fault you have a problem. And they are trying their best to help you solve it.

Even in the best case, when there's good communication between yourselves and your team, the relationship can become strained when a treatment fails. If you let this linger, anger and depression can result.

Too Close or Too Far

"Frequently lacking other social support, the infertile couple may become enmeshed with staff members and overly dependent on them. On the other hand, patients may distance themselves from the staff because they feel betrayed or have no more energy to pursue treatment. . . ."

—A. G. Sadler, R.N., M.S., and
C. H. Syrop, M.D., "The Stress of Infertility;
Recommendations for Assessment and
Intervention," 1987

Let's say you've done everything your team has told you to do. You've followed doctor's orders—and there are many of them. You've endured the big procedure you've been dreading for months. But you still receive that frightful call . . . the one that tells you your blood test has just come back negative. You're still not pregnant, after two years of trying, after six months of diagnostic work, after eight months of IUI, and after a painful and costly ART procedure. How are you supposed to feel? Who are you supposed to blame? Let's be honest. If you were in a saner mindset, you'd see that your doctor and his team did everything they could to make it a successful procedure. But five minutes, five hours, and sometimes five *days* after receiving that call, you still feel that they might have been able to do something differently, to have somehow made that procedure successful.

At times like these you should keep in mind that your doctor and the health care team he works with are human. While they are trained as professionals to understand your frustration and anger during this difficult time, they're not going to welcome constant rudeness, hostility, or confrontation. If this pattern begins, they too may show signs of either enmeshment or distancing. They may attempt a flurry of treatments, all with low success rates, just to get you off of their backs. Or, they may distance themselves from you by being less available for appointments, or by being less supportive when you do reach them. None of these options is going to work to your long-term benefit, so if you have a basic belief in your doctor and his team, don't abuse them. They're doing everything they can—given the available medical technology—to get you pregnant. Know your doctor is looking for the right formula, the magic recipe that will get you pregnant. And accept the team's humanity, especially during this sensitive time in your life. As the old saying goes, "Don't bite the hand that feeds you."

On the other hand, you should reassure yourself—by constantly doing your homework—that your doctor is, in fact, doing all he can to properly treat you. You can regain some measure of control by learning to be a participant in your own care. Ask your doctor each step of the way, "Where are we going? What is this therapy supposed to accomplish?" and "What do my results tell you?"

When appropriate, communicate your fears, frustrations, and concerns . . . especially if you think you're being poorly handled by someone on the medical team.

I Can't Control It

I remember getting scanned by my doctor. She had adjusted my Pergonal prescription that month, in the hopes of stimulating more follicles. As soon as my ovaries came up on the screen, she said, "Couldn't you have given me a couple more? We want a baby here." I couldn't believe it. Here I was doing everything I could to get pregnant, following her regimen, praying for more follicles, and she was blaming me for not making more. Like I had some control over it!

—Cheri, age 38

Cheri was understandably sensitive to her doctor's words. First of all, she too was disappointed that she didn't produce more follicles. And she was hurt that her doctor would blame her. While it wasn't the correct thing to say, her doctor was really voicing her own frustration at her lack of control, and her disappointment at not seeing the number of follicles she was hoping for. Both doctor and patient had the same goal. And both were being frustrated by the same enemy. The doctor's mistake was in revealing her human side. Point these things out to your doctor. You will probably feel better once you do. Remember, good communication between you and your doctor can only serve to help make your treatment experience more positive. Among other things it empowers you, by giving you some input into your own care. A secure physician won't feel threatened by your questions. He won't assume you're questioning his skills or integrity. Instead, he'll welcome your inquiries, since they'll help him to see how you're feeling about your treatment, and the options he's choosing.

In some cases, when your physician is open to discussions, you may still find yourself intimidated and uncomfortable questioning his reasons for making certain treatment decisions. There are a number of possible reasons for this. First, since he holds the key to your becoming pregnant, you may be subconsciously afraid of upsetting him. "After all," says that little voice inside your mind, "if you make him angry, he may stop giving his best efforts to making you pregnant." Move past those fears. Communicate your feelings. Your doctor is a professional, who understands that asking questions is not the same as criticizing. He needs to know what you're thinking, especially if you don't understand the treatment protocol he's using, or if you feel discouraged about something he is—or isn't—doing. He understands that at times you're going to be frustrated. He will be too. Putting these feelings of frustration out in the open will help to relieve them. Just be sure you don't do it by berating him, or blaming him for things that aren't within his control.

Another thing that happens to some women is that they begin seeing their infertility doctor as being beyond human. Even when you and your husband can't achieve a pregnancy, he still has the ability to do it. It's positively godlike. When you start having feelings like this, it's time for you to reexamine your doctor's role in the endeavor the three of you are engaged in. Remember that he's in charge of only a small piece in the overall picture. He's there to help you get pregnant. He'll be using *your* physical resources to accomplish this. Once a pregnancy *is* achieved, and your infertility doctor is out of the picture, you and your partner will have a truly momentous lifelong job ahead of you—nurturing both the pregnancy and the child it produces. Don't fall into the trap of overvaluing your doctor's role in this process. Doing that will only reinforce negative feelings about your own worth that your condition may have fostered. And feeling worse about yourself, can only make your struggle harder.

A third type of doctor-patient problem can occur if your doctor is of the opposite sex. You may go beyond seeing him as "godlike" and develop a more far-reaching fantasy . . . a sexual fantasy. Don't be surprised if this happens. You're ripe for it. Your sex life with your partner has undoubtedly suffered during your infertility treatment. Your coupling with your husband has apparently failed. And at this vulnerable time, you find yourself having extremely intimate contact and conversations with your doctor almost daily. It's easy to see how, under these circumstances, you could make the jump from seeing him as the "helper" who is aiding you and your partner in your quest, to the man who could actually assure you a pregnancy. In your desperation, you might begin to transfer your feelings of love from your partner to your doctor. Very often you won't be consciously aware of this switch.

Frequently you'll discover it through your dreams. Perhaps you'll replay the meetings between you and your doctor, imagining new dialogue. Perhaps you'll even imagine having sex with him. You may be concerned and feel guilty about these things that are popping out of your subconscious. Don't be. This is a natural reaction in your situation. These fantasies commonly present themselves, either consciously or subconsciously. Just be careful to avoid acting out on them. Don't misinterpret things your doctor says or does during your appointments. Don't try to make your waking life conform to your dreams.

——————

"A common scenario for women undergoing infertility treatment is to develop strong positive feelings toward their doctor. Oftentimes women may also have sexual feelings that present themselves in fantasies and/or dreams. These women should not feel guilty about these desires, as long as they do not act on them."

> —*Eva Ritvo, M.D., Assistant Professor*
> *Department of Psychiatry*
> *University of Miami—School of Medicine*

——————

If you think you're falling victim to some of these feelings, you may want to try to attend appointments as a couple. This will help you to keep your feelings in perspective. And having both of you there is also a good way to ensure that all the technical information your doctor is conveying will be heard and remembered.

This is especially true for your initial consultation, and for those appointments when treatment results are going to be available and explained. Having each other's support is not only worthwhile, it can serve to bond the two of you in your quest for a baby. If your mate can't come, it's a good idea to have a friend or close family member accompany you. This is a stressful time in your life. You're feeling rattled and confused. You need another pair of ears to help you take in, and interpret, the information you're receiving from your team.

SECONDARY INFERTILITY . . . IN A CATEGORY ALL ITS OWN

"Secondary infertility" describes your condition when you find that you and your husband have become infertile after already having had a biological child together.

Coming Up Empty . . . The Second Time Around

I was pregnant with our son the first month we tried. We were thrilled, since we had heard that some people have a tough time conceiving. Two years after Kyle was born, we decided to try again. Now, two years after that, we still have no more children. I can't believe I am one of those people who desperately wants a child, albeit a second one. Kyle wonders why he is the only one in his class who doesn't have a brother or a sister. And I do too.

—*Cathy, age 28*

The causes of secondary infertility are the same as those of primary infertility; the only difference is that they surface later. Most likely, your secondary infertility is caused by a physical problem that has developed since the birth of your first child. Or it may be a condition that wasn't serious enough to leave you infertile the first time around, but has now worsened to a point at which it is preventing you from conceiving.

Just as most people believe that having a baby is a birthright, they also believe in the right to have as many as you want. So when the ability to have more is taken from you, you go through the same emotional reactions that you experience with primary infertility. When you hear about other babies being born, or see new babies being breast-fed or in strollers, you will probably have a difficult time with it. It doesn't matter that you have already had the pleasure of doing it once. That experience has passed, and you desperately want to re-create it. Of the many emotional reactions common to both primary and secondary infertility, guilt is the one that overlaps the two most often. You may experience guilt for not being satisfied with the child you have, or for not being able to provide your child with siblings. And your most serious feelings of guilt may be for spending so much emotional and physical activity on your treatment for secondary infertility, that you're not giving enough to your present parenting experience.

It's Affecting My Child

After months of my five-year-old daughter asking me why we haven't given her a baby sister or brother, I finally explained to her that we were trying, and a doctor was now helping us. When she was on summer break, I was forced to bring her with me to the infertility clinic. So many times, I had to say no to invitations to picnics and days at the beach, because of treatment that only added to my frustration and my disappointment at being infertile. At the clinic, she saw the nurses take my blood and teach me to give myself my own shots. Now she asks me if all babies come from mommies taking medicine in their bottoms.

—*Marianne, age 33*

———

When you want more babies and you're meeting up with difficulties, it's natural to turn to those around you for support. But when you have secondary infertility, you'll probably get less sympathy from your friends, either because they're skeptical about the fact that your infertility actually exists, or because they feel that you've already had a parenting experience, and should be satisfied. You'll probably be asked, "What's so bad about not having it again?" This is what makes people who are suffering from secondary infertility stand apart from other infertile people. In a funny way they're caught between both worlds—the infertile and the fertile.

One way to get around this is to look for support groups made up of people with secondary infertility. If you join a group made up of primary infertility sufferers, you may feel as if you have to apologize in order for you to be accepted and supported. After all, you've already had the parenting experience they may never be able to enjoy.

How to Cope with Your Emotions

It's one thing to understand why you're not feeling like yourself. . . . Obviously, infertility brings a lot of emotional stresses, none of which you asked for. It's another thing again to learn how to deal with them. McDanields, Hepworth, and Doherty, in their article "Medical Family Therapy with Couples Facing Infertility," give some very good pointers that you can use to maintain your emotional well-being as you work on getting pregnant. We've incorporated some of them into a ten-point plan, which advises you to:

- Discuss your "secret"
- Define what being infertile means to you
- Educate yourselves
- Develop a realistic financial plan
- Try to normalize your sex life

- Avoid placing blame
- Don't let your infertility crisis take over your life
- Acknowledge the loss of easy reproductivity
- Explore your thoughts about life with and without a child
- Consider professional/psychological help

DISCUSS YOUR "SECRET"

Communication is the key to unraveling much of the frustration you and your partner may have as you go through infertility treatment. As we have said before, it's important to understand that both of you have arrived at this place preprogrammed with your own experiences and viewpoints. Because of this, your reactions to being infertile are going to be different. The only way you'll be able to understand each other's feelings, is through openly communicating. Once you do, you'll be able to support each other's reactions. You need to be able to tell each other when it hurts, and when things feel better. To do this, you need to find ways to continually update each other about how you're feeling.

One way to do this is by making infertility decisions together. For example, you can jointly decide whom you trust enough to share the news of your infertility problem. Consider that close family and friends care about your well-being, and will most likely be there to support you.

There are several positive reasons to bring other people into your secret. When you discuss your problem with them, they may suggest some things that you haven't considered, or they may bring thoughts or fears that you've been trying to ignore to your attention. And when you communicate what is going on in your relationship to people outside of your marriage, you're forced to move away from your denial and focus on the problem. It not only helps to decrease your isolation, it lets your friends and family members know why you've been acting so distant. Finally, by letting your family in on your secret, such questions as "When are you going to give me a grandchild?" will diminish. Normally, when you reveal your emotional crisis to the people who love you, your network of support increases tenfold. And as this familial support increases, pressure decreases.

When you do bring people into your secret, you need to set some ground rules for them. Let the people around you know what sorts of questions are safe to ask, and where your comfort zone ends when you're discussing your infertility. It's appropriate for you to set these boundaries, since this is your problem. Your confidantes should understand that at times you'll have a need to talk about your problem, and at other times you'll want to avoid the painful issue. It's your responsibility to clarify, for those close to you, what is helpful and comforting, and when and how discussions and updates can be had.

You and your partner will also need to make some decisions about how you plan to deal with your greater world . . . the circle of people who don't really need to know about your personal business. Discuss who those people are, and decide what you plan to tell them when inquires are made. And prepare yourselves before you attend social occasions to deal with the pushy intruder who feels closer to you, than you do to them.

Caged by a Cousin

I remember attending a cousin's wedding, where I was cornered in the bathroom by one of our family's biggest busybodies. She started asking me, "Are you thinking about having a family?" When I nodded, she said, "You better get on with it, you're not getting any younger." When I then told her that Bill and I are would love to start a family, but we've run into some difficulties, the story began to get juicy for her. She might as well have been reading a copy of "Star" magazine. She started firing questions at me. "Is it Bill? Is it you? What are your chances? You wouldn't consider carrying somebody else's baby, would you?" I could feel the heat rising in my body. I felt so helpless, so humiliated. I started answering some of the questions, but then I couldn't stand it any longer and just excused myself and ran out of the bathroom. I ran out of the party room, and found a place behind some trees. I stood there and just bawled.

—Amy, age 37

Prodding like this can increase your despair and reinforce your feelings of pain and isolation. To avoid this, you should learn to turn the tables when you find yourself in situations like these. Make the person who's moving in on you be defensive, instead of offensive. For instance, Amy could have responded with, "It really bothers you that we don't have children." Or, "Tell me, exactly why do think this is your business?" Or, if you have a career, "Was it hard for you to have given up your career to have kids?" These are just a few of the many things you can say to a pushy person. The goal is to make them be the one who's uncomfortable, instead of you. Always be armed with responses, so you can remain calm and in control.

DEFINE WHAT BEING INFERTILE MEANS TO YOU

Each one of you has your own interpretation of what being infertile means. The way you define it grows out of the way it impacts you personally. Each of you has come to where you are with different expectations for your life. Reach deep down inside yourself, and find what being infertile means in relation to those life goals.

Has parenting always been a part of your life's expectations? To what extent? After the initial questions of your diagnosis and prognosis have been answered, you may want to revisit those life goals, and discuss them with your partner. Is being a biological parent, and *only* a biological parent, a part of your expectations? You and your partner should understand each other's answers thoroughly. Get down to the basics of what's really essential to making your lives meaningful. Once you do, you may find that having a baby isn't as high a priority as you thought. Or, maybe it has such importance that you're willing to make lifestyle changes, such as opting for a career that's less demanding, if that's what it takes to improve your chances of success.

EDUCATE YOURSELVES

As we have said before, one of the biggest stumbling blocks with infertility is the sense that you have no control over your situation. A good way to combat that is by becoming an expert in your infertility problem. You can use the information you gather to reassure yourself that you're receiving the correct treatment. This will help you to feel as if you do have some control over your body and your future. Research your problem by reading books, pamphlets, and the information that's published by Resolve and the American Society for Reproductive Medicine. Use your new knowledge as the basis for constructive discussions with your medical team.

Discuss the information you've gathered with your partner. Decide which treatments you will try, and set some limits at which you will consider stopping, if need be. A clear understanding of each other's expectations will help to diminish stress between the two of you. Avoid the disappointment of trying to live up to unrealistic goals, by agreeing to revisit them periodically, and be willing to change them if necessary.

Encourage your partner to join you during your diagnostic workup, even if he or she isn't being assessed. This way your partner remains actively involved in the treatment, and has opportunities to ask questions. Understanding the biological basis of your problem can often help you to depersonalize it. By realizing you have a medical condition common to thousands of people, you can shift your energy away from your sense of failure and blame.

These steps can help you to feel as if you are somewhat in charge of your experience. You may not have had any control over creating the problem, but you can exert some as you try to fix it.

DEVELOP A REALISTIC FINANCIAL PLAN

You may be amazed by the cost of infertility treatment when you begin it, but that doesn't stop you. Most likely you have some sort of savings put aside for "a rainy day," and in the beginning you think that your medical expenses couldn't possibly blow through it. But as time passes, ongoing treatment can begin to suck that savings account dry. Spending beyond your limits magnifies the stress you're already under as you try to get pregnant.

As a physician I have no right to tell couples how much they can afford to spend on their infertility treatment. But over the years I have always felt uncomfortable with couples that become so desperate that they take out second and third mortgages on their homes, or borrow money from family and friends to support the costs of their infertility treatments.

For some, the choice that has to be made is between one more procedure and the annual vacation. Others have to endure the blow of still not being pregnant after going through the last procedure that they can afford. At that point, they're left without the time or funds to explore alternatives, such as adoption.

Couples in this situation have to live with the possibility that they were forced to remain childless because of financial reasons. Don't let this happen to you. Develop a realistic financial plan from the beginning. Clearly define the total you have to spend. Compare it to the costs of various procedures, and make your decisions wisely. Take into account the fact that some procedures may have to be repeated several times. Do the things that are appropriate for your condition, but don't put undue pressure on your already stressful life by not realistically thinking through a long term plan. If treatment has to stop suddenly, the pain, anguish and disappointment you'll experience could be devastating.

TRY TO NORMALIZE YOUR SEX LIFE

By now you know that it's normal for infertility to negatively affect your sex life. Some of you may be embarrassed or ashamed to talk about your feelings having to do with sex. You're going to have to conquer that reticence. At least you have a running start. Now that you're going through infertility treatment, you're *forced* to discuss sex, at least from a medical standpoint. But you must learn to discuss your most intimate thoughts with your partner, as well. Make sure you've separated the concepts of fertility and potency in your own minds. Learn to support and respect each other's emotional reactions, especially if your partner is told that his or her infertility problem is severe. Give each other both time and space when it is needed. And most of all, try to maintain and protect the tenderness, the passion, and the joy that you once shared before infertility treatment invaded your intimacy.

One way to do this is by taking some time off. By doing this, you can exercise some control over your sex life, away from the intrusions of medical treatment. Even though you don't want to deviate from trying to have a baby, sometimes it's necessary, to strengthen your sexual relationship. If this means taking a break from treatment for a month, so that you can go back to making love without schedules or interruptions, try to do it. If you find that you just can't, look for a quick fix . . . take a romantic weekend away, or buy some "toys" to help bring back a sense of fun to the sexual experience. Rejuvenate your passionate relationship, whatever it takes. Don't let it go beyond repair. Remember, infertility is temporary. After it's resolved, you'll want your sexual relationship to continue on. So protect it!

AVOID PLACING BLAME

When you hear the news that you, as a couple, are infertile, each of you will immediately take it inside of you and begin to formulate your feelings about it, based largely on your past experiences. This tendency to internalize the problem and mull it over on your own can be a dangerous one. Many times, especially when only one partner is responsible for the infertility, strong feelings of blame and guilt can result. One party will blame, and the other will feel guilt. If these feelings are held inside, and this split persists, it can separate the relationship into two warring halves.

It's His Problem, Not Mine!

My husband's sperm count is so low that I've had to endure several procedures, all of which so far have failed. It's so unfair that I have to undergo all this invasive work just because he came up short. And it makes me even angrier when I tell people that we're having difficulty getting pregnant, and everyone assumes it's my problem. But it's not! It's his!

—Lucy, age 26

Lucy's thinking is bound to put her relationship in jeopardy. Sure it's unfair that while her husband is the one who has the infertility problem, he doesn't have to undergo invasive medical treatments. But it's a fact of life. He didn't plan to have the problem, nor wish for Lucy to have to go through physical pain. No doubt he's distressed that she has to undergo those treatments.

Infertility too often becomes a game of fingerpointing. Yet no matter what its source—whether both partners or just one—once it's been discovered, an infertility problem becomes a problem for *both* of you. And it's up to *both* of you to work together to solve it, in order for a baby to arrive. Laying blame only slows this process down.

Internally blaming her husband just intensifies Lucy's anger and frustration. Assuming he's aware of her inner feelings, which he probably is, they only make him feel even more guilty, inadequate, disappointed, and helpless. Lucy has to accept that the problem is theirs together . . . it happened to them as a unit, not individually.

It's much healthier for your relationship if you join forces in trying to cope and conquer. To do that you must stop internalizing. Instead, communicate, to try to understand each other's feelings. Once you look outside yourself, you can work together toward your common goal. Luckily for Lucy, she is able to do something about their infertility problem. What she seems to be forgetting is that before infertility treatment came into being, there was nothing either partner could do to resolve these situations.

DON'T LET YOUR INFERTILITY CRISIS TAKE OVER YOUR LIFE

Most crises are temporary. Infertility can be an exception. Not only can this crisis be rather lengthy, in some cases it can persist for your entire reproductive lifetime. Because of that, it's important to limit the space you're going to give it. Confine infertility to its own small area within the totality of your life, so that its pain doesn't dominate your everyday existence. Make sure you continue pursuing the pleasurable things you did before. Maintain your hobbies and social activities. Strive to find some additional goals, ones that you have control over. Do your best to control your treatment by empowering yourself with knowledge to balance your life. And then, learn to accept the lack of control that remains. While this can be frustrating and difficult at times, it's a natural part of life.

"Your control during a medical crisis is usually quite limited. Part of the maturation process is learning which aspects of the medical crisis are within your control and which are not. This acceptance helps you to handle situations more appropriately. When you learn how to accept and manage problems, not just solve them, your feelings of competence can increase."

—Eva Ritvo, M.D., Assistant Professor
Department of Psychiatry
University of Miami—School of Medicine

ACKNOWLEDGE THE LOSS OF EASY REPRODUCTIVITY

By now you have to accept that you are having difficulty getting pregnant. Most likely, that difficulty won't change without treatment, if it changes at all. This means that all the dreams you've always had—of making tender love, falling easily into pregnancy, and delivering a beautiful child—are gone. At the very least, pain, embarrassment, and inconvenience have intruded on your dream. In the worst case, you'll never hold that baby in your arms at all.

You've lost a birthright. It hurts and that's normal. Grieve that loss, like you would any other serious loss. If you don't, you'll be reminded of it every time you see children, or hear other people discussing them.

If your problem is severe or incorrectable, then you really are grieving the loss of the biological child that will most likely never be born. You might consider doing things that actively acknowledge this, such as writing a good-bye letter to your unknown child. Discuss with your partner how each of you pictured your "fantasy child." Then move on to discussing how each of you has to let that child go.

Even if your problem *is* correctable, you're letting go of the normal act of making a baby. Acknowledge that, and let yourself be sad that you've been cheated of a piece of the pattern of life that most people take for granted.

EXPLORE YOUR THOUGHTS ABOUT LIFE WITH AND WITHOUT A CHILD

Once you've been dealing with an infertility problem for some time, you've hopefully learned the difference between your internal and external desires. But have you ever made yourself analyze how much of your need to have a child is internally motivated, as opposed to externally motivated? Are you longing to have a child to fulfill a life dream? Or is it just something that you feel you should have done by the time you've reached your age? Are people pressuring you to have a child, telling you you'll miss out if you don't? Or does the desire come from the very core of your being?

Discuss your thoughts about these questions with your partner. You may find out some surprising things. Sometimes, people who never really felt a strong desire to have a child begin to obsess on it when the possibility is taken from them. Caught up in that obsession, they lose any sense of their true desires. Why not revisit the self you were before this all started, and ask it whether having a baby is as important to you as you have begun to believe. Maybe that old self will be able to let go of the dream easily. Or maybe it will insist that having a child is the most important thing to you, that it always has been and always will be. If that's the answer you get, you've found out that you'll never be able to bring your infertility experience to a close, unless you do everything possible.

From these discussions, you can discover whether each of you really has the will to continue treatment. Only you and your mate know these answers. You must work hard—both within yourselves as individuals, and outside yourselves as a unit—to bring them to the surface.

CONSIDER PROFESSIONAL/PSYCHOLOGICAL HELP

You've only got to look back toward the beginning of this chapter to Mennings's definition of a crisis, to understand how you can feel that your infertility situation is beyond your personal ability to cope. The thoughts and feelings surrounding your infertility may be churning in your head, drowning out much of your clear thinking. Your life may seem to be off-balance, out of sync, as if you are living in a state of disequilibrium. Maybe you're even feeling so challenged that you no longer know what to do.

You're not crazy. This is a normal and understandable reaction to infertility. You may just need a little help in handling the unfamiliar emotional stresses that you're experiencing. Even your doctor may suggest that you seek outside counseling—either individually or in a group. But he can't do that if he isn't aware that you're in need of support. And he won't be, if you hide your emotional crisis from him.

I'm Not Crazy

"Patients are self-conscious about their feelings and sensitive about the medical staff's opinion of them. They are afraid of being criticized for being troublesome or of being considered crazy, so they avoid bringing their feelings to anyone's attention."

—P. P. Mahlstedt, Ed.D.
"Psychological Issues of Infertility and Assisted Reproductive Technology," 1994

Probably you're expecting your doctor to focus primarily on the medical aspects of your problem, you're not expecting emotional guidelines or support. As a result, the issue of outside help won't surface, unless it's obvious to your doctor that you're having extreme difficulty coping with your pain—or if you simply ask about it.

Sheri Found Support

I chose not to let anyone know I was going through infertility. Then something happened that told me I needed help. I responded very inappropriately to a dear friend who had just had a C-section. She was upset, and I was extremely unsympathetic. That wasn't like me. When I told this to my doctor, she recommended a support group. I vividly remember my first session. We went around the room, and everyone told why they were there. I wasn't sure why I was. But as time passed, it became clear to me how much I needed the support. I met some of my best friends there. I started hearing other people's stories, some worse than mine, and they made me feel lucky by comparison. I learned more about others' problems, which helped me not to obsess over my own. We even joked about our own experiences, which helped to lift my depression. The world started looking brighter. When going through infertility, I really believe finding emotional support is as important as the treatment itself.

—Sheri, age 35

Take the first step. Ask your doctor if he would recommend that you seek outside counseling. Most likely he'll turn the tables on you, and have you ask that question of yourself. Suffice it to say, if you're experiencing emotional stress similar to what we've described, and if the question of professional help has entered your mind, it might be worth investigating.

Thinking About Therapy

While infertility usually creates an emotional crisis for you and your partner, it also affects the relationships around you. For this reason, if you're looking for someone to talk to who can give you help, you might consider going outside your close circle of family, friends, and co-workers. Recognize that these people give you their opinions and advice from a subjective point of view. They can't help it. And sometimes you need the informed, objective point of view of an uninvolved individual.

This person should be trained to listen to any and all of the feelings you have, with both sensitivity and objectivity. When they do this, it allows you to say anything you want, without worrying about whether they're judging your feelings and thoughts. It's also a good idea for this person to be familiar with the medical aspects of infertility.

You're taking a journey toward a baby, and you will be faced with many difficult decisions along the way. A therapist can help you make those decisions. They can help you to decide who, and what, to tell. They can guide you in setting limits on unhelpful, and often intrusive, questions and advice. A therapist can aid you, as a couple, to explore the effects of your infertility on all aspects of your lives together, particularly in the areas of deepest pain and conflict. And a therapist can give you the tools to help you feel better about yourselves, both as individuals and as a couple. The role of the professional therapist is to help you decide what is best for you. And to keep the contents of your sessions in complete confidence as you make those decisions.

BUT THERAPY ISN'T FOR ME

There are many of you who feel that, no matter how difficult the struggle, talking to a complete stranger is just not for you. In the past you've been faced with conflicts and crises, and you've been able to work your way through them yourself, or with the help of people who love you. If this is how you feel, then talking to an outside professionally trained person is most likely an option you're not going to take. But before you totally discount the idea, ask yourself: What are you afraid of? What harm can come of it? Is the idea of needing psychological help just too demeaning for you right now, when you're already struggling with a shaky self-image because of your infertility? Might you learn something about yourself from a person who is an expert in the field . . . who can help you sort out your emotions, your conflicts, and give you tools to help ease the pain?

Granted, it may feel uncomfortable at first to talk to someone about your relationship, your medical condition, and your innermost thoughts and feelings. But once you pass through this awkward stage, you might find the experience to be extremely worthwhile.

Deciding to see a therapist is a difficult decision. Finding the right one for you can be even harder. With help from Linda Callahan, an experienced therapist, we'll try to point you in the right direction.

INDIVIDUAL THERAPY VS. GROUP THERAPY

Psychological help for infertility is usually found in two very different forums. Which one you'll prefer depends on the issues you're going to tackle.

Individual therapy—seeing a therapist one-on-one—is the first option. You and your partner could also go to sessions together under this format. Individual therapy is an appropriate choice when you're trying to examine your past histories—which might include psychological disorders prior to infertility diagnosis—as well as your present personal and psychological issues.

Your other option is a support group setting. There, discussions that are guided by a facilitator include every member of the group. Hearing and understanding what other people are going through—how they are making decisions, and how they are coping—can be a very beneficial experience. Of course, people within a support group must make an ethical commitment amongst themselves to keep private whatever is discussed, and one of the facilitator's jobs is to ensure this commitment. Support groups are of particular help to people with isolation issues, since it quickly becomes clear that everyone in the group is experiencing more or less the same things.

Each of these methods of treatment can be a good choice. It's up to you to decide which format you're most comfortable in.

THE DIFFERENT DISCIPLINES

There are a number of types of professionals who offer help with infertility problems. These include:

- Psychiatrists
- Psychologists
- Marriage, Child, and Family Therapists
- Social Workers

Each group has its own requirements for training, degrees, and licensing.

Psychiatrists have a doctorate in medicine (an M.D.), a license to practice medicine, and should be board certified in psychiatry and neurology.

Licensed Clinical Psychologists have a doctorate in philosophy (a Ph.D.) or psychology (a Psy.D.), awarded for studies in either clinical psychology, counseling psychology, or health psychology.

Marriage, Child, and Family Therapists have a master of arts degree (an M.A.) in psychology, or in marriage, child, and family therapy, and a license in marriage, family, and child counseling (M.F.C.C.).

Social workers have a master's degree in social work (an M.S.W.), and a license in clinical social work (L.C.S.W.).

While there is little variation across the United States regarding the degree requirements for professionals, each state has its own licensing boards. Whichever type of therapist you choose, it's important that they be licensed to practice in the state where you live. This ensures that they have passed the written and oral exams required by the state board that governs their licensing, and that they have the education and experience required to practice as a therapist.

Of course, you still need to keep in mind that a person's qualifications don't necessarily guarantee good treatment, or the kind of treatment you are looking for. That's why the best way to find a good therapist is often through recommendations from people you know and trust.

HOW TO FIND A GOOD THERAPIST

A good place to start is with your doctor. He should be able to recommend therapists who are experienced in working with couples facing infertility. The hospital that your physician is associated with may already have support groups for patients and couples. And if you are interested in individual therapy, the facilitator of these groups may be able to help find the right therapist for you. Resolve—the infertility support group—may be able to refer you to therapists in your area who are known by this organization. In addition, Resolve sponsors support groups in a number of cities throughout the country.

Each type of therapist has a professional association with both national and local chapters. You can go to the American Medical Association (AMA), the American Psychological Association (APA), the Association of Marriage and Family Therapists (AMFT), or the National Association of Social Workers (NASW), to obtain referrals.

It's not a good idea for you to see the same therapist who is treating one of your friends or family members. But if a friend or a family member wants to give you a recommendation, that still may be helpful. You can call their therapist to get the names of other therapists in your community that share similar treatment styles and philosophies.

THE COST OF THERAPY

Infertility is costly. Therapy associated with infertility is no exception. Before you interview professionals, you'll want to be clear on how you are going to pay for your therapy. Generally speaking, psychiatrists have the highest fees; psychologists the second highest; social workers and marriage, family, and child therapists the lowest.

Most mental health professionals charge a set fee, but many are willing to alter their prices on a sliding scale, based on your ability to pay. Some take insurance, others don't. You will have to call your insurance company ahead of time to find out what your coverage for psychological treatment is. Find out what their limits are on the size of fee they will cover, what portion of the fee they will pay, and for how many visits. Armed with this information, you'll find that many therapists are willing to negotiate a fee that's a combination of your insurance payment and a contribution from you.

Universities and state colleges that offer degrees in the various psychological disciplines we've mentioned often have clinics where their graduate students work as interns under the supervision of licensed professionals. Because you are seeing "therapists in training," these clinics offer reduced fees. In many of them, the experienced and licensed clinicians who are there to supervise the interns also have office hours for private consultations, and may charge a fee that is on a sliding scale. At the very least, university and college clinics can give you referrals to professionals who are already licensed and in private practice.

Finally, the many Resolve support groups that have been organized in cities and states throughout the country charge very reasonable fees. The cost per couple for a ten-week group session ranges between $100 and $300. If you are interested, call or write to Resolve to get more information.

SELECTING THE RIGHT THERAPIST FOR YOU

So you've done your research. You now have the names of a few therapists that sound like good possibilities. How do you decide which one is best for you? You do it by interviewing them, thoroughly enough so that you can decide, based on their answers, who you want to employ. Don't be shy about doing this. Take the attitude that you are the consumer, and that you must be satisfied before you contract for their services. Remember how important your choice is: you're looking for someone to help you and your partner through one of the most difficult transitions in your life. With these things in mind, it's time to start making some phone calls to see who really sounds right for you.

Rule number one is that you must feel comfortable working with your therapist. Remember this as you talk to each one. Trust your feelings. If your styles don't match during this first conversation, they probably won't later.

Rule number two is that you're looking for someone who's specifically qualified to work in the area of infertility. There are some questions that will tell you whether your prospects have this experience and skill.

Ask them if they are skilled and experienced in working with couple relationships.

Ask them if they understand the issues involved in infertility. Have they had experience working with people affected by a severe loss in their life? Are they familiar with grief issues?

Ask them if they have a background in working with people facing medical crises. Are they able to understand the procedures and medications required to treat infertility? Do they have an understanding of the physical and psychological effects of these procedures and medications? If not, are they willing to educate themselves on their own time?

Be sure to ask the professionals you're interviewing what degrees and licenses they have, and find out where they received their training. Then ask what their specialty is: couples, families, or individual therapy. Ask if they've had experience with infertility patients, and if so, what they think the main issues are for the individuals and couples involved. Then ask how they feel infertility impacts a couple's relationship with their friends and family members.

As you listen to their answers, you will begin to get a general sense of whether you feel comfortable talking to this person, which will tell you whether or not you would like to make an appointment. Take notes, so you can compare and contrast the different people you speak to. If you aren't sure from the phone call, particularly because you didn't get a chance to ask all of these questions, don't worry. It might be a good idea to have one session with someone you feel right about. While you're there, you can ask more questions, and get a better in-person sense of them. If you end up feeling the therapist isn't right for you, all you've wasted is fifty minutes and a one session fee.

Many therapists with infertility expertise have been infertility patients themselves. If a therapist tells you that he or she has had personal experience with infertility, ask them how long it has been since they resolved their infertility. In other words, have they actually solved their problem? Do they have a child, or have they decided to live child-free? If this person is still in treatment, or is in the process of adopting or finding a surrogate, they are still emotionally involved in the process, and will be less able to be objective about you and your problems. If this is the case, ask them if they could recommend another therapist who has already resolved their infertility problem. Or maybe one who has never experienced it firsthand. After all, a therapist who is an expert on depression doesn't have to be a former depression patient.

Your therapist must be objective. There are therapists who have resolved their own issues and have a child, but who still remain highly opinionated regarding the treatment and resolution of infertility. Avoid this at all costs. If a therapist offers personal information about their own infertility, in hopes that you may relate it to the way that you are feeling, you must avoid this too. A therapist's self-disclosure is rarely helpful to the patient. You, as a patient, should not be aware of what your therapist's infertility problem was, or how they chose to resolve it. Knowing this will constrain you. You will feel that you should conform to what your therapist concluded was the right thing to do. You won't be free to be yourself. It's only human nature to withhold your thoughts, if you think you'll offend your therapist or be judged by them. If you spend your therapy time saying what you think your therapist wants to hear, you're wasting your money. It would be much more productive to look for someone who can focus objectively on your unique circumstances, thoughts, and feelings.

Any competent therapist can help you negotiate most of the emotional minefields that threaten your journey through infertility. However, because of psychiatrists' training as doctors, they are in a unique position to understand the medical aspects of infertility treatment. You won't have to spend your expensive therapy hours educating a psychiatrist about the procedures and reactions to medications you're experiencing.

On the other hand, psychiatrists are expensive. If you can't afford one, there are other professionals who have had the training you require and may offer advantages a psychiatrist does not. Although psychologists, social workers, and marriage, family, and child therapists lack extensive medical training, many are familiar with infertility medications and how they affect you physically and emotionally. They are also keenly aware of how medical treatment affects your relationships with your doctor, spouse, family, and friends. To find these therapists, look for a specialty in medical family therapy, or family systems medicine. They have been trained in a biopsychosocial model of treatment, which recognizes how infertility affects the individual on the biological, psychological, and social levels.

When doing your interviewing, listen for signs that a therapist understands all of the different areas in which infertility impacts your life and your relationships. Most important, trust yourself. You will know when you have found the right person. It will simply feel right.

Some Alternative Roads to Well-being

A number of psychological experts believe that infertility treatment should not only medically repair the cause of your problem, but should simultaneously bring your psychological health into balance as well. In some cases, they would tell you, when your doctor medically treats your problem to the best of his ability, but you still meet with no success, the underlying cause of this failure can be traced to the mind. Many studies have shown that our emotions significantly affect our health. So it follows that restoring a balance between your mind, your body, and your psyche *might* be helpful. Of course, you must be careful in the way you apply this principle, since a number of other problems are tied to structural physical causes, which can't possibly be altered by your attitude.

RESTORING A BALANCE

There are a number of "alternative" types of psychological therapy that try to address this issue. Many of them have one thing in common. They try to help you regain physical health by restoring the balance between your body and your mind.

"By reawakening the body's own biological intelligence, a balance is restored between the mind, the body, and the emotions, simultaneously."

—*Michelle Leclaire O'Neill, Ph.D., R.N.*

Dr. O'Neill, for one, studies the interaction and communication between the psyche, the nervous system, the immune system, the endocrine system, the reproductive system, and other bodily systems. She believes that, "when we deny our true selves, we are not in harmony." In her experience some cases of infertility, especially unexplained infertility, can be a manifestation of an imbalance between our mind, our body, and our spirit. Another way of looking at this is that when you try to force your body to do what your mind, deep down, doesn't want it to do, the body rebels.

Rather than looking at infertility in a negative way, Dr. O'Neill views it as an opportunity to advance psychological growth that's being suffocated by unresolved conflicts. She tries to help patients move away from the hopelessness and fear that a life-challenging diagnosis often brings. She substitutes the idea that beneficial things can grow out of it that will alter the lives of not only the patient, but his or her family, in constructive ways. One thing that sometimes stands in the way of this happening is a patient's belief that he or she is a victim. It's hard for a "victim" to assert himself, because "victims" are usually acted *upon*. So if you've fallen into the victimization mindset, you'll have to step beyond it to progress.

Let's assume that you do, and that you are ready to move on. Dr. O'Neill starts from the premise that our beliefs and attitudes affect our emotions, which can then affect our health. So it would follow that by influencing our beliefs and attitudes in new directions, we can also change our health. This is particularly true if there are negative emotions or conflicts lodged in your subconscious, as you are struggling to get pregnant. Take the example of the career woman who looks at her biological clock and decides that it's time to have a child. She's actually ambivalent about being a mother, but she knows it's now or never. So she goes through the motions of trying to get pregnant. She learns there are some minor corrections needed to make her fertile, and she makes them. Still, time passes, and she doesn't become pregnant. Due to her goal-oriented personality, her need to become pregnant turns into an obsession. What she must do is listen to herself. If she, in fact, really wants to become a mother, she must prepare for the baby. In Chinese the uterus is called the "palace of the sun." It is sacred. You must calm down, be quiet, and invite the soul of the baby into this welcoming place in your body. When this woman is mentally prepared and ready to be a mother, she may possibly be able to affect the health of her body, and the baby will come.

There are a number of different alternative treatments that try to help patients do this. Dr. O'Neill combines six steps that lead to a conscious well-being, with a two-year health plan. Diet, exercise, environment, purpose in life, social support, creative thinking, meditation, self-hypnosis, imagery, and the study of your dreams are just a few of the techniques she uses. She also suggests that you must make a real commitment to reducing your stress; Gregorian chant from the Benedictine monks, or any other "chant" music can help to soothe you. And she advises you to have fun. Return to the enjoyable things you did before infertility altered your well-being.

Please note that Dr. O'Neill's treatment is just one of many psychological therapies that have been created to assist infertility treatment. There are any number of treatment centers around the country that offer other positive thinking philosophies which are said to help in infertility. If these types of holistic remedies appeal to you, they may be worth investigating. However, it is important for you to keep in mind that not all mental health professionals agree that your own "negativity" might be the reason for your infertility.

"The mind body connection is an intriguing area of study. While there may certainly be a link between your mental state and fertility, this link is poorly understood. It is important for couples to remember that these relationships between the mind and the body are not clinically proven. While you must attend to your mental health, it is important not to blame yourself or your spouse for your infertility. To do so simply increases your burden."

—Eva Ritvo, M.D., Assistant Professor
Department of Psychiatry
University of Miami—School of Medicine

TRADITIONAL CHINESE METHODS OF HEALING

Traditional Chinese medicine (TCM) is thought to be effective for psychological and emotional problems, as well as for physical ones. It views each person as an energy system in which the body and mind are unified, each influencing and balancing the other. Western medicine attempts to isolate and separate a disease from the other aspects of a patient. Chinese medicine emphasizes a holistic approach, and treats the person as a whole.

The importance that mental well-being plays in Chinese medicine becomes obvious when you examine the three separate approaches every TCM treatment involves. Acupuncture is used to release endorphins, the body's natural painkillers. The release of these chemical secretions gives you a feeling of well-being. They help you to relax, and to regulate all of the systems in your body. Western scientists have observed that the meridian points used in acupuncture show a variety of unique bioelectrical properties, and that stimulating them causes definite physiological reactions in brain activity, blood pressure, heart rate, and immune system response. It has also been demonstrated that fluid extracted from these points contains high concentrations of DNA, RNA, amino acids, and many other hormones, such as adrenaline and cortisone. After an hour-long acupuncture session, which will cost between $60 and $100, it is common for you to feel extremely peaceful, as if you had just taken a week's vacation in Hawaii. This sensation will last for several days after the session is over.

Chi gong therapy can also be a part of TCM treatments. Chi gong involves meditation, breathing, and imagery exercises that assist in health and general well-being. Traditional Chinese medicine believes that the better a person's overall health is, the better their chances for fertility.

The final facet of TCM treatment is herbal therapy. There are at least 100 different herbs that can be prescribed for infertility. They are taken mostly in the form of teas, but are sometimes given as pills, capsules, or powders. It's rare to prescribe the same combination of herbs to different individuals; the recipe you're given depends on your constitution, and the timing of your cycle. Medicinal teas require some simple cooking procedures. Their taste can be bitter, but most people do get used to them. A week's supply of herbal medications should cost somewhere between $20 and $30.

If you decide to pursue Chinese medicine, you will first need to have a thorough consultation, which will go far beyond the type of medical history that your Western doctor takes. Understand that much of this technique has been practiced for more than 4,000 years. The traditional Chinese medical doctor examines you as a whole person. He's not just looking at the symptoms of your condition, he's examining your entire physical and psychological context. He pays attention to the subtlest disturbances in your health. Because there are so many small variations in the person as a whole, treatment for the same illness can be different for each patient. Taking into account the nature, severity, and duration of the problem to be treated, your Chinese medical doctor will design a program tailored to your unique clinical portrait.

While it can be used on its own, the great majority of patients use TCM as an addition to the Western medical treatment they're receiving. TCM has been shown to be of help with endometriosis, uterine fibroids, tubal blockage, premature menopause, male infertility, sperm antibody conditions, poor ovulation, and luteal phase defects.

For example, if you don't ovulate normally, your hypothalamic pituitary ovarian balance (which we discussed in Chapter Two) can possibly be corrected by herbal therapy. You might want to explore this with an herbalist or a doctor of oriental medicine. It appears that pregnancy occurs equally frequently with Eastern and Western approaches to this particular problem. While there haven't been any controlled studies to date, the anecdotal information that is available indicates that success rates are approximately the same whether ovulation defects are corrected through the use of herbs or of ovulation-induction drugs. As for male infertility, there have been reports that Eastern philosophies have had a positive affect on them, as well.

———

I remember the month when I stopped taking Clomid and started getting acupuncture along with my husband. When I went in for my ultrasound, we were all shocked. I had more eggs ready for ovulation than I had with the drugs. And then we tested my husband. He, too, had a dramatic increase in his production of sperm. We were sold from that minute on.

—Melinda, age 32

———

When compared cost-wise to Western drug treatments, holistic alternatives are usually cheaper. Unfortunately, while more and more data is developing that shows certain types of situations are conducive to a holistic approach, it is often difficult to find Western physicians who accept Eastern medical philosophies. Nevertheless, if you do decide to experiment with alternative therapies, you should continue to see your doctor so that he can monitor, with ultrasound, the physiologic changes that occur, and can do hormonal evaluation.

If you're interested in pursuing traditional Chinese medicine, there are two national organizations you can contact to learn more, and to see whether any centers are located near you. They are The American Association of Oriental Medicine and the National Commission on Certification of Acupuncturists.

Reaching Your Infertility Resolution

By now you've been on your journey for what seems to be an unbearable length of time. If you'd been traveling in miles, you would have circled the globe. You're tired. Your body aches, both mentally and physically. And you're emotionally depleted from all of the difficult decisions you've had to make along the way. But you've learned a lot about yourself, as a person, and as part of a couple. You've also grown a lot. You've had to survive things you didn't think you were capable of. You've had to pull yourself back up and move on, after each failed treatment. And in the process, you've slowly gotten stronger in accepting your situation.

Acceptance is the final stage of grief or mourning. It's the point at which you are finally ready to accept the reality of your infertility. To some of us the word *acceptance* has the connotation of giving in. It shouldn't. In reality, it's the doorway through which we walk into a new and energized future.

MOVING TO THE NEXT STEP

"Acceptance, the final stage of mourning, is characterized by replenished energy and readiness to view the future with hope rather than despair. At this point the couple can begin to negotiate the available options. . . ."

—Linda Callahan, M.A.
"The Crisis of Infertility and Its Effect
on the Couple Relationship," 1992

For most of you, acceptance will come about in a slow and gradual manner. This is especially true if you've experienced unexplained infertility, since you've tried so many approaches and are probably still grappling for answers.

Often the decision to clearly accept the reality that your infertile condition isn't going to change, and to comfortably move on, is triggered by what seems like an insignificant event. The most commonplace thing can push you over the top into a new way of thinking. For instance, let's say you've been in treatment for years, when someone close to you hurts you one more painful time. You decide that's it. Maybe it happens when your doctor suggests another treatment, and you find yourself completely stripped of the energy and the will you need to try it. At that point your doctor may convince you that there's no reason to continue on your present path. Or you could be offered an advancement in your career that forces you to choose between moving up and continuing in treatment. You suddenly decide that enough is enough. In each of these examples, you're entering the final stage of your grieving. You're facing the fact that it's time to move on. It's this that pushes you toward resolution.

"Resolution is an end point that occurs only after considerable time— time to accept that infertility has been a reality in your life, time to respond to the fear and pain it has inflicted upon you, and time to gather the strength to weather the crisis. Resolution means that you have finally put into perspective all those months or years of trying to have a baby."

—L. P. Salzer, L.C.S.W., "Surviving
Infertility—A Compassionate Guide Through
the Emotional Crisis of Infertility," 1991

As you begin the process of resolution, you're at a crossroads. Not only do you have to decide what to do, you have to decide when to do it, especially if you still have some doubts about stopping at all. It might help if you talk to other people who have made the decision to end treatment. See how they feel about it now. Or maybe you could put things into a set time frame. For example, you could decide that you will stop treatment by your next birthday, and then work on your resolution process in the interim. And of course it's always a good idea to consult with a psychological professional, who can guide you as you make the right decision.

Keep in mind that for some, the crossroads comes early in treatment. For instance, you may learn early on that it is impossible for you to carry a child. Maybe you've begun premature menopause. Or that it's impossible to have your own biological child, since your husband has been found to have no sperm. In these cases the decision to move ahead to another option has to be faced at the time of the diagnostic workup. This places you in an odd situation. You know you should make a decision about what to do next, but you haven't had time to complete your grieving process and mourn the loss of your fantasized biologic conception and birth. Don't be rushed. Take the time you need to work through acceptance before you move on to considering the many worthwhile options that are still available to you.

As we've said, acceptance isn't resignation; it's an opportunity to move on to other possibilities. For you as an infertility patient, these include:

1. egg donation, if the female partner can't produce her own eggs
2. donor insemination, if the male partner can't produce any sperm and ICSI is not a possibility
3. surrogate parenting, if the female partner can't carry a pregnancy
4. adoption
5. child-free living

No matter which you choose, you may still have difficulty accepting the fact that your family will be different from the "traditional" family. But by going through the infertility process, you've had to face the fact that having a traditional family has never been an option for you. The choice is now one of finding the alternative that best fits you, both as individuals and as a couple. So as you investigate these options, you should also examine your feelings. Here are a few of the many questions that you should consider.

1. What are my reasons and motivations for becoming a parent?
2. How important is the physical experience of pregnancy to me?
3. Would I be comfortable carrying a baby from an anonymous donor?
4. Can we both accept that one partner may be a biological parent, while the other is not?
5. Would it be better to adopt, and if so, what are our needs?
6. Can we accept the thought of living child free?

Infertility is an unfortunate condition that rocks the very foundations you were raised on. It forces you to take the time to assess yourself, and to figure out what you most want and need in your life. These things are very personal; only you and your partner can know what's best for both of you.

Perhaps, if you're fed up with treatment, you're still not sure whether stopping is the right decision. After all, when you began your diagnostic workup, you told each other that you weren't going to quit until you had succeeded in having a baby. Recognize that as time has passed, and you've met with no success, your feelings may have begun to change. This change represents how you've grown through the process. But how can you know whether you've changed enough to be able to relinquish your original dream?

"When the desire to parent is greater than the desire to have a genetic offspring. This is when the door opens to nongenetic alternatives."

—*Carole Lieber Wilkins, M.A., M.F.C.C.*

For most of you, when you are truly ready to forge ahead, you will know. Jill certainly did.

I moved away from infertility treatment gradually, first by looking at the idea of options in general, then by taking consistantly closer steps. The process took time. At first I wasn't ready at all for adoption. I could have kept on with treatment. It was like rolling the dice. I would tell myself that if the thing we were doing didn't work, *then* I'd be ready. But every time we failed there'd be something else out there to keep me going.

But my husband is older than I am. I began to realize that he was more sick of the in vitro than I was. He was sick of me being on the drugs. He was sick of the constant doctor appointments. He was sick of the whole thing. And when I thought about it, I didn't want to do this for another five years, and then have a child when he was too old to play with it. Finally he dragged me to an adoption agency. And then we met with a lawyer. Two days later, on Mother's Day, I found out my latest in vitro cycle hadn't worked; I wasn't pregnant. But the same day the lawyer phoned and told us they'd found a baby for me. It was a boy, and it had already been born. And as he said it I realized I wasn't ready for this. Everyone else was so excited, and I didn't want to let go of the dream of this biological child I had in my head, the little boy I had wanted to give to my husband . . . the little boy who would always be a part of him. I felt angry that I was being forced to look at this. And when the biological mother tested positive for drugs, I felt relief, because I wasn't ready yet psychologically.

Three days later there was another phone call, and another baby. This one came through friends that had heard we were going through the adoption process. And again this situation sounded great. But when we met with the girl's lawyer, I started crying. I couldn't stop thinking that there were still frozen embryos that could be used. Maybe the next in vitro cycle was going to work. So I backed out again. When those babies were getting thrown at me, it made me realize more and more that I wasn't ready to let go of my biological child yet.

Then in July I heard about my baby's birth mother. I was honest with her lawyer about my frozen embryos. He understood. He reassured me that if my in vitro worked, I could back out of the adoption. And when I met the mother it felt better, but I still carried this disappointment around. So I went through another frozen cycle. At this point she was six months pregnant. This cycle didn't work either, but at about the same time I found out, she had an ultrasound. When I found out the baby was a girl, it started to become my baby. All of a sudden I started becoming more and more excited and possessive.

It forced me to let go of the dream of the little boy I had wanted to have. You have to take the time to mourn for your biological child. It's like a death in the family. And when you're at the point at which you can say "I've mourned for my child . . . I've let it go . . ." you're ready for adoption. Once you mourn for your biological child, that fantasy is gone. You have to remind yourself that a lot of times the reality doesn't live up to your fantasies.

My idea now is that everyone's baby comes to them through whatever vehicle is appropriate. You come to the point at which you understand that God has given you this child to take care of. It doesn't matter how biologically or genetically this came to you, it's your baby.

You want to go out there and tell all those women who can't give up on infertility treatments to let go. I have, because this child is a jewel.

If you, like Jill, reach a decision that it is time to move away from infertility treatment, and toward another option, you will then have to deal with a very basic issue—what being a parent means to you.

How much of what you're looking for relates to the experience of raising a child? And how much is linked to your need for genetic and biological links? A clear understanding of your feelings about these things can help you to make your decision.

THE DESIRE TO PARENT

Your desire to parent can grow from a number of different things. Does it come from a need to make your extended family happy, or a need not to break with tradition? Is it because it's the nineties and having a family is the thing to do? Is it because you had a bad childhood, and you want to give a better one to your kids? Or is it simply because you've always imagined you would have children? There are many possible reasons for your desire to parent. By examining them, you should be able to recognize which are most important to you. These may direct you toward a very clear path. For example, if you are very caught up in the idea of continuing your genetic family line, you can quickly eliminate adoption, and some types of donor situations, from your thinking.

Some reasons for wanting to parent aren't genetically linked. They're tied up in fulfilling emotional needs for you or your partner. For example, a lack of self-esteem, a poor self-image, or a number of other insecurities can be contributing factors in your need to have a baby. Perhaps a baby represents a family that you can be in charge of, a unit where you can control the moving pieces. Or maybe you're subconsciously looking toward children to reflect your financial stability and your success in life, thereby making you feel worthwhile.

If you've been subconsciously feeling inadequate, children can represent to you a way to become accomplished, thus making you more satisfied with your life. What better way could there be to prove that you're an adequate adult, than to have children? If you've never experienced a loving relationship, particularly as a child, you may think children will make you feel loved and needed. And by loving your children, you can make up to them for what you never had.

Or maybe you just love children, and have always looked forward to the responsibilities of loving, guiding, and giving. If that's the case, keep in mind that parenting is a lifetime commitment with no guarantees. The experience may never live up to your expectations.

After you've discussed both these possibilities, and others, you'll have a better idea of which facets of parenting are essential to you. Make sure that you and your partner understand each other's needs, and that you can reach a complementary fit between them. Don't leave any conflicts on the table. They may come back to haunt you later. For example, if the decision leans toward donor sperm, make sure you are both in agreement. You don't want to find out in later years that your husband is resentful about the choice you made. He could feel disconnected from the child—both as a father and as a nongenetic parent. Once you're sure you're in agreement, you can clearly choose your next course of action.

Never forget that once you've made the commitment to be a parent, it doesn't really matter in the long run whether you gave birth to your child or not. Once you take on the responsibility of raising children, your child's genetic origin has little to do with this lifetime experience. The goal is simply to be a good parent. But having children using donor sperm and donor eggs offers some special challenges in this regard.

DONOR TECHNOLOGIES . . . I'VE GOT A SECRET

Assisted reproductive technologies let you create a pregnancy using donor sperm, donor eggs, donor embryos, and even donor uteri. The hope is that once you get pregnant using one of these alternatives, and you relish in the joy of the birth of your baby, any possible misgivings you might have had about the process will be overlooked. If you have any doubts as to whether this will happen for you, there are some questions that you might ask yourself. Will the fact that you're not biologically related to your child affect your ability to love him or her, or to accept his or her limitations? How much do you want to know about your anonymous donor? Would you feel more comfortable using a donor who's known to you? Who, if anyone, will you tell about how your child was conceived?

Happily, these things can almost universally be resolved. But as thrilled as they might be, all donor parents still face one difficult decision. While it is true that this technology offers couples the opportunity to experience almost every aspect of reproduction, there are those who feel it also gives them the ability to mask the truth. This thinking is somewhat new, because the ability to perform these technologies is also new. This masking can, in the eyes of some experts, cause psychological damage to donor insemination children. Should the child know? And if so, when? Will the knowledge about the way they were conceived be enlightening or confusing?

Unlike adoption or surrogacy, sperm donation and egg donation can remain a secret. This secrecy is the biggest issue surrounding these options. How will you deal with it? When the idea of working with a donor is presented to you, you may feel that keeping your child's genetic origin a secret is a viable possibility. But eventually, as time goes on, your feelings may sway more in the direction of being honest with your child about his or her genetic makeup. When that happens you will probably be able to tell your child how they were conceived, but you will still be able to give them little or no information about the actual donor, should you wish to do so. During the many years that sperm donation has been in effect, the medical profession has generally done it on an anonymous basis in order to protect sperm donors from legal questions of paternity. This also shields the recipient father from society's lack of acceptance of male infertility. And egg donation, too, is usually done with some degree of anonymity for the donor. Today, openness in sperm and egg donation is beginning to grow. One of the reasons to decide ahead of time whether you will want to tell your child about his genetic donor, is that you can look for a program that offers full disclosure.

If you are going to tell, the next question becomes, when? Very young children can't possibly understand the technologically sophisticated process that led to their conception. So if you start talking about it in the early years, the language you use must be simple, and the process must be put in terms that a young child is able to grasp. You will probably find that if you introduce the subject early on, your child will continue to ask you a series of ever-more-specific questions as he or she gets older. Children explore concepts as they are ready to hear them. By the time they are teenagers or young adults, they should be able to comprehend fully the steps that led to their conception. Since privacy about this issue is important to most parents, you might want to hold off telling your child until he or she is old enough to protect your secret about his or her conception and genetic makeup. The only drawback to this is that you may be risking your child's anger. If this is the decision you make, you may want to keep a journal or file. When you finally do tell your child, you can use it to explain why you waited so long.

If, on the other hand, you feel you want to keep the issue a secret, both partners must feel completely comfortable with that decision. Talk it out with your partner. Make sure you clearly understand your own feelings as well as your partner's. Be aware that as the years go on, guilt and anxiety can creep up, accompanied by the uncomfortable feeling that you are lying to your child. After you search your soul and thoroughly evaluate all the issues, you may feel that it's worth it to carry this burden. Just know ahead of time that you may have to pick up this load.

To help relieve yourself of some of its weight, you may decide to tell your child, and those around you, a larger truth. You can let them know that you had a serious infertility problem, and that you went through an enormous ordeal to have a child. Then it's only the details that you're not revealing. But be prepared. There could come a time when your child finds out the truth by accident, through blood types, eye color, or a disease you've developed that your child fears getting. And the possibility always exists that after time and growth, one partner will have a need to share the truth with the child. Life is filled with surprising turns. You just have to understand that this may be one of them. With this possibility in mind, it can be helpful to imagine what it would be like to tell your child . . . how you would cope if you were forced to tell.

If you and your partner decide that you want to tell your child the truth of his genetic makeup, but you don't know when, you may try to confide in others who are close to you, and look to them for support. Be aware that by asking a friend to be sworn to secrecy, you are giving them a burden, a burden they might not want to carry. Add to that another fear—once you tell the truth, you can never take it back. So where can you go to find support, to help you and your partner discuss your issues, *without* obligating family and friends? You go to a professional. One who is trained and experienced in this area. One who will help you, in complete confidentiality, address your feelings and conflicts, and will guide you to the right choices for you.

As you can see, donor situations bring along a number of highly charged questions as part of the package. But when you've decided you definitely want to parent, and are given the option of having a child that has at least half the genetic makeup of your couple, you'll probably want to go ahead, despite these problem areas. It's normal to experience a fear of the unknown as you begin the process. Because of this, it might be helpful if you take a few months to adjust to your choice before starting the medical work. During this time you should examine your feelings, your concerns, and your fears, and you should discuss them freely between you and your partner. It's natural to worry about what will be taking place within your doctor's laboratory, whether he is performing a procedure with your sperm, your embryos or the chosen donor's. It's natural to worry about the health of your baby, whether it's genetic makeup is yours or another's. And it's natural to worry how the baby is progressing within the uterus, whether it's your uterus or another woman's. If you understand ahead of time that many of the fears you feel are just a normal part of having a baby, it will help you to proceed with the confidence that, together, you are unquestionably doing the right thing.

SURROGACY . . . WHOM DO YOU TRUST?

While surrogacy is an alternative that carries with it the possibility of a baby, it also involves you in an emotional interaction that is different from any other infertility treatment. Whether you become involved with conventional surrogacy, in which the infertile woman is not the genetic parent, or with gestational surrogacy, in which both halves of the infertile couple are genetically linked to the child, you'll be facing one common issue. You must put your faith and trust in an unrelated third person, to nourish, protect, and carry your fetus to delivery.

In this chapter we have dealt with trust and openness within your coupling. In surrogacy that trust, openness, and intimacy now has to be extended to a third party. Your surrogate may not have been known to you before conception, except on a limited medical and psychological basis. But a unique bond forms between you, your partner, and your surrogate during gestation. This bond is hard to understand or describe, but is an extremely powerful one.

Touched by an Angel

I really cried, seeing her in pain as she pushed my baby out. I wanted to trade places with her so badly. It's hard feeling indebted to someone, especially when you'll never be able to pay them back. This is going to sound screwy, but sometimes I wish that she'd get sick and need a bone marrow transplant, and that I was a perfect match. I'd feel as if I'd repaid her. All my life I've wanted to believe in angels. Now, nobody can tell me there's no such thing. I know she's human, but to me, she's my angel.

—Claudia, age 32

Because surrogacy pulls together people who otherwise would never have known each other, confidence in your match with a surrogate is of the utmost importance. How do you know who is the right match? Follow your intuition. Medically, the candidates will all have been screened from a health as well as a psychological viewpoint. The only issue that will remain is whether this is a person with whom you can share an intense, bonding relationship throughout pregnancy, and a special relationship for the rest of your life.

Take your time in choosing a surrogate. Make sure you are comfortable. Any small issues that make you uneasy before pregnancy can become magnified tremendously during the stress of pregnancy and delivery. It takes a special woman to be a surrogate. It also takes a special couple to utilize this medical alternative. If you feel this is you, do your homework and listen to your feelings during this process.

ADOPTION

Maybe you've examined your heart and found you have a need to parent, but you and your partner have decided, for a variety of reasons, that assisted reproductive technologies are not for you. You then may want to look in the direction of adoption.

In the beginning, when you learned of your infertility, adoption probably couldn't have been farther from your mind. Then one day you realized that you were able to bring yourself to discuss it. As a result of your growth, of your acceptance of your condition, and of your understanding of your need to parent, it had become a possibility worth examining.

We never knew all these people had adopted kids. It's like coming out of the closet. Once people knew, we started getting all these phone calls. If you open the door and let people know you're interested, they only want to share what joy adoption's brought to them.

—*Jill, age 35*

If you're considering adoption, be forewarned. Though it isn't always, it can be a difficult, tedious, and lengthy process. This is especially important to you, since your patience has already been worn down during infertility treatment. Realize that when you begin looking into adoption, you're beginning a whole new reproductive process. It brings with it many of the same feelings that you experienced with infertility. You'll have a lack of control over when a baby becomes available, over the child's genetic background, and over the birth mother's pregnancy experience. Worse yet, she might change her mind. And by the time she does, you may already have invested your emotional energies in receiving the child. But let's say she doesn't change her mind, and you are going to receive your baby. Then you'll probably begin to worry about whether you'll bond with it appropriately.

Can I Make Him Mine?

When the phone rang to say that a baby boy could be ours in a few months, I became very anxious. Would I be able to truly love this baby boy, as if he were my own flesh and blood? Would my parents? Would I always be thinking, deep down, that he really isn't mine, and that I wished that he was?

—*Cindy, age 37*

Fears about bonding are one of the most common worries among people approaching adoption. Rest assured that if you truly believe and feel that you are the child's mother and father, the bonding that takes place will be natural and strong, no matter what the child's genetic origin is. There's very little gain to be had by worrying about the quality of your bonding. After all, since you'll never know any other form of parenting, you'll never have anything to compare it to. And your child will never have grown up in any other kind of family either.

". . . the bonding that occurs between a parent and baby is an 'emotional glue' that transcends the blood relationship. Your feelings for your child—whether adopted or biological—can be equally intense. It may be hard to recognize this, however, until you have experienced it."

—*L. P. Salzer, L.C.S.W.*
"Surviving Infertility," 1991

As you approach the option of adoption, make sure you have first reached some sort of resolution to your infertility. That you have learned to accept your infertility, and the limitations it makes on your life. That you have come to terms with the fact that you cannot, and/or will not, pursue the other options offered by donors and surrogates. Be sure that both you and your partner have closed the chapter on genetic immortality in the book of your life together. This is such a final decision, it can be very difficult.

You must also understand and accept that adoption is going to be a slightly different experience than biological parenting. Nothing about your child's arrival will resemble that other experience. You will have to plan how you are going to communicate the concept of adoption to your child. And you will have to be able to live with the fact that your child's birth parents will always exist. If you can accept these things and be comfortable with them, you're ready for adoption. It's neither a better nor a worse experience than biological parenting, it's just a different one. Remember, if there's one thing your infertility has taught you, it's that you have the strength to face your feelings head on, and the tools to resolve them.

CHILD-FREE LIVING—ANOTHER ROAD TAKEN

You've accepted your infertility, and examined your reasons for wanting to parent. Maybe, to your surprise, you discovered in doing so that living child-free is an appealing option for you. Maybe you learned that the needs that were going to be filled by having a child could be resolved in other ways. For instance, you may have been trying to have a child to fulfill the traditional expectations of others around you. And when you examined your personal desires, you discovered you didn't have the same traditional expectations. You had no need to live on in family members beyond your generation. Or maybe you were socialized to believe that children would make your marriage whole. But as you investigated further, you found that your life was already complete. With a good marriage and a fulfilling career, you felt no need to have children.

Having made this decision, you may find thoughts of a lonely old age filling your worry box. This is a very bad reason to have children. How many stories have you heard in which parents and children no longer speak once the children are mature? Even in the best relationships, children and grandchildren shouldn't be depended on to single-handedly stave off your loneliness during old age. Even if you did have children, it would be up to you to build a network of people around you during your lifespan.

One of the best parts of deciding to put aside the idea of children is that you free yourself from the emotional roller coaster of infertility. Choosing to remain child-free lets you begin to live your life again, and in ways that are not available to most of those with children.

Will you regret your choice later? It's possible. But there's less chance of that happening if you've carefully examined beforehand exactly what it is you really want out of life. If you are a victim of infertility, have suffered through treatment, and are now leaning toward a child-free life as your resolution, make sure you have mourned the loss of your fantasized biological and adopted children. If you don't take the time to grieve over this loss, your resolution won't be complete and you may be left with strong regrets. Do the work now, so that you don't suffer in years to come.

One nice thing about this decision is that it's not necessarily final. You can always revisit the subject at some later date. This is especially true if you or your partner are still unsure about the decision. Resuming treatment and examining adoption options remain as available alternatives if they're pursued within a reasonable time frame. But beyond a certain point, it's not a good idea to keep using this lack of finality as a fallback.

Child-free living is not for everybody, but it represents a wonderful option for many of you. Your life can be rich, filled to the brim with varied interests, a fulfilling career, great travel plans, and the pursuit of your many talents. If you make this choice, embrace it, like all of the alternatives offered, with vigor and the confidence of knowing you did the right thing.

I'VE HAD MY BABY . . . WHAT'S LEFT TO RESOLVE?

Acceptance and resolution are stages you will have to go through if you're not successful in your quest to have a child. And to the surprise of many, they're also phases you will have to go through if you do succeed in becoming parents.

You are the fortunate ones. After so much time and so much effort, you were rewarded for your hard work. You received that longed-for call from the nurse to inform you that you were pregnant. Then you enjoyed nine joy-filled months of pregnancy, which ended with a beautiful new-born cradled in your arms. Although you may feel as if this resolved your infertility, technically it did not. Resolution is achieved emotionally, not physically. Still, if your journey ends with a baby, does it really matter?

Twins and my Resolution

I thought that I had resolved my infertility problem when I gave birth to healthy boy and girl twins. But the effects of the past four years stay with me. I look at life a little differently now. I'm more conscious of my body's functions. I sometimes feel guilty for having these wonderful babies, when others I've come to know through the treatment process don't. And I still feel extra sorry for anyone I meet who discovers they have an infertility problem. If I forget for just a moment, it seems it's always that time when I'm asked, "Do twins run in your family?" Often I found myself staring at each child and wondering how I could be so lucky. Had it not been for my doctor and his treatment, they wouldn't be here. It's almost like someone is going to take them away from me. I'm amazed at how deep my scars are. But as time has passed, I'm beginning to believe that mothers in general think about how lucky they are. It's one of life's great experiences, no matter how you get there.

—Lisa, age 36

It does matter. Whether your infertility resolution involves a life with children or without them, whether it means children with half your genetic makeup or adopted children, your life will never be the same. And the scope of these life changes will reflect the severity of the infertility problem you've gone through. It will leave you with scars, reminders of wounds that have healed and are healing still. These scars don't necessarily mean that you have, or have not, resolved your infertility. They simply represent the fact that a crisis did exist in your life. For most of you, your healing process will be going on for years to come.

Some Final Thoughts

The emotional and medical aspects of infertility can't be addressed separately, they need to be looked at as two halves of a whole. Both aspects must be dealt with on a daily basis, and both must be taken into consideration as you make the many turns along your personal road. Sometimes you may feel lost in a very technical, medical maze. Don't be shy about expressing your emotional reaction when this happens, both to your partner and to your doctor. Remember, when you choose your doctor, look for someone you will be comfortable talking to openly. As you go through this difficult process, you'll need all the support you can get. From everyone!

Approach treatment positively, and with an open mind. Don't be afraid to laugh. Educate yourself and set sensible limits. Try to be optimistic, but at the same time, realistic.

If the day finally comes when you decide to stop, sit down with your doctor, and together review the road you've traveled. As you relive the many things you've tried, you'll be able to say to yourself that "you did the best you could." And that is all that anyone can do.

15

Controversies in Reproductive Medicine

Reproductive medicine is no stranger to controversy. As early as 1968, when the idea of producing an in vitro baby was still no more than a dream in the minds of a few doctors, it stirred public debate. A cover article published in *Life* magazine that year claimed that scientists were considering attempting fertilization and embryo growth outside the human body. It went on to condemn this possibility as an unethical and immoral attempt to tamper with the processes of nature. During that same period, a complete ban on any type of experimental work in human in vitro fertilization was announced by the National Institutes of Health and supported by the federal government.

Public hostility toward reproductive medicine reached a peak in the late seventies and early eighties, as actual work in in vitro fertilization began taking place. Religious and Right-to-Life groups demonstrated almost daily in front of Eastern Virginia Medical School, as the Jones Institute worked inside to create the first American breakthrough from in vitro fertilization. In Los Angeles, as we attempted to produce our first in vitro birth, we tried to keep a low profile, but still received negative comments and criticism when we announced our initial success.

We dealt with this sort of backlash by trying to educate the various groups that objected to our work. By doing that, we were able to convince most of them that what we were doing was life-promoting, rather than life-threatening. Still, the discussions we had, showed us the complexity of the moral and ethical issues we were dealing with, and the way in which they reached into the very essence of human life. The questions that were asked then seem important still. And as research and technology have advanced, new questions, both primal and complex, have been added. Some of them may touch on issues you will have to deal with as you undergo treatment. Others are important enough to bear thinking about, even if you don't have to face them personally.

When Does Life Begin?

The biggest controversy that exists in the arena of reproductive medicine is the question of when, and where, life begins. Some religious groups are convinced that it happens as soon as the egg and sperm fuse— at the very moment of fertilization. Other segments of society—mainly the scientific and medical communities—feel that life, as we perceive it, begins at some point after sperm and egg fusion. The farthest swing of the pendulum is to those people who believe that life doesn't really exist until the moment that a baby is actually delivered, alive and kicking.

Specialists in reproductive medicine have long tried to grapple with this knotty question. The National Ethics Committee that was formed in 1984 set out to outline moral and ethical guidelines for these emerging medical technologies.

I was one of 12 individuals who were chosen by various organizations, and assigned the daunting task of creating a document that would be used as an ethical standard for reproductive technologies in the United States. Our group was made up of physicians, scientists, and ethicists, as well as clergy. One of our first goals was to determine, in some manner, the point in time at which a new life begins. The ethics commission spent months reviewing various religious and scientific documents that discussed the initiation of life. The conclusion we finally reached reflected all of our individual viewpoints and areas of expertise.

The committee's report, which was published in 1986, concluded that life, as we know it, begins 10 to 14 days after conception. This is the point at which the neural tube, or embryonic pole, is developed, and the human embryo, if divided into separate cells, will no longer generate a separate fetus from each of them. At this point, the fetus has reached unity. Past this point of development, there is no way it could be anything but a single baby.

While not everyone agrees with this decision—some religious groups take particular exception to it—it is the standard that scientists are now required to adhere to as they make decisions in areas such as genetic research on embryos. But, in reality, the doctors who work in the area of reproductive medicine normally interpret the beginning of life in an even stricter fashion. While they feel free to discard sperm cells, or eggs that don't fertilize, embryos are protected from the moment that they fertilize. This continues throughout their development, up until the time that they either produce a baby or demonstrate that they're not viable and won't continue to grow and develop.

Taking Embryos to Court

Given this widely held belief that life begins very early in embryonic development, a number of issues having to do with their handling have now entered the courts. The ownership of embryos is one area that has had a great deal of exposure in the legal system. And the parental rights that might, or might not, attach to embryos have been legally challenged on a number of occasions as well.

In some of these cases it has been suggested that embryos should have legal protection, just as a child would during a custody battle. But as we write this, the courts have not yet taken that step, and embryos are still being viewed as property rather than as people, during legal proceedings contesting parental rights or legal custody.

Custody battles over embryos have arisen in a number of contexts. In cases of divorce, where the couple has frozen embryos in storage, courts have had to make a decision on how to award them, as well as the right to use them, to one of the divorcing parties. In California, parental rights to an embryo were questioned when a surrogate carrier became pregnant with an embryo produced from another couple's egg and sperm, and then challenged their rights to the child after it was born. Her claim that she, as the gestational parent, had rights to the child was dismissed by the court. Of course, the decision might not be so easily made in the case of a surrogate who is also an egg donor, who *does* have a genetic relationship to the child.

Keep in mind that before you undergo any procedures that result in frozen embryos, you must fill out consent forms, in the off chance that after you've produced extra embryos you die suddenly. The consent form directs your doctor how to deal with the embryos. Your choices are handing the embryos over to research, donating them to another couple, or having them thawed and destroyed. This system was set up so that all embryos are accounted for. None is left abandoned, or free for the picking.

In the future, there will be more and more legal cases involving the misuse of embryos. In some countries, such as Australia, it is already a criminal offense to handle them improperly, and the United States may move in that direction as well. If it does, it will be driven by revelations such as the case at the University of California at Irvine, in which this well-known fertility center allegedly took embryos created from the eggs and sperm of infertile patients and transferred them, without permission, to unrelated couples. Surprisingly, since no state or federal laws govern embryo stealing, there's some question as to whether there can be criminal prosecution for these actions. Obviously, laws need to be developed which protect both rights of genetic parents as well as the rights of the embryo, which is for all intents and purposes an unborn child. Until this is done, cases like this will remain in legal limbo.

Who's Watching the Lab?

The mishandling of eggs and embryos that apparently took place at U.C. Irvine might have been avoided if the federal and state governments, in cooperation with medical societies, would agree on guidelines for licensing and regulating in vitro laboratories. As of the present, there is no central registry to which data from in vitro laboratories must be reported. And if physicians and scientists continue to fight the idea, there won't be one anytime soon.

Regulation problems exist on a state level as well as on a national one. Most states have kept their heads in the sand on the issue of standardizing and licensing in vitro laboratories. It is beyond comprehension to think that laboratories that do urine tests are required to have licenses, be inspected, and undergo annual reviews (in most states), while laboratories that generate embryos that grow into new human lives have *no oversight or licensing requirements*. The College of American Pathologists (CAP) and the Clinical Laboratory Improvement Amendment (CLIA) govern and regulate pathology laboratories throughout the United States. But they have yet to establish standards for reproductive embryology laboratories. As things stand now, literally anyone can set up an IVF laboratory and run it without supervision. This lack of regulation leads to difficult problems, such as the recent case in The Netherlands in which a woman, after trying to become pregnant for five years, succeeded through in vitro fertilization to give birth to twins. One looked like its blond, blue-eyed parents. The other was black. The laboratory apologized for its "regrettable mistake."

We've pushed for standardized laboratory licensing for in vitro laboratories for over ten years. As consumers, you too should insist that federal and state government agencies work in concert with the medical and scientific communities in establishing guidelines that will protect both embryos and patients from unscrupulous activities and potentially harmful medical procedures.

Sperm and Egg Donation . . . to Know or Not to Know

Donated sperm has been used for over 40 years in this country, traditionally behind a veil of anonymity. While one sperm bank in California does give donor insemination children who have reached the age of 18 access to information concerning their biological fathers, the vast majority still maintain total secrecy. The reason cited for this is usually the potential legal ramifications that might follow upon full disclosure. The recipient might request child support from the donor. The offspring might make claims to his estate. A child born to a single mother might seek out the donor father for support if she dies. Or attempts by the offspring to seek out the donor might just be embarrassing or uncomfortable.

The code of secrecy that applies to egg donation is not quite so strong. Unlike sperm donation, egg donation is done with varying degrees of secrecy, largely depending on the medical center that is involved. In some, such as ours, couples are given the option of knowing the donor if they choose to, and donors and recipients are even allowed to interview each other and make a decision based upon their meeting. In other clinics, the recipient couple is always unknown to the donor, even when they know who she is, have seen photographs of her, and have her name and her historical and medical background. And in still other clinics, couples are limited to strictly medical information about donors, and donors know nothing about recipient couples.

Much of the reluctance to get into totally open situations is due to fears of what legal ramifications there might be in the future. Will donors someday have additional rights to their natural born offspring, even though they simply donated egg or sperm? Until this is clarified, donations will continue to be done through a one-way mirror type of situation, which protects the recipient couple. New clinical approaches to donation will evolve only as far as legal guidelines do.

Whether you tell the child about its origins is another area of controversy with donor sperm or eggs.

Where Did I Come From?

"Do we tell the child?" is probably the most commonly asked question, when I talk with couples who are discussing the possibility of donation. While there is no best answer to this dilemma, one good approach was given to me by a couple who was consulting with me about egg donation. They had previously adopted two children, and strongly believed in telling the child from day one . . . even before the child could understand . . . even before the child could be cognizant of what adoption meant. They suggested that you talk about it as you would anything else. You make it a natural, normal part of growing up. You say that you used eggs from someone else, because mommy's didn't work. By starting to discuss this from a very young age, you can help the child to feel that there is nothing very different or odd about it.

And What About Surrogates?

The use of another woman's reproductive system to carry a pregnancy for infertile couples has been controversial from the very beginning. In the earliest days of conventional surrogacy, when pregnancy was achieved through artificial insemination using sperm from the male in the infertile couple, this already complex issue was further complicated. Since the egg that was used to create the fetus was the surrogate's, she was not only a carrier, she was also the genetic mother of the child. Because of these close biological links, this type of surrogacy was fraught with legal problems, the worst case scenario being the surrogate who decided after carrying a pregnancy that she didn't want to turn the child over to the couple who had contracted for her services. Once it became possible to create an embryo in vitro, and eggs other than the surrogate's could be used, the issue of genetic connection was removed. With this new type of surrogate, known as a "surrogate gestational carrier," the legal aspects of the process cleared up dramatically. In most cases where surrogate gestational carriers are used, the egg and sperm come from the infertile couple, making them the genetic parents of the child. The surrogate gestational carrier is limited to providing a safe and healthy environment into which the embryo can be transferred, and where the fetus can grow and develop.

Nevertheless, controversy around this issue still exists. In some countries around the world—Australia, France, and England, for example—the use of both gestational and conventional surrogates is a criminal offense. In some states within the United States, being a surrogate is illegal, while in others the process is so well accepted that state laws have been passed to protect the rights of the genetic parents of the child which is produced.

The main source of objections to surrogacy is that it coerces women into being "wombs for hire." It's hard to ignore this aspect of the process, when in most cases surrogates are women of modest means, being hired by couples with far more money than they have. This has become even more evident in recent years, as a shortage of gestational surrogates has created a situation in which the price of their services is escalating. In this new market-driven environment, surrogates may become bargaining chips that go to the highest bidder.

From an ethical standpoint, surrogates should be compensated for the time and labor involved in carrying the pregnancy. But they shouldn't be viewed as objects to be purchased for a nine-month interval. As more and more couples require the services of gestational carriers, and they continue to become more in demand, they will be able to insist on higher compensation for their services. If this continues, an industry standard may have to be set at some point that will guarantee surrogates fair compensation for the time and labor involved in carrying a pregnancy, but which will protect couples of average means from being priced out of the market.

Ovarian Cancer and Fertility Drugs

Fertility drugs have been used to induce and control ovulation for almost 40 years without major complications. During that long time period, over 300 scientific articles have been published concerning possible health risks related to their use. With just two exceptions, none of those published studies demonstrated a relationship between fertility drugs and any type of female cancer—be it of the breast, ovaries, uterus, cervix, or vagina. But those two isolated exceptions still managed to stir up a storm of controversy.

Both dissenting articles were published in the early nineties. The first, released in 1992, reanalyzed previously published data, and used it to demonstrate a formerly undetected relationship between fertility drugs and ovarian cancer. This article, which was authored by Alice Whittemore, claimed that women who took fertility drugs had a 27 times greater risk of contracting ovarian cancer than women who had never used fertility drugs.

This claim, which frightened women across the country, was based on poor research techniques. The type of study Whittemore did is called a met-analysis. It draws on the conclusions of previous articles, without looking at the original data on which those articles were based. Whittemore's risk factor was drawn from the fact that nine women in the groups that had been studied had been found to have ovarian cancer. But since Whittemore didn't have the original data, she didn't know what types of drugs these women had taken—clomiphene citrate, human menopausal gonadotropin, estrogen, progesterone, prednisone, or aspirin—what quantity of the drugs had been taken, or the period of time over which they were used. Despite her lack of information, she compared these ovarian cancer cases to a group of infertile patient controls. In order for her to have an appropriately matched control group, at least six or seven of this group should have been exposed to fertility drugs, but only one of the twenty-three women in her control group had been.

After publication, a number of experts in ovarian cancer and statistics reanalyzed Whittemore's data. They took the flaws in her group's technique into account, and were satisfied that the data, if compared to an appropriate control group, wouldn't demonstrate any increased risk of ovarian cancer related to the use of fertility drugs.

The second negative study concerning ovarian tumors and fertility drugs was published in 1994. It studied a group of almost four thousand women who had taken clomiphene citrate, and then followed them for up to twenty years after their fertility drug use. It found eleven ovarian tumors, four of which were malignant, and seven of which were what is called "borderline"—in other words, they had some abnormal cells which while not yet cancerous, could become so.

A finding of four malignancies in a group of about four thousand women is no higher than the expected incidence in the general population; about one in every thousand women will have ovarian cancer in her lifetime. Thus, the risk of ovarian cancer was not elevated by clomiphene citrate use, according to this study. But a finding of seven borderline tumors of the ovary in this size population was considered to be significantly elevated.

When the seven women with borderline tumors were analyzed separately, it was found that some had taken a very prolonged course of clomiphene citrate. In fact, all seven had taken Clomid for at least twelve months. So what the study strongly suggests is that *prolonged* exposure to clomiphene citrate will very likely increase the risk of benign, or borderline, tumors of the ovaries. This recent study has created less controversy than Whittemore's, as the data was analyzed extremely well, and the factual statistical comparison has been found to be sound. Therefore, the study's conclusions concerning clomiphene citrate have been accepted.

Its message concerning clomiphene citrate use has been recognized by physicians and patients alike—prolonged exposure should be avoided. Today, when using clomiphene citrate, we rarely go beyond four to six cycles, and we rarely do those cycles in four to six consecutive months. As a patient, you need to be aware of these findings, and discuss them with the physician who's treating you, as you decide on your treatment plan.

The bottom line with fertility drugs is that they should be used judiciously. They shouldn't be used if the need for them is minimal. And if they are used, they should be limited to the smallest amount necessary to accomplish the clinical outcome you're looking for. By using drugs this way, outcome can be improved, while risks are diminished.

Studies looking for a relationship between other fertility drugs and ovarian cancer are ongoing today. To date, no data has been found or published that would suggest an increased risk with the use of human menopausal gonadotropin. As this research continues, you can be assured that there will be more and more information available as to any potential problems that may arise with the use of drugs for controlled ovarian hyperstimulation.

Is the Environment Hitting Men Below the Belt?

The possibility that male fertility is decreasing as a result of environmental pollution is fiercely debated. The case of the disappearing sperm first came to light in the early eighties, when researchers compared current sperm count findings to similar studies from the thirties. They discovered that among healthy and "fertile" adult males, the average sperm count had declined by about 40%, from 120 million sperm cells per milliliter of semen to about 70 million.

This finding was confirmed in September 1992, when a group of statisticians at the University of Copenhagen published an analysis of 61 male fertility studies that had been done between 1938 and 1990. After reviewing the medical records of 15,000 European men, these researchers found that average sperm counts had decreased by 42%, from 113 million to 66 million sperm cells per milliliter.

Their conclusion was widely disputed, since it appeared from their findings that the decline had occurred before 1970, and that sperm counts had actually increased in the two decades since. So skeptical French researchers began to analyze sperm bank records, in an attempt to discredit the Danish report. Instead they found that the average sperm counts of Parisian men had declined by one-third between 1975 and 1995. The French doctors also noted a significant decrease in the vitality of the men's sperm.

While some researchers still disbelieve these findings, others are convinced that a variety of widely used pesticides are feminizing male fetuses and embryos by mimicking estrogen. They base their theory on the fact that similar reproductive problems have been found in wild birds, reptiles, and fish that live in, or near, heavily contaminated waters. Other biologists maintain that even if the general population is being exposed to increasing levels of pollution, the small concentrations of man-made chemicals found in the diet of the average man are far less than those in contaminated waters where animal irregularities have been seen, and these chemicals are harmless.

As this debate rages on, you might want to play it safe. One precautionary step you can take is to refrain from eating fat from beef, fish, or any other animal, since most pollutants accumulate there. And limiting your consumption of fat is a good general health rule anyway. You can also cut your risk by avoiding exposure to pesticides and petroleum products, many of which are known to mimic estrogen, and to disrupt human hormones.

IVF vs. Tubal Surgery

If you are a patient with a diagnosis of tubal factor infertility or pelvic factor infertility, you will eventually need to make a decision between surgery and assisted reproductive technology. Since this choice is somewhat controversial among physicians, it's not surprising that it may be a difficult one for you as well. Even though IVF is less invasive physically, it's more invasive financially. Yet some doctors choose IVF simply because it's physically easier on the patient, without considering its financial impact.

If your condition *can* be corrected surgically, your decision becomes an easy one. Pregnancy outcome is one factor that is clearly against IVF. The chances of pregnancy average around 20% to 25% per cycle following distal surgery, the same percentage IVF offers. However, IVF only gives you one chance to conceive, where if your tubes are surgically corrected and are potentially functional, you've gained a chance of pregnancy that repeats itself month after month after month.

The decision becomes more difficult if your doctor tells you there's a possibility that surgery won't be able to correct your problem. If your tubes are badly damaged, IVF—even though it is more expensive and it is not covered by insurance—becomes the realistic choice. But while IVF can bypass this sort of difficult pelvic or tubal factor problem, it's an expensive procedure, which isn't covered by most insurance carriers. So some couples who can't afford IVF, but who have coverage for tubal reconstructive surgery, will still choose surgery. Even though the damage is significant and the odds are low, it's the only alternative they have.

This is when the issue of surgery versus IVF becomes a thorny one for physicians. They have the quandary of knowing what is right medically, but being forced into giving the least beneficial treatment because it's the only one the patient can afford. If third-party payers were required to cover assisted technology, as they do surgical treatment, appropriate choices could be made without jeopardizing the patient or compromising the ethics of the physician. If mandated coverage for IVF doesn't come to pass some time in the near future, more and more ineffective surgery is going to be performed on patients who don't really need it.

High Cost vs. Low Success Rates

The cost-effectiveness of infertility treatment, or the lack thereof, is one of the issues that has been tried and judged in the lay press over the years. The high cost and low success rate of assisted reproductive technologies have been particularly scapegoated. As we have seen in the past decade, advancing the success in human reproductive disorders has been accompanied by an ever-increasing cost and an ever-increasing concern about the manipulation and unethical use of these technologies. This was illustrated several years ago with public exposure of several clinics across the country that were exaggerating success rates with in vitro technology, in order to improve patient recruitment and income generation.

A more recent scandal, occurring in Southern California, concerned the use, and misuse, of egg and embryo donation—taking them from couples who had not given their permission, and giving them to couples who possibly paid an increased fee to receive these high quality embryos, which would give them a better chance to generate a pregnancy.

Why have costs escalated in this area of medicine? Are doctors causing it, or is this inflation consistent with what's happening in other industries? The answer, hopefully, is that it *is* consistent, but sometimes I wonder. Is the fact that doctors have become too greedy the reason the majority of reproductive specialists have openly opposed third-party reimbursement for infertility services? Are Ferraris and summer homes their right? Does it matter that the success rates with IVF haven't advanced in the last decade, as long as their net worth has grown significantly? How many specialists have put back into research as much as they have taken out of their patients' pockets in failed infertility treatments?

The answers to these inflammatory questions are extremely discouraging. What started as an honest attempt to learn about basic human reproductive function has turned into one of the largest medical industries of our history. The "scientific breakthroughs" of today—the 60-year-old woman who delivers a baby from egg donation, or the grandmother who carries her daughter's embryo to term—are designed for media attention rather than for improving general scientific or clinical outcome. Where are the basic experiments that are necessary to improve embryo quality and success rates for the 35-year-old woman with tubal disease—a much more typical infertility patient? If success rates for her improve, the media doesn't care, and the doctor or clinic that has achieved them doesn't have a flood of new patients coming to the door. It's the clinic that gets a 65-year-old woman pregnant that is swamped with patients.

The basic issues that started Edwards, Steptoe, Johnston, Lopata, Trounson, Jones, and me down this road almost two decades ago must not be forgotten. Many of those questions that were asked then, are still being asked today. We must continue to look for answers that improve the cost-effectiveness of human reproductive treatment, or it will cease to be an alternative for the majority of the many millions of people, worldwide, who suffer from this disorder.

More Controversies to Come

Reproductive medicine is such a fast-changing field, it's almost guaranteed that as soon as we deal with the controversies that are before us today, new ones will surface. What might they be?

One controversy that has already begun to surface concerns whether eggs should be removed from unborn fetuses and donated to infertile women. This could be viewed as the egg bank of the future.

Genetic manipulation of embryos is another source of debate. Some question whether this can be done safely, without making unforeseen changes in the natural order of things. Others worry about when it will be done. While many can accept that it might be used to correct genetic abnormalities that would alter a child's quality of life, others fear that it will be done for more superficial reasons. Will genetic engineering give us the ability to produce the "perfect child"? And once we have the ability to choose certain genetic characteristics that make a more hardy or more viable baby, will we begin to discard embryos that don't reach that standard? . . . Will we select the best and lose the rest? Assuming science gives us that ability, would it be moral for us to exercise it? These thoughts are not so far-fetched. Already, with the availability of sperm selection, some families are using technology to select the sex of their children. Isn't it safe to assume that they would use technology to select other attributes, as well?

The use of genetic technology will have to be addressed once we see the effect that correcting defects has on human life. The issue is fraught with so many potential difficulties that rigid oversight and regulation will be a necessity.

We've discussed only a few of the many areas of controversy that exist in reproductive medicine today. It's possible that you will be faced with some of them during your own treatment. If you are, you should discuss them in detail with your physician. Decisions should be made once you've been given detailed information. Absorb that information, think about it, and then rediscuss it. Through understanding and knowledge, controversies can disappear.

16

The Future of Reproductive Technologies

The advancement of technology has always come at a cost, both financial and emotional. When Galileo proclaimed in the early seventeenth century that the earth revolved around the sun, the inquisition branded him a heretic and put him on trial. Not much had changed by the mid-sixties, when breakthroughs in IVF were announced. They, too, were greeted with condemnation and protest from a public that felt starting life in a laboratory was tantamount to tampering with God's work. Today, this bias against reproductive medicine remains so strong that you, or a member of your family, may have been met with it during your struggle to have a child. It's unfortunate that this sort of prejudice can make an already traumatic situation even worse. And beyond causing this sort of personal pain, the narrow-mindedness of certain individuals and groups has greatly limited the ability of reproductive scientists to do the sort of clinical research that would, hopefully, give you and others the resources to have a family when you desire, with a minimum of physical, emotional, and financial invasiveness.

One of the most important things you can take from this book is the ability to educate and inform other people about what's actually happening in the field of reproductive medicine, and in the process, help them become more accepting of it. From the very beginning, researchers in the reproductive area have attempted not only to advance the knowledge and success rates in their field, but also to provide a structure within which both investigators and patients can feel comfortable that they are using technology in ethical ways. The public's "need to know" is particularly important in the area of future reproductive technologies. Success with reproductive technologies is stagnant right now. The only way for physicians to improve clinical outcomes with these very expensive and invasive procedures, is by continuing to experiment, and yet public protest has delayed work in some of the very areas that promise the most advancement.

Some potential techniques that seem threatening today may actually become medical necessities in the future. An open mind, and an open dialogue, can help to ensure both the progress of science and the protection of human beings. One of the most important things we need to do in order to continue this advancement is to keep the public informed about technologies as they emerge. We need to work together to educate religious groups, legislators, and consumers about the necessity for research in the field of reproductive medicine.

As you will see, some techniques that hold out the promise of help are nearing reality right now. Others lie further in the future.

What's in the Works Now?

FREEZING THE HUMAN EGG

It's just one more example of sexual inequality! Mature sperm can be frozen, thawed, and go on to produce healthy embryos and babies, while mature eggs stubbornly continue to resist this process. For almost ten years, since the first success with human embryo freezing, scientists have made freezing mature, unfertilized human eggs a high priority. Women of reproductive age, when faced with the loss of their ovarian function as a result of chemotherapy, radiation therapy, or surgical removal of the ovaries due to various types of cancers very often long to preserve their reproductive potential to be used at a later, more appropriate time. Men with this dilemma are able to store their sperm, comforted by the knowledge that it can be used when the moment is right. Women don't have this comfort zone. If they're not yet prepared to have children at the time of their surgery, they're simply out of luck. For, while eggs can be collected from them prior to their treatment, those eggs can't be safely frozen and stored unless they have first been fertilized and become an embryo. And in many cases—when a woman isn't yet married, for example—that's simply not practical.

The roadblock standing in the way of successful egg freezing is a microscopic bit of cytoplasm called the mitotic spindle. At the point when eggs are retrieved from the mature follicle for use in vitro fertilization—in the hours just prior to ovulation—the genetic material within them is fully formed, and ready to combine with the genetic material from the sperm cell. This genetic material is contained in the area of the egg cytoplasm called the mitotic spindle. The mitotic spindle is a very small structure found on the surface of the egg cytoplasm, which contains 46 chromosomes that are lined up and ready to match with the 23 chromosomes that will be coming from the sperm cell. Immediately prior to entrance of the 23 chromosomes from the sperm, the 46 chromosomes of the mitotic spindle divide and throw off 23 chromosomes, leaving 23 to join with the sperm's component. Unfortunately, the mitotic spindle is extremely sensitive to temperature changes. Its functioning can be interfered with by cooling or freezing.

Researchers have tried to get around this in a number of ways. They've used different types of protective materials, different types of freezing protocols—they've even tried "snap freezing" mature eggs. To date, all of these technologies have shown very little success. While there have been five or six births reported worldwide after human eggs were frozen and thawed prior to fertilization, this represents an extremely low level of success given the number of attempts that have been made, and the dollars invested, to produce them.

Recently, investigators in Korea, England, and Australia have tried a new approach to human egg freezing. They've collected immature eggs from the ovaries, frozen them, and then matured them in vitro after thawing. Once the eggs have been matured, in vitro fertilization takes place, followed by an embryo transfer. The use of this freezing, thawing, and in vitro maturation technology has been very limited, but it has produced a live child on several occasions. While this method is still in its experimental stages vis-à-vis human eggs, it has been used for some time by cattle breeders, who have developed in vitro environments that allow immature bovine eggs to develop and mature as if they were still in the follicle.

Though the freezing and thawing of immature eggs has shown some success, it still presents doctors with a number of obstacles. The first is the loss of eggs that occurs during the in vitro maturation process. Initial clinical studies indicate that only 50% to 60% of thawed eggs will mature correctly in vitro. And of those, only half will fertilize, even if routine in vitro fertilization is assisted with ICSI. These high rates of egg loss, and failed fertilizations, show that the technology is still very crude, and only marginally successful.

The second impediment to this technology—the difficulty involved in collecting immature eggs—has greatly limited this research. Immature eggs are almost impossible to retrieve using current methods for egg recovery. So in order to obtain immature eggs, the ovary, or a piece of the ovary, has to be surgically removed. For women who are losing their ovaries surgically anyway, this doesn't present too much of a problem. For these women, immature egg collection may provide a way to maintain their future reproductive potential. But for other women, the dilemma of immature egg collection poses a real problem. In most of the experimental cases where immature egg freezing has been attempted, women who were losing their ovaries to surgery, donated their eggs to women who were trying to conceive.

Another source of eggs, which has been considered for cryopreservation, is the immature oocytes that are found within the ovaries of aborted fetuses. After about the fourth or fifth month of fetal development, the ovaries contain millions of these immature eggs. Collecting, freezing, and then thawing these immature fetal eggs for in vitro maturation was first debated in England, where it was roundly condemned from an ethical standpoint. When discussed in the United States, the possibility of removing ovaries from aborted fetuses for use as future "egg banks" was again denounced because of ethical considerations. The only place where this possibility has not been discounted for clinical research is Asia—primarily China and Korea—where this work is currently ongoing. Whether the role of fetal ovaries will ultimately be accepted in this potential future technology is a question that still remains to be answered.

PREIMPLANTATION GENETIC ANALYSIS

As we write today, researchers already have the ability to determine certain genetic abnormalities while a potential in vitro fetus is still in the embryonic state. They do this by removing a cellular sample from the embryo, prior to transferring it into the uterus. From this cellular material they can determine whether or not the embryo carries certain genetic abnormalities.

The number of things which can be screened for in this way is currently rather limited. Determining whether an embryo is a male or a female by counting its X and Y chromosomes is relatively easy to do. But going beyond that, to diagnose inherited diseases, is more difficult. As of yet, scientists have only been able to identify the gene sequences for a limited number of diseases. And in order for this knowledge to be useful, they must develop a probe for each sequence in question, which will analyze the embryonic DNA to see if that particular sequence is present. Since very few of these DNA probes currently exist for the human genome, screening an embryo for the multitude of genetic abnormalities that exist, or even having the ability to safely and accurately do a karyotype analysis of an embryo—to look at its chromosomes' number and appearance—is still somewhat limited.

One very real question is whether this manipulation and genetic study of embryos prior to implantation is all that important. Certainly, in families that have a strong history of genetic abnormalities such as hemophilia or muscular dystrophy, or other disorders such as cystic fibrosis or Tay-Sachs disease, it could be invaluable to know whether a particular embryo carries these flaws. But this gives rise to the next important question—what to do with the embryo if it is determined to be harboring a genetic disease? Would that embryo be rejected and discarded? Most researchers feel that this would be ethically appropriate, since the embryo is genetically abnormal anyway. However, other segments of society, especially pro-life organizations, feel that discarding an embryo is tantamount to aborting a fetus, and should be condemned. This points up the fact that any time genetic studies involve human embryonic material, legislative guidelines will more often than not need to be developed to control the use of technology.

Although there are now very few abnormalities that we can screen an embryo for, and the ability to perform a complete analysis of genetic abnormalities in the embryo isn't available, in the near future we will probably advance to a point at which we can analyze an embryo, genetically, as routinely as we now analyze an early pregnancy with chorionic villus sampling or with amniocentesis. While the ethical issues this raises have yet to be totally agreed upon, there is at least one very important reason to continue this research. One of the goals of preconception genetic diagnosis is to improve the methods that are used for in vitro fertilization. By looking at embryonic abnormalities through genetic testing, researchers may be able to determine whether the type of ovarian stimulation that's used to promote multiple follicle development, or the culture environment in which embryos are grown, are predisposing embryos to certain genetically based problems. Finding the answer to these questions may help doctors to improve the quality of the embryos these follicles produce.

Future Possibilities

MY BROTHER, MYSELF . . . CLONING HUMAN BEINGS

The word *clone* strikes a note of fear in many. Science fiction has given us the image of groups of identical beings, spawned from the single cell of a prototype, marching in lockstep into the future. Is cloning fiction? . . . or is it a reality? Cloning, in the strictest scientific sense, is the creation of a new structure based on the duplication of the DNA in a single cell. So cloning in the human context would, by definition, mean replicating a human sperm or a human egg—in other words, multiplying it to produce a number of identical sperm or eggs. As doctors, we are told to "never say never" about anything in medicine, but I feel safe in saying that the development of this type of technology to clone human gametes is something that will never happen, due to its difficulty. However, there is a variation on cloning that might very well take place.

In this version of "cloning," an egg and sperm are used to produce an embryo in vitro. The cells of the embryo are then separated, to create a number of identical individual embryos. Since the embryo which is separated isn't a single cell, this isn't true cloning. But it is quite similar.

This experiment has been performed with a number of mammalian species, and embryos that have been split have successfully developed, been born, and gone on to produce their own offspring. It has been used most frequently in the cattle industry. Bovine embryos have been split at the morula stage—80 to 100 cells—and have gone on to become identical twin calves. Or embryos have been separated at the four-cell stage, to produce quadruplets. The same experiment was performed with human embryos by investigators at George Washington University in 1993. They took a human embryo at the four-cell stage of development, and separated the cells into four individual embryos. They gave each embryo an artificial zona pellucida. Then they observed whether the separated embryonic cells would continue to grow and develop individually. They did. There is still a great deal of research to be done before this process has practical use for human reproduction. In the bovine experiments, there have been problems such as low birth weight, especially in four-cell embryo separation. But the 1993 human "cloning" study brought on such an outcry from religious and ethics groups that this area of investigation has literally come to a halt.

Hopefully, it will be resumed at some time in the future, as it would be of great benefit to infertile couples who have difficulty producing multiple embryos for IVF transfer. The ability to replicate a single embryo would certainly improve the chances of producing a pregnancy for these people. Using the technology of embryo separation and multiplication, everyone who could produce even one embryo, would suddenly have the ability to freeze multiple embryos from a single cycle. Given the cost of in vitro cycles, and in most cases the lack of third-party payment for them, this would be a great advantage to most infertile couples. The ability to use the "cloning" technology would allow physicians to make ART procedures more affordable, and to improve their clinical outcomes.

Unfortunately, as with any other developing technology, the public's understanding of what is going on needs to keep step with the experimental process. Contrary to popular opinion, the process of taking an embryo and making it into four identical embryos does not involve any sort of genetic manipulation. It's actually similar to the creation of fraternal twins from a single egg and sperm. While the appearance of the people produced from the cloned embryos may be the same, their thoughts and behaviors aren't. If human embryo cloning had been discussed realistically, and people were made to understand that the process is merely a separation and natural multiplication of identical embryonic cells, public outcry might have been avoided. It may not be so hard for the general public, and for ethical and religious groups, to accept this technology once they fully comprehend it.

SAYING GOOD-BYE TO THE UTERUS

Today, women who lose their uterine function must use a gestational surrogate carrier to have a baby brought to term. But within our lifetimes, it may be possible for embryonic development to be started through in vitro fertilization, and to then take place completely outside of the uterine environment, up through the time of delivery!

Scientists are bringing this possibility ever closer by extending the extrauterine survival of fetuses at both ends of their developmental spectrum. The ability to maintain neonatal survival after premature birth has improved dramatically over the past ten years. Babies that are delivered prematurely after as little as 22 to 24 weeks of pregnancy, weighing as little as one to two pounds, survive and develop outside the uterine environment on a regular basis today.

At the other end of the spectrum, nonhuman embryos have been maintained in an in vitro environment for as long as two to three weeks before their development ceases. Currently human embryos can only be cultured in vitro for a much shorter five- to six-day period, after which they need to be attached to a source of nutrition. Up until now, that connection has always been made to the mother. However, experiments have been undertaken in recent years that have tested the potential for in vitro embryos to attach to a culture container, or to a cellular matrix within a culture environment, instead of to a human host. As these experiments proceed, scientists are beginning to be able to extend embryo growth and development—and then *fetal* growth and development—outside the uterus, further and further into the early stages of pregnancy.

Work is currently being done in some centers to determine the ability of large animal fetuses to survive when removed from the uterus at the end of the first trimester—after around 12 to 14 weeks. These experiments have illustrated our ability to maintain fetal survival outside of the uterus at these early stages. As this technology advances, we will progressively be able to maintain normal fetal development and health outside the uterus starting earlier and earlier in a pregnancy. Ultimately, it may be possible to have an embryo form in vitro, and for its entire fetal growth and development to occur in a nonhuman, artificial, extracorporeal environment. Certainly, we are far away from being able to do that today, but if this technology does advance, the uterus would literally no longer be necessary.

Obviously, this type of technology has the potential to be misused. For instance, fetuses could be grown for the sole purpose of producing certain organs—such as hearts, lungs, or ovaries—to be used for medical procedures. This type of abuse would need to be protected against before this technology can be used with human embryos. As is true in all of the areas that we are discussing in this chapter, controls will have to be extremely well thought out.

DESIGNER BABIES

Another popular hook for science fiction and suspense novel writers is the suggestion that in the future, human genetic traits will be controlled and selected by scientists. From a factual standpoint, sometime soon it will probably be possible to select and exclude certain genetic traits from embryos. The human genome mapping that has been going on for the last decade will eventually identify the entire human "genetic map," and once that is done, different problem areas, or different traits, can be addressed individually on an embryonic basis. This ability to select and control certain aspects of genetics will probably happen within our lifetime.

How often it will actually be applied remains to be seen. Obviously, not everyone will want to use this technology, but if the ability to medically predetermine the genetics of offspring exists, the tendency to misuse that technology will be high. One of the great fears regarding this technology is that everybody will desire the same types of genetic characteristics. Once we are able to identify the various gene sequences that make up body build and constitution, and the body's phenotype—things such as its height, weight, hair color, and eye color—it will be a short time before these areas can be manipulated. This could remove some of the differences that make human life so variable and interesting. Do we really want all of the men in our population to be six-foot-four? Do we want all of the women to be five-foot-eight and weigh 110 pounds?

Will we use our ability to make genetic choices to preselect our children's potential careers and lifestyles, based on our own interests at the time of their conception? Why not program an embryo to become a seven-foot-four child, so that you can ensure a future NBA star? The answer is that your seven-foot-four offspring could just as easily want to be a violinist. We can't genetically preselect his mind, desires, or social interests. Because of this, manipulating the physical characteristics of our children is an area that could be fraught with extreme disappointments.

Conclusion

While technologies such as the ones we've discussed are now only theoretical, in the future they will be clinically usable. As they continue to evolve, a tremendous amount of time, effort, and interest needs to be given to considering the possible negative uses to which they might be put. Even though physicians don't like to be governed by nonmedical bodies, they are going to have to accept the fact that legislative activities go hand in hand with their ability to explore and develop new areas of technology. They should remember that the public's fears do have some basis. When a story like the University of California at Irvine's reproductive health center scandal hits the front pages of newspapers across the country, concerns raised by the public, as well as by state and national legislators, literally turn back the timetable on advances in areas ranging from genetic technology to embryo/egg donation technology . . . for good reason. Scandals like this one show why doctors should not only be accepting of ethical and legislative oversight, but should be heavily involved in helping to formulate the structure of the necessary bodies. Even though licensing and legislation may play a more and more prominent role in research, they needn't diminish or detour the advance of knowledge in the treatment of human reproductive disorders.

The right to procreate is a basic human right. The liberty to do so using technologies that are available today, or will be in the future, should also be a basic human right. Infertility is a human disorder, in the same way that heart disease, kidney disease, or bladder disease is a human disorder. And the ethical use of assisted reproductive technology should be just as acceptable as the high-tech treatments that are used to combat those other diseases. The advancement of science in the reproductive area—in fact, in *all* areas of medicine—needs to be supported more than ever in today's environment of criticism and bias.

The future holds what it holds. Neither we, nor anybody else, can tell you exactly what will be happening technologically in the arena of reproductive medicine. But if the future holds nothing more than a new understanding and acceptance of the fact that infertility is a human condition and disorder, just like any other human condition or disorder, it will be brighter for the ever-increasing number of men and women who are infertile.

Terms We Used in This Chapter

Cloning: growing cells in the laboratory that are genetically identical to each other.

Extracorporeal fertilization: another term for in vitro fertilization; fertilization outside of the female's reproductive tract.

Mitotic spindle: the 46-chromosome structure found within the cytoplasm of the egg prior to fertilization.

Phenotype: the outward appearance of a person's genetic makeup. For instance, brown hair, blue eyes.

General Glossary

Abdominal ultrasound aspiration: a procedure used to remove the egg from the ovary, with visualization by external ultrasound viewing. This was the original procedure developed to replace laparoscopic collection of eggs for IVF. During this procedure the aspirating needle is passed through the abdominal wall into the ovarian follicle to collect the egg.

Acrosome membrane: a covering over the head of the sperm which contains enzymes that when released from the membrane will allow the sperm to penetrate the egg.

Acrosome reaction: the breakdown of the acrosome membrane that changes the sperm into a cell that can penetrate the egg.

Adenomyosis: a condition in which the cells of the uterine lining (endometrium) invade the muscle of the uterine wall. This is similar to endometriosis, which is found on surfaces of the pelvic organs.

Adhesions: bands of scar tissue that can attach the surface of various organs to each other—for instance, a fallopian tube to the surface of an ovary.

Agonist: a drug or chemical that is designed to perform the same function as the natural, or parent, compound. For instance, Lupron is a synthetic preparation of gonadotropin-releasing hormone, but lasts longer and performs longer than the parent compound.

Ampullary: the outer or distal end of the fallopian tube. It is also the widest part of the fallopian tube.

Androgens: male sex hormones produced by the testes and ovaries that give rise to male characteristics.

Anorexia: an aversion to food.

Anorexia nervosa: a mental disorder in which an aversion to food and obesity becomes an obsession.

Anovulation: failure to ovulate.

Antibody: a protein substance produced by the body in response to a stimulating substance (antigen).

Antigen: any foreign substance that causes the body's immune system to produce antibodies against it.

Asherman's syndrome: a condition where scar tissue forms in the uterine cavity that interferes with normal uterine lining development. Usually this is associated with the loss of the menstrual period following a D&C.

Assisted hatching: a windowlike opening made in the zona pellucida of the embryo to improve implantation or attachment of the embryo to the uterine lining.

Assisted reproductive technologies (ART):   a term used to identify procedures such as IVF, GIFT, and ZIFT.

Asthenospermia: a term used to describe sperm that has poor mobility or progressive movement, i.e., low-motility sperm.

Autoimmune dysfunction: a disease or dysfunction that occurs because the body's immune system attacks and destroys its own tissues.

Balanced translocation: the crossover of genetic material from one arm of a chromosome to the other arm. The person with a balanced translocation is clinically normal, but can pass the abnormal translocation on to offspring.

Basal body temperature chart (BBT):   a daily record of the body's temperature at rest. When ovulation occurs, the body's temperature will rise 0.6°F to 0.8°F above baseline.

Bicornuate uterus: a malformation of the uterus resulting in two separate cavities, each with a connecting fallopian tube.

Bipolar disease: blockage at both ends of the fallopian tube.

Blastocyst: the time in embryonic development where the embryo consists of the cells that will make the placenta and those which will form the fetus.

Blocking antibodies: protective antibodies that are formed by the mother's immune system in response to her embryo during implantation.

Bulimia: a disorder involving binge eating and self-induced vomiting.

Capacitation: a change in the sperm cell that occurs after ejaculation and during the passage through the female reproductive tract, which enables the sperm to penetrate the egg.

Carbon dioxide test: an antiquated test used to determine whether there is any blockage of the fallopian tubes.

Cervical mucus: a mucus secretion produced by glands in the cervical canal under the influence of estrogen.

Cervix: a narrow opening that connects the uterus to the vagina and produces mucus that allows the sperm to enter into the uterus.

Chlamydia: a bacteria that is considered to be sexually transmitted, which may be an underlying cause of infertility.

Chocolate cysts: ovarian cysts filled with degenerating blood which resembles melted chocolate. This occurs when endometriosis invades the ovary and bleeds cyclically, creating the cyst.

Chromosome: the structure in each cell's nucleus that hold the parents' genetic information in the form of DNA (deoxyribonucleic acid).

Cilia: the hairlike projections inside the fallopian tubes that move the egg and/or embryo toward the uterus.

Cleavage: the process of embryo cell division.

Clomiphene citrate: a synthetic hormone that stimulates a woman to ovulate. Clomiphene citrate can also be used in men to improve sperm production. The brand names of this substance are Clomid and Serophene.

Cloning: growing cells in the laboratory that are genetically identical to each other.

Coagulum: nonliquefied ejaculate that is present upon emission.

Computer-assisted semen analysis (CASA):   the measurement of sperm number, shape, and movement by computer technology.

Computerized axial tomography (CAT):   a diagnostic X-ray procedure that utilizes computers to project an image on film.

Congenital abnormality: a malformation that takes place during fetal development.

Conization: the surgical removal of abnormal cells on the surface, or within, the cervical canal.

Corpus luteum: the cyst that forms after a follicle releases its egg. It produces estrogen and progesterone during the second half of the ovulatory cycle.

Crohn's disease: inflammatory disease of the small bowel.

Cryocautery: the destruction of abnormal cervical cells by freezing.

Cryopreservation: storing of tissue or cells by freezing.

Cryptorchism: failure of the testicles to descend into the scrotal sac.

Culture medium: the fluid solution used for growth of cells or tissue in vitro.

Cumulus oophorus: a sticky mass of cells in a cloudlike pattern that surrounds the egg at the time of ovulation.

Cytoplasm: the material within the cell that is fluidlike and contains the microscopic structures that relate to cell function.

Dehydroepiandrosterone sulfate (DHEAS):   a hormone made by the adrenal gland that has androgen (male hormone) effects.

Deoxyribonucleic acid (DNA):   the material in each cell nucleus that contains each individual's genetic code.

Dermoid: a usually benign tumor of the ovary that can contain hair, teeth, and bone fragments—also known as teratoma or germ cell tumor.

Diethylstilbestrol (DES):   a man-made estrogen originally used to prevent miscarriages. Is known to cause abnormalities of the cervix, vagina, and uterus of the unborn fetus.

Dilatation and curettage (D&C):   opening the cervix and removing the contents of the uterine cavity by scraping or suction.

Directional motility: a term used to denote sperm that can move in a straight line.

Dominant follicle: the largest follicle of a follicle group; the dominant follicle contains the egg that will ovulate.

Donor insemination: an insemination with sperm other than the husband's. Donor insemination is used for pregnancy initiation.

Doppler stethoscope: an instrument that can detect the movement of red blood cells in a blood vessel, and then determine the velocity of that blood flow.

Down regulation: the use of GnRH agonist to stop the pituitary gland from producing and releasing FSH and LH, causing the ovaries to stop developing follicles and estrogen. Thus the ovaries are "down regulated."

Dysgenesis: faulty formation of any cell or organ.

Dysmenorrhea: painful menstrual periods.

Dyspareunia: painful intercourse.

Dysplasia: abnormalities in the cell layers covering the cervix, vagina, or vulva.

Ectopic pregnancy: a pregnancy (embryo) that implants outside the uterine cavity. Most commonly this occurs in the fallopian tube, but can occur in the ovary or abdominal cavity.

Egg aspiration: the removal of the egg from the follicle during the in vitro fertilization procedure.

Egg donation: aspiration of eggs from a woman volunteer to be used to impregnate another woman.

Egg production protocol: the use of various combinations of drugs (i.e., clomiphene citrate, Metrodin, Humegon, etc.) to stimulate multiple eggs to ovulate.

Ejaculate: the fluid (semen) that carries the sperm cells out of the male's reproductive tract.

Ejaculatory duct: the tubes that connect the testicular system to the urethra in the penis for the release of sperm during orgasm.

Electron microscopy: an instrument that can magnify structures 50,000 to 100,000 times.

Embryo: a term used to describe the time from the fertilization of the egg until the eighth week of pregnancy.

Endocrinologist: a physician who specializes in diagnosis and treatment of problems relating to hormones or endocrine gland abnormalities.

Endometrial biopsy: sampling or removal of a piece of the uterine lining (or endometrium) for microscopic study.

Endometrial polyps: an overgrowth of normal endometrial tissue, forming a protrusion into the uterine cavity.

Endometrioma: a cyst in the ovary caused by endometriosis; sometimes called "chocolate cysts."

Endometriosis: a disease in which normal endometrial cells get outside the uterus, stick to the surface of organs, and cause inflammation and tissue damage.

Endometritis: infection or inflammation of the uterine lining (the endometrium).

Endometrium: the lining of cells inside the uterus that is sensitive to estrogen and progesterone stimulation.

Epididymis: the coiled tubules attached alongside the testicles that act as a storage system for the sperm prior to ejaculation.

Estradiol: an estrogen formed and released by the ovarian follicle during ovulation.

Estrogen: a category of female hormone that is necessary for female characteristics.

Estrogen replacement therapy (ERT): the use of various types of estrogen to alleviate postmenopausal symptoms and diseases (i.e., osteoporosis).

Extracorporeal fertilization: another term for in vitro fertilization; fertilization outside of the female's reproductive tract.

Fallopian tube: a narrow tubular structure connected to the uterus that carries the egg from the ovary into the uterus after fertilization.

Fecundity rate: the ability of a woman to become pregnant during any given month that ovulation occurs. It is described as a percentage figure, i.e., 25% per month.

Fertilization: entrance or penetration of the egg by the sperm cell.

Fibroids: a benign tumor made up of fibrous tissues found in the uterus.

Fimbria: fingerlike projections on the end of the fallopian tube that pick up the egg after ovulation.

Fimbrioplasty: a surgical procedure to reconstruct the fingerlike projections on the end of the fallopian tube.

Flare-up regimen: one of the types of drug protocols used to stimulate multiple follicle production.

Follicle: a small fluid-filled sac contained within the ovary that prepares the egg for ovulation. The follicle is also the estrogen production factory in the female.

Follicle aspiration: see Egg aspiration.

Follicle-stimulating hormone (FSH):   a protein hormone produced and released by the anterior pituitary gland. FSH stimulates follicle growth in the female and sperm production in the male.

Follistatin: A small protein hormone found in the follicle fluid that controls follicle growth.

Galactorrhea: a milklike production from the breast of a woman who is either not nursing or has never been pregnant. Galactorrhea may indicate a benign tumor in the pituitary gland.

Gamete intrafallopian transfer (GIFT):   a surgical procedure whereby the egg and the sperm are laparoscopically placed into the fallopian tube.

Gametes: the reproductive cells of the male and the female, i.e., the egg and the sperm.

Germ cell: the precursor of other cells, i.e., the spermatid is the precursor cell of the sperm cell.

Germinal cell aplasia: a congenital condition in which the cells that are necessary for formation of gametes are not present.

Gestational surrogacy: the use of a woman to carry a genetically unrelated embryo for an infertile couple.

Gonadotropin-releasing hormone (GnRH):   a small protein hormone produced in the hypothalamus, responsible for controlling the production and release of FSH and LH.

Gonadotropins: the protein hormones FSH and LH; they stimulate ovarian function in the female and testicular function in the male.

Gonads: the glands that produce the male and female gametes (i.e., the egg and the sperm).

Gonorrhea: a sexually transmitted bacterial infection that can cause tubal damage in the male and the female.

Granulosa cells: the cells within the ovarian follicle that make estrogen and progesterone during the ovulation cycle.

Hamster penetration assay/Hamster test: see Sperm penetration assay.

Hatching: the final event that the embryo must complete before implantation can occur. Hatching of the embryo is a breaking out of the zona pellucida in order to implant in the endometrial cavity.

Hemizona assay test: a test used to determine whether sperm binding or attachment to the zona membrane of the egg is normal.

Histones: a simple protein found in the cell nucleus that contains a high proportion of basic amino acids.

Hormone replacement therapy (HRT):   see Estrogen replacement therapy.

Human chorionic gonadotropin (hCG):   a hormone produced by the placenta during pregnancy. It is used as an LH replacement during ovulation-induction therapy to cause egg release.

Human menopausal gonadotropin (hMG):   one of the "fertility drugs," made up of FSH and LH. HMG is made from the urine of postmenopausal women.

Hyaluronic acid: the bond, or glue, that holds granulosa cells in a tight mass around the mature egg cell.

Hyaluronidase: an enzyme that is found in the sperm membrane, which is released during fertilization so that the sperm can separate the granulosa cells from the egg.

Hydrosalpinx: closure of the fallopian tube at the fimbriated end, which results in a fluid-filled saclike structure.

Hypospadia: a congenital defect of the penis in which the urethral opening occurs on the underside rather than at the end of the organ.

Hypospermatogenesis: low sperm production.

Hypothalamus: the midportion of the brain that produces GnRH and other hormones that control the pituitary gland.

Hysterosalpingogram (HSG):   an X-ray study in which a dye visible by fluoroscopy is injected into the uterine cavity to determine the shape of the uterus and patency of the fallopian tubes.

Hysteroscopy: a surgical procedure that uses a small telescope placed through the cervical canal to view the interior of the uterine cavity.

Idiopathic: any condition that has no known cause.

Immunophenotype: an individual's profile of natural killer cell activity as it relates to the immune system.

Implantation: the attachment of the embryo to the endometrial lining of the uterus.

Incubation: maintaining a controlled environment to allow cell growth and development.

Infertility: the lack of conception after six months of unprotected intercourse.

Inhibin: a protein hormone that interferes with the activity of FSH.

Interstitial: the portion of the fallopian tube that travels through the muscular wall of the uterus to connect the endometrial cavity to the fallopian tube.

Intracytoplasmic sperm insemination (ICSI): the injection of a single sperm cell into a mature egg.

Intramural: any structure within the wall of another structure, i.e., intramural fibroids.

Intrauterine device (IUD): a small, inert, usually plastic device placed in the uterine cavity to block implantation of an embryo.

Intrauterine insemination (IUI): placement of sperm into the uterine cavity.

In vitro fertilization and embryo transfer (IVF-ET): the procedure in which the egg is removed from the ovary, fertilized in the laboratory environment, and the resulting embryo placed into the uterine cavity.

In vitro mucus penetration test: a test used to determine whether sperm mucus interaction is normal; commonly done with bovine mucus and human sperm.

Isthmus: the most muscular part of the fallopian tube; the isthmus is connected directly to the uterus.

Kallman's syndrome: a congenital condition in men in which the hypothalamus fails to produce GnRH, resulting in lack of FSH and LH production and lack of sperm production.

Karyotyping: counting and identifying the genes in a person's cells.

Killer cells: the cells in the immune system designed to attack rapidly growing masses of cells.

Klinefelter's syndrome: a chromosomal and developmental abnormality in the male that causes the individual to have female characteristics, and male sterility.

Laparoscopy: a surgical procedure in which a telescope is inserted through the abdominal wall to view the inner organs.

Laparotomy: a surgical procedure in which an incision is made through the abdominal wall in order to view the inner organs.

Leydig cells: the cells in the testicles that manufacture testosterone.

LH surge: the large release of LH from the anterior pituitary that causes the release of the mature egg from the follicle.

Loop electrocautery excision procedure (LEEP): a procedure used to remove abnormal cells from the cervical area using an electric cutting wire; similar to a conization.

Luteal phase: the second half of the menstrual cycle; the luteal phase begins with ovulation and is characterized by elevated levels of estrogen and progesterone.

Luteal phase defect: inadequate production of hormone from the corpus luteum, or poor response of the endometrial lining to hormonal stimulation, which interferes with implantation.

Luteinizing hormone (LH): protein produced and secreted from the anterior pituitary gland, which is involved in ovulation.

Macrophage: cells arising from the bone marrow that kill or remove unwanted cells from the system, i.e., bacteria or tumor cells.

Magnetic resonance imaging (MRI): an imaging device that does not use X ray or ultrasound, yet gives a clear picture of our internal organ systems.

Menarche: the onset of menstrual function.

Menstruation: the cyclic shedding of the endometrial lining of the uterine cavity, indicating lack of pregnancy.

Methotrexate: a chemotherapy agent that destroys placental cells. Commonly used for the treatment of early ectopic pregnancies.

Microfertilization: see Intracytoplasmic sperm insemination.

Micromanipulation: the use of high magnification and hydraulically controlled instrumentation to achieve fertilization in vitro.

Microscopic epididymal sperm aspiration (MESA): aspiration of the epididymis to procure sperm for use in microfertilization.

Microsurgery: a surgical procedure in which magnification and tiny instrumentation is used in order to improve reconstructive surgical outcome.

Miscarriage: loss of a pregnancy prior to the 20th week of gestation.

Mitotic spindle: the 46-chromosome structure found within the cytoplasm of the egg prior to fertilization.

Müllerian ducts: the fetal structures that fuse to form the uterus.

Myomectomy: the surgical removal of fibroids (myoma) from the uterine body.

Myometrium: the muscular wall of the uterus.

Nucleus: the part of the cell that contains the genetic profile.

Oligozoospermia: low sperm number.

Oocyte: another term for egg.

Oocyte donation: see Egg donation.

Oocyte maturation inhibitor (OMI): a protein found in the follicular fluid that keeps the egg from maturing.

Osmolarity: the pressure created by a liquid due to the concentration of various particles within it.

Ovarian dysgenesis: a congenital condition caused by an abnormality in the second X chromosome, resulting in sterility in the female.

Ovarian failure: a condition in which the ovaries are either devoid of follicles and eggs, or they are nonresponsive to FSH stimulation.

Ovarian stimulation: the use of fertility drugs to either regulate single egg ovulation or multiple egg production.

Ovaries: the female organs responsible for the production of sex hormones and eggs.

Ovotestes: a congenital abnormality characterized by the presence of gonads that are a mixture of testicles and ovaries.

Ovulation: the release of the egg from the follicle.

Ovulation induction: the stimulation of follicle growth and egg release through the use of fertility drugs.

Partial zona dissection (PZD): a form of micromanipulation in which the zona pellucida is opened to allow sperm to swim through.

Pelvic cavity: the lower part of the abdomen; the pelvic cavity houses the uterus, ovaries, and fallopian tubes.

Pelvic inflammatory disease (PID): infection or inflammation of the female reproductive organs, usually caused by a sexually transmitted disease.

Penis: the male sexual organ.

Percoll separation: a liquid gradient that is used to filter the semen during sperm washing, prior to in vitro insemination.

Pergonal: a mixture of FSH and LH that is used to stimulate ovarian follicle activity. The most common source for production of this drug is postmenopausal women's urine.

Peritoneum: the silky lining that covers the inside of the pelvic abdominal cavity.

Perivitelline space: the space between the zona pellucida and the surface of the egg cytoplasm.

Petri dish: the plastic or glass container in which embryos grow and develop during in vitro fertilization procedures.

Pharmacologic: above natural physiologic levels.

Phenotype: the outward appearance of a person's genetic makeup. For instance, brown hair, blue eyes.

Physiologic levels: hormonal levels that are identical to those produced naturally by a person's system.

Pituitary: a small gland at the base of the brain that secretes hormones that control our endocrine organs.

Pituitary adenoma: a benign growth that causes the pituitary gland to be overproductive of certain hormones.

Pituitary macroadenoma: a benign growth in the pituitary gland that exceeds 10 mm in diameter.

Placenta: a spongy structure surrounding the fetus that serves as a conduit between the mother and fetus during pregnancy.

Polar body: an extrusion of material from the cytoplasm of an egg. It usually contains unused sets of chromosomal material.

Polycystic ovarian syndrome (PCOS):   the development of multiple ovarian cysts due to an imbalance of hormone in the ovary.

Postcoital test (PCT):   a test used to determine whether sperm/mucus interaction is normal, i.e., whether the sperm can move properly through the cervical mucus.

Preimplantation genetic diagnosis: a removal of an embryonic cell prior to implantation to determine whether the genetic makeup of the embryo is normal.

Presacral neurectomy: the removal, or cutting, of the nerves that carry pain sensation from the uterus.

Progesterone: the hormone produced from the corpus luteum after ovulation. It is also the hormone responsible for maintenance of early pregnancy.

Prolactin: the hormone produced from the pituitary that prepares the breasts for lactation.

Pronuclear oocyte sperm transfer (PROST):   another term for ZIFT.

Pronuclear stage: the stage in embryonic development that occurs after sperm penetration of the egg.

Pronuclei: structures that look like moon craters on the surface of the egg; the presence of pronuclei indicates fertilization.

Prostaglandin: a hormone that is produced by the endometrium, which causes the uterine muscle to contract.

Prostate gland: a walnut-shaped gland that provides fluid for semen during ejaculation.

Prostatic urethra: the portion of the male urethra that goes through the prostate gland.

Proximal (or corneal) block: obstruction of the fallopian tube at the junction of the tube and the uterus.

Puberty: the point in human development when sexual maturation occurs.

Receptor: the site on a cell surface where a hormone attaches to express its function.

Relaxin: a hormone that may be involved in uterine muscle activity.

Rete testis: a network of canals that drains the sperm from the seminiferous tubules.

Retrograde ejaculation: ejaculation of the sperm into the bladder, instead of through the prostatic urethra.

Retrograde menstruation: the back-flow of menstrual blood and tissue into the pelvic cavity.

Rokitansky syndrome: the congenital absence of the uterus.

Salpingitis: inflammation of the fallopian tubes.

Salpingitis isthmica nodosa (SIN):   a type of tubal disease that causes obstruction; usually found in the proximal portion of the fallopian tube.

Salpingostomy: a surgical procedure where an opening is made in the fallopian tube either to alleviate an obstruction or remove a tubal pregnancy.

Scrotal sac: a saclike structure that cradles the testes.

Seminal fluid: the liquid that carries the sperm out of the male reproductive tract.

Seminal vesicles: the glands that produce the majority of the seminal fluid.

Seminiferous tubules: the tiny tubules within the testes that are necessary for sperm production.

Septate uterus: a fibrous division of the uterine cavity.

Sertoli cell: the cells within the testes that are involved in sperm cell production.

Sexually transmitted disease (STD):   a disease or organism that can be transmitted by sexual contact.

Sperm: the male reproductive cell.

Spermatocyte: an immature sperm cell.

Sperm penetration assay (SPA):   a test utilizing hamster eggs to measure the ability of the human sperm to fertilize.

Sperm washing: a technique used to separate sperm cells from seminal fluid.

Stenotic: a narrowed opening.

Subcutaneous injection: the placement of medication immediately beneath the skin.

Submucosal: immediately beneath the endometrial layer of the uterus.

Subserosal: immediately below the silky outer lining of the uterus or other pelvic structures.

Subzonal sperm insemination (SUSI):   a micromanipulation technique whereby the sperm is injected into the perivitelline space of the egg.

Supra ovulate: the stimulation of multiple eggs to ovulate.

Syncytiotrophoblasts: the cells that form the placenta.

Testicle: the male reproductive organ.

Testicular feminization: a syndrome in which the individual appears to be female, but her ovaries are testicular tissue.

Testis: singular for testicles.

Testosterone: the male hormone.

Teteratospermia: sperm that has an abnormal shape.

Transvaginal ultrasound aspiration: a technique used to aspirate eggs from the ovary for in vitro fertilization.

Tubal embryo transfer (TET):   the placement of the embryo into the fallopian tube after in vitro fertilization.

Turner's syndrome: a genetic abnormality in which the female has a missing chromosome and no ovarian function.

Ultrasound: an instrument that emits pulsed sound waves that are reflected off solid tissues to give an image of internal body structures without the use of X ray.

Urethra: a small tubular canal that carries urine in the female, and urine and seminal fluid in the male.

Urofollitropin (FSH):   urinary FSH that is used to stimulate follicle growth and development; Metrodin.

Uterine didelphys: duplication of the uterus; a double uterus.

Uterosacral ligament: the major supporting ligament of the uterus. A common area of involvement with endometriosis.

Uterus: a muscular organ with a hollow cavity lined with a layer of cells called endometrium. The function of the uterus is to protect and nourish the developing embryo/fetus.

Vagina: a canal in the female that connects the external sex organs with the cervix and uterus.

Varicocele: dilated veins around the testicle, most commonly on the left side, which can cause sperm abnormalities.

Vas deferens: the tube that connects the epididymis (sperm storage area) to the prostate gland; the pathway for sperm to leave the testicular area.

Vasectomy: a surgically created obstruction of the vas deferens, which is used as a method of male sterilization.

Vasovasostomy: reversal of a vasectomy by reconnecting the vas deferens.

Vitelline membrane: the membrane that surrounds the egg cytoplasm, which the sperm fuses with prior to penetration of the egg cytoplasm; located under the zona pellucida.

Wolffian ducts: the embryonic structure that forms into the fallopian tubes during fetal development.

Zona pellucida: the outer protein covering of the egg that the sperm first comes in contact with during fertilization.

Zygote: a fertilized egg.

Zygote intrafallopian transfer (ZIFT): placement of a fertilized egg into the fallopian tube; see PROST or TET.

Resources

ORGANIZATIONS

American Association of Oriental Medicine
433 Front Street
Catasauqua, PA 18032
(610) 433-2448

American Association of Tissue Banks
1350 Beverly Road, Suite 220A
McLean, VA 22101
(703) 827-9582

American College of Obstetricians and Gynecologists
409 12th Street SW
Washington, DC 20024-2188
(202) 638-5577

American Society of Andrology
309 West Clark Street
Champaign, IL 61820
(217) 356-3182

American Society for Reproductive Medicine
1209 Montgomery Highway
Birmingham, AL 35216-2809
(205) 978-5000
email: asrm@asrm.com

The American Surrogacy Center
638 Church Street NE
Marietta, GA 30063
(770) 426-1107

American Urological Association, Inc.
1120 North Charles Street
Baltimore, MD 21201
(301) 727-1100

The Clinical Laboratory Improvement Amendment (CLIA)
Administered by the Department of Health and Human Services
Health Care Financing and Administration
75 Hawthorne Street, Fourth Floor
San Francisco, CA 94105-3901
(415) 744-3722

The College of American Pathologists (CAP)
325 Waukegan
Northfield, IL 60093-2750
1-800-323-4040

Endometriosis Association
8585 North 76th Place
Milwaukee, WI 53223
1-800-992-3636 (in U.S.)
1-800-426-2363 (in Canada)

International Council on Infertility Information Dissemination
(INCIID)
P.O. Box 91363
Tucson, AZ 85721-5251
(520) 544-9548

National Adoption Center
1218 Chestnut Street
Philadelphia, PA 19107
1-800-TOADOPT not in PA
(215) 925-0200 in PA

National Adoption Information Clearinghouse
1400 Eye Street NW, Suite 600
Washington, DC 20005
(202) 842-1919

National Commission on Certification of Acupuncturists
1424 16th Street NW # 501
Washington, DC 20036
(202) 232-1404

National Committee for Adoption
1930 17th Street NW
Washington, DC 20009-6207
(202) 328-1200

Resolve
1310 Broadway
Somerville, MA 02144-1731
(617) 623-1156
Fax: (617) 623-0252
Helpline: (617) 623-0744
http://www.resolve.org

Serono Symposia, USA
100 Longwater Circle
Norwell, MA 02061
1-800-637-7872

Society for Assisted Reproductive Technology (SART)
1209 Montgomery Highway
Birmingham, AL 35216
(205) 978-5000
email: asrm@asrm.com

The Society of Reproductive Endocrinologists (SRE)
1209 Montgomery Highway
Birmingham, AL 35216
(205) 978-5000
email: asrm@asrm.com

The Society for Reproductive Surgeons (SRS)
1209 Montgomery Highway
Birmingham, AL 35216
(205) 978-5000
email: asrm@asrm.com

USEFUL PERIODICALS

Fertility and Sterility
American Society for Reproductive Medicine
1209 Montgomery Highway
Birmingham, AL 35216-2809
(205) 978-5000, Fax (205) 978-5005
http://www.asrm.com/profession/fertility/fspage.html
email: asrm@asrm.com

Fertility Weekly
1087 Crooked Creek Road SE
Eatonton, GA 31024
1-800-705-7185, Fax (706) 484-1813
http://www.holonet.net/homepage/fwabout.htm
email: kkey@hendersonnet.atl.ga.us

INCIID Insights
International Council on Infertility Information Dissemination
P.O. Box 91363
Tucson, AZ 85752-1363
(520) 544-9548, Fax (520) 509-5251
http://www.inciid.org
email: INCIIDinfo@aol.com

Infertility Helper
36 Norwood Road
Toronto, Ontario M4E 2S2 (Canada)
(416) 690-9593
http://www.helping.com/family/iy/iy.html
email: helper@helping.com

Newsletter of Resolve National
1310 Broadway
Somerville, MA 02144-1731
(617) 623-0744, Fax (617) 623-0252
http://www.resolve.org
email: resolveinc@aol.com

Index

A

Abdominal ultrasound aspiration, 345

Abnormal sperm shapes (teratospermia), 96, 113

Abortions, 171, 175, 195

Acceptance stage, 435–439

Acrosome membrane, 44–46, 50, 98

Acrosome reaction, 45, 50, 96, 247, 331

Acupuncture, 253, 433

Adenomyosis, 191, 194–195, 205, 230

Adhesions, 109, 155, 256–262, 266–268, 277

Adoption, 72, 437–439, 444–446

Adrenal gland problems, 78, 119

Adrenocorticotropic hormone (ACTH), 153

Age, assisted reproductive technologies and, 5, 13, 310, 312–314

Agonists (*see* Gonadotropin-releasing hormone agonists)

AIDS (acquired immune deficiency syndrome), 249

Alcohol use, 2–3

Alternative approaches, 252–253, 430–435

American Association of Tissue Banks, 250

American Hospital Association, 227

American Society for Reproductive Medicine (ASRM), 60, 61, 63, 71, 222, 259, 335, 340, 348

Ampullary portion, 23, 31, 207, 208, 214, 230

Ampullary reversal, 222, 223

Androgens, 123, 127, 150, 152, 153, 163

Anesthetics, 144

Anorexia, 163

Anorexia nervosa, 149

Anovulation, 121, 163, 271, 277

Antibodies, 288–294, 300

Antibody testing, 351–352

Anticoagulants, 289

Antidepressants, 121, 144

G

H

I

O

P

T